ATLAS OF
GASTROINTESTINAL
ENDOSCOPY

ATLAS OF
GASTROINTESTINAL
ENDOSCOPY

Editor

Emmet B. Keeffe, MD

Professor of Medicine
Chief of Clinical Gastroenterology
Medical Director, Liver Transplant Program
Stanford University Medical Center
Stanford, California

Contributing editors

R. Brooke Jeffrey, Jr, MD

Professor of Radiology
Chief of Abdominal Imaging
Stanford University Medical Center
Stanford, California

Randall G. Lee, MD

Professor of Pathology
University of Pittsburgh Medical Center
Pittsburgh, Pennsylvania

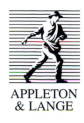

APPLETON
& LANGE

Developed by Current Medicine, Inc.
Philadelphia

Current Medicine

400 Market Street
Suite 700
Philadelphia, PA 19106

Managing Editor . . . . Lori J. Bainbridge
Development Editors. . . . . . . Ira Smiley and Paul Arthur
Editorial Assistant . . . . Debbie Singer
Indexer. . . . . Maria Coughlin
Art Director . . . . Paul Fennessy
Designer. . . . . Patrick Ward
Illustration Director. . . . . Ann Saydlowski
Cover Illustration. . . . . Wieslawa Langenfeld
Typesetting. . . . . Ryan Walsh
Production. . . . . Lori Holland, Sally Nicholson

Library of Congress Cataloging-in-Publication Data

Atlas of gastrointestinal endoscopy / editor, Emmet B. Keeffe;
   contributing editors, R. Brooke Jeffrey, Jr., Randall G. Lee.
      p. cm.
   Includes bibliographical references and index.
   ISBN 0-8385-0448-5
   1. Endoscopy—Atlasses. 2. Gastrointestinal system—Diseases—
Diagnosis—Atlases. I. Keeffe, Emmet B. II. Jeffrey, R. Brooke.
III. Lee, Randall G.
   [DNLM: 1. Gastrointestinal Diseases—diagnosis—atlases.
2. Endoscopy, Gastrointestinal—atlases. WI 17 A87917 1998]
RC804.E6A87 1998
616.3'307545—dc21
DNLM/DLC
For Library of Congress   97-45781
                                       CIP

Although every effort has been made to ensure that drug doses and other information
are presented accurately in this publication, the ultimate responsibility rests with the
prescribing physician. Neither the publishers nor the authors can be held responsible
for errors or for any consequences arising from the use of information contained herein.
Products mentioned in this publication should be used in accordance with the prescribing
information prepared by the manufacturers. No claims or endorsements are made for any
drug or compound at present under clinical investigation.

Printed in Singapore by Imago

10 9 8 7 6 5 4 3 2 1

Preface . . . .

ADVANCES IN GASTROINTESTINAL ENDOSCOPY, coupled with ever improving radiologic imaging and more sophisticated interpretation of biopsy samples, have revolutionized the practice of gastroenterology. The *Atlas of Gastrointestinal Endoscopy* was created to satisfy requests from gastroenterologists to gather an outstanding collection of endoscopic images to highlight the many advances in endoscopy.

The *Atlas* contains approximately 900 high-quality endoscopic images, with companion radiographic and histologic images. As editor, I solicited the assistance of an expert imaging radiologist, Brooke Jeffrey of Stanford University Medical Center, and experienced gastrointestinal pathologist, Randall Lee of the University of Pittsburgh Medical Center, to help select appropriate radiographs and photomicrographs to accompany the endoscopic images. All three of us were impressed by the high quality of the materials contributed by numerous authors whose names appear in figure courtesy lines. We augmented their contributions with additional illustrative images. We added some endoscopic, radiographic, and histologic materials to further display the use of diagnostic or therapeutic endoscopy in the management of specific diseases. We also included selected schematic figures and tables where appropriate to complement the endoscopic, radiologic, and histologic images.

The word "endoscopy" refers to the inspection of a body cavity using an endoscope. "Gastrointestinal endoscopy" refers to the use of endoscopes to visualize the upper and lower gastrointestinal tract, including the biliary tract, gallbladder, and pancreas. From its early origins more than 50 years ago, using rigid endoscopes with primitive illumination to visualize the esophagus and stomach from above and rectum and sigmoid colon from below, gastrointestinal endoscopy has undergone remarkable growth and had a dominant impact on the practice of gastroenterology. The evolution from a relatively primitive diagnostic procedure for the first 25 years of the short 50-year history of endoscopy to an expanded diagnostic and complex therapeutic procedure has been made possible by improvements in endoscopic instrumentation and pioneering clinical outcomes research. The earliest endoscopes relied on an electric light source for illumination. The modern era of endoscopy dawned in the 1950s with the discovery of fiberoptics and development of a flexible fiberscope. In the late 1980s, video endoscopes with improved optics and ease of use further expanded the capability to diagnose the cause of gastrointestinal symptoms, to treat benign and malignant disease, and to pictorially document endoscopic observations. Endoscopy has dramatically changed the management of important and prevalent diseases such as esophagitis, peptic ulcers, gallstones, colonic polyps, and malignancies of the entire gastrointestinal tract, including the biliary tree and pancreas.

This *Atlas of Gastrointestinal Endoscopy* chronicles the most important developments and current state of the art in the use of diagnostic and therapeutic endoscopy. This book would not have been possible without the assistance of many individuals. I wish to thank Mark Feldman of the University of Texas Southwestern Medical Center at Dallas, and Abe Krieger, President of Current Medicine, for the opportunity to edit this volume. In particular, I thank my contributing editors, Brooke Jeffrey and Randy Lee, the numerous authors who contributed to make this volume possible, and the developmental editors, Ira Smiley and Paul Arthur.

Emmet B. Keeffe, MD

Contents . . . .

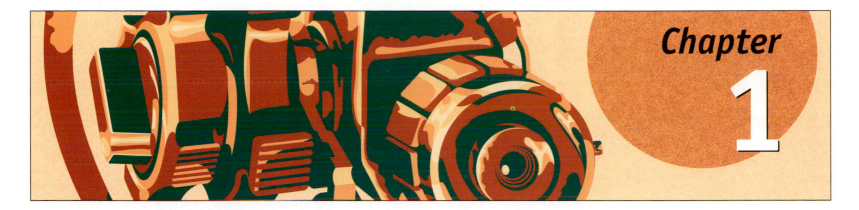

Esophagus

 Normal Anatomy

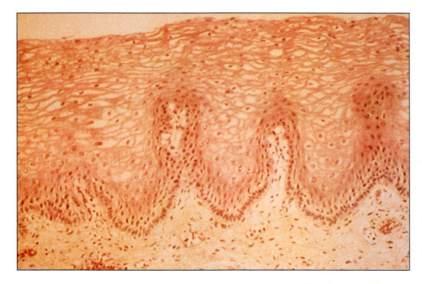

Figure 1-1. Normal histology of the esophagus. The lining of the esophagus is a partially or nonkeratinized stratified squamous epithelium that overlies the connective tissue of the submucosa and the thick circular and longitudinal muscle layers (not shown). (*Courtesy of* Sambastiva Rao, MD.)

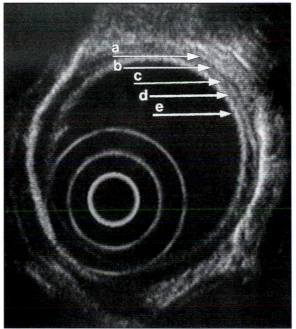

Figure 1-2. Endoscopic ultrasound of the esophagus. This endosonographic image of the esophageal wall demonstrates the five-layer structure that is seen throughout the gastrointestinal tract. These layers correspond to the mucosa adventitia (*a*), muscularis (*b*), submucosa (*c*), and mucosa (*d* and *e*). Because of balloon filling, the layer structure is not recognizable in all parts of the circumference. (*Courtesy of* Arvydas Vanagunas, MD.)

Rings, Webs, and Diverticula

Esophageal web

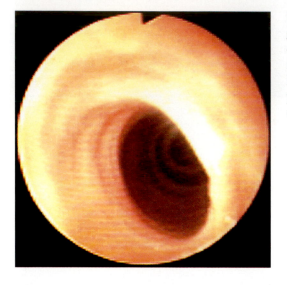

Figure 1-3. Endoscopic view of esophageal webs. Ring-like structures in the esophagus are generally known as *webs*; they can be single or multiple. In most patients no underlying etiology is apparent. It may, however, be associated with graft-versus-host disease in bone marrow transplantation and with some dermatologic diseases, such as epidermolysis bullosa and mucous membrane pemphigoid. This figure is from an otherwise healthy elderly patient with dysphagia. Endoscopic testing revealed multiple esophageal webs. Esophageal dilatation relieved his symptoms. (*Courtesy of* Wallace C. Wu, MB.)

Epiphrenic diverticulum

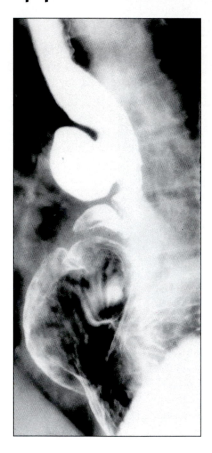

Figure 1-4. Esophagram of a patient with multiple epiphrenic diverticula and achalasia. This is a known association; the diverticulum is presumably caused by the underlying motility disorder. Pneumatic dilatation is thought to be contraindicated in this situation because an increased risk of esophageal perforation may exist. The patient had Heller's myotomy and multiple diverticulectomy. (*Courtesy of* Wallace C. Wu, MB.)

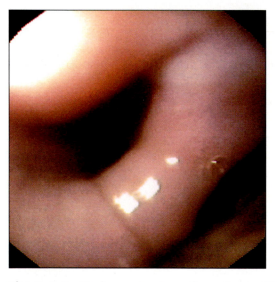

Figure 1-5. Endoscopic view of a patient with a large epiphrenic diverticulum. Two lumen can clearly be seen, one representing the diverticulum and the other the esophageal lumen. (*Courtesy of* Wallace C. Wu, MB.)

Schatzki's ring ·

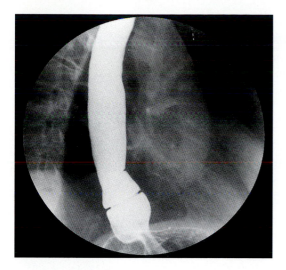

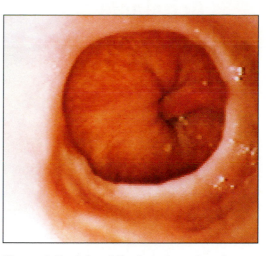

Figure 1-6. Schatzki's ring on barium esophagram. Esophageal webs and rings are thin esophageal stenoses typically composed of only mucosa. Rings formed at the gastroesophageal junction, as described by Schatzki, are usually silent but become symptomatic when the internal diameter is less than 13 mm. (*From* McBride and Ergun [1]; with permission.)

Figure 1-7. Schatzki's ring viewed endoscopically. (*Courtesy of* Gulchin A. Ergun, MD, and Peter J. Katirilas, MD.)

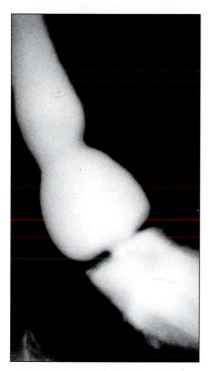

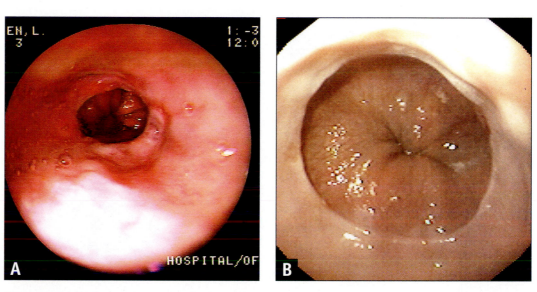

Figure 1-8. Esophagram of malignant stricture, demonstrating the use of contrast radiography in preparation for therapeutic esophageal endoscopy. Contrast radiography is an important part of the work-up of a patient with dysphagia and provides the best measure of lumen caliber. In addition to defining the location of the lesion and probable cause, it also helps clarify the best therapeutic approach, including the method of dilation, the need for fluoroscopic guidance, the need for biopsies or brushings, and aids in follow-up examinations. Barium esophagram may also identify a motility disorder as the cause of the dysphagia. (*Courtesy of* R. Lee Meyers, MD, and Eugene M. Bozymski, MD.)

Figure 1-9. Endoscopic views of Schatzki's rings. Acid-peptic strictures and Schatzki's rings are the most common strictures requiring dilation. Although in most instances endoscopic examination allows obvious distinction between the two, variation in air insufflation and the differences in magnification over short distances between the lower esophageal sphincter and the endoscope can make the assessment of the lower esophagus difficult in some patients. A subtle peptic stricture may be missed endoscopically, or, alternately, may be confused with a Schatzki's ring. Contrast radiology can be a more sensitive technique for demonstrating subtle rings and strictures and for calibrating the lumen more precisely. (*Courtesy of* R. Lee Meyers, MD and Eugene M. Bozymski, MD.)

Achalasia

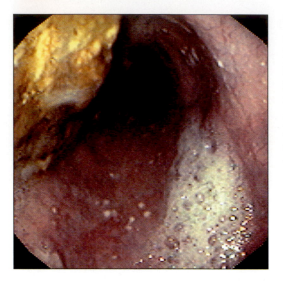

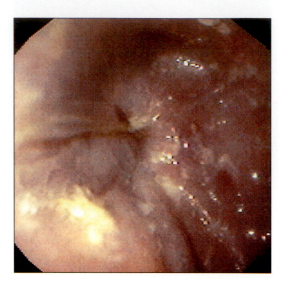

Figure 1-10. Endoscopic view diagnostic of achalasia. Achalasia can occasionally be diagnosed by endoscopy. This image is from a patient who had a markedly dilated esophagus with a large amount of retained ingested food. In a patient with chronic history of dysphagia, this finding is diagnostic for achalasia. In addition, the tightly closed lower esophageal sphincter, which may be difficult to intubate, may show a rosette appearance. (*Courtesy of* Wallace C. Wu, MB.)

Figure 1-11. Classic endoscopic rosette appearance of the gastroesophageal junction in a patient with documented achalasia. This finding is caused by the tightly closed lower esophageal sphincter. (*Courtesy of* Wallace C. Wu, MB.)

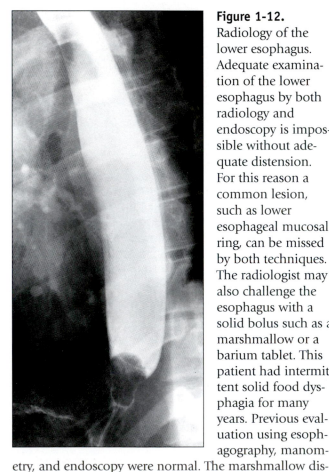

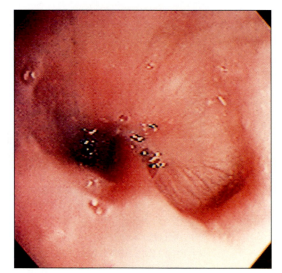

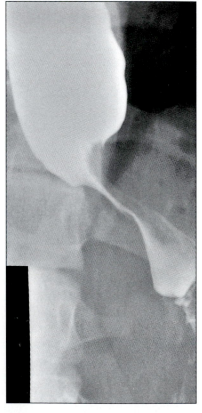

Figure 1-12. Radiology of the lower esophagus. Adequate examination of the lower esophagus by both radiology and endoscopy is impossible without adequate distension. For this reason a common lesion, such as lower esophageal mucosal ring, can be missed by both techniques. The radiologist may also challenge the esophagus with a solid bolus such as a marshmallow or a barium tablet. This patient had intermittent solid food dysphagia for many years. Previous evaluation using esophagography, manometry, and endoscopy were normal. The marshmallow distended the lower esophagus and brought out the lower esophageal mucosal ring. In addition, impaction of the marshmallow reproduced the patient's symptom. Esophageal dilatation rendered this patient asymptomatic. (*Courtesy of* Wallace C. Wu, MB.)

Figure 1-13. Endoscopic view from a patient with achalasia of the lower esophageal sphincter (LES). Note that the region of the LES is tightly closed. Usually a small amount of pressure is needed before the endoscope pops into the stomach. Above the LES there is a wide-mouth diverticulum known as the *epiphrenic diverticulum*. (*Courtesy of* Ravinder K. Mittal, MD.)

Figure 1-14. Barium swallow in a patient with achalasia of the esophagus. This study shows a dilated esophagus in a patient with achalasia of the lower esophageal sphincter. (*Courtesy of* Ravinder K. Mittal, MD.)

Foreign Body Impaction

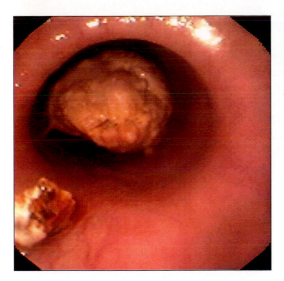

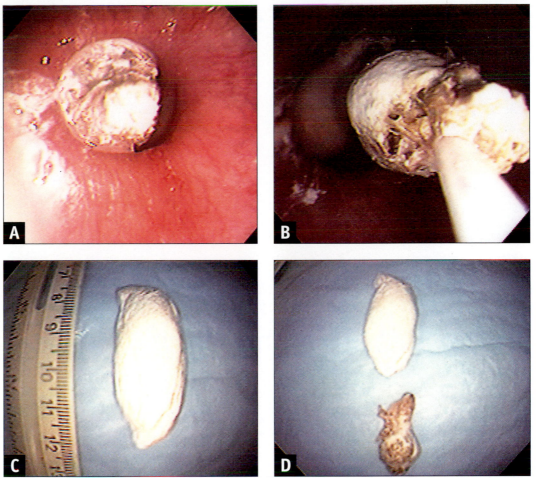

Figure 1-15. Endoscopic view of meat impaction. Foreign body ingestion with esophageal impaction by items other than food is more common among children. In adults, it tends to occur only in psychiatric patients. Food impaction, particularly of red meat or raw fruits and vegetables, however, may occur in patients with esophageal diseases. This figure is from a patient who is suffering from meat impaction. He had given a history of intermittent solid food dysphagia. The offending bolus was removed endoscopically. The patient was then found to have a lower esophageal ring 9 mm in diameter. After undergoing esophageal dilatation, the patient became completely asymptomatic. (*Courtesy of* Wallace C. Wu, MB.)

Figure 1-16. Results when barium and barium-soaked cotton balls are swallowed by a patient with food impaction, seen endoscopically. This patient is a 46-year-old woman with B-ring above a hiatal hernia. **A**, A barium-soaked cotton ball in the midesophagus (a large amount of liquid barium was already suctioned); **B**, extraction of the cotton ball with barium pool below in the esophagus above the impaction; **C**, 4.5 cm × 2 cm cotton ball "mass" removed from the esophagus; **D**, 3.0 cm × 1.5 cm meat impaction with cotton ball. (*Courtesy of* Matthew S.Z. Bachinski, MD, and Roy K.H. Wong, MD.)

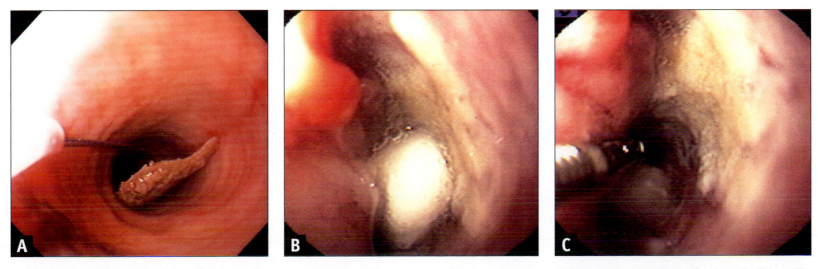

Figure 1-17. Endoscopic views of various objects causing impaction. Food, particularly meat, and small pieces of bone are common. **A**, A chicken bone within the esophageal lumen and mild trauma in the esophagus proximal to the impacted bone. **B**, Squamous cell carcinoma of the esophagus as the underlying abnormality causing narrowing of the esophagus. **C**, Subsequent impaction of a theophylline pill that required removal endoscopically with forceps. (**A**, *Courtesy of* Dr. P. McNally, Eisenhower Army Medical Center; **B**, *courtesy of* Dr. K. Yamamoto, Madigan Army Medical Center; **C**, *courtesy of* Matthew S.Z. Bachinski, MD, and Roy K.H. Wong, MD.)

Gastroesophageal Reflux Disease

Reflux esophagitis

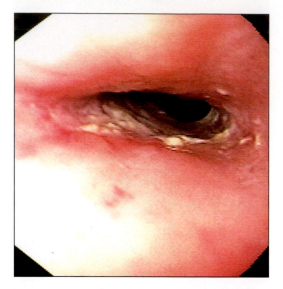

Figure 1-18. Erosive esophagitis: endoscopic view. The hallmark of reflux esophagitis on endoscopy is the presence of one or more erosions within the distal esophagus [2]. Although the finding of such lesions is neither sensitive (occurring in less than 50% of those whose heartburn is explored endoscopically) nor specific (because they can occur with other esophageal injuries), the diagnosis is established by the chronicity of symptoms coupled with the typical nature of the lesions and in the absence of other definable causes (*eg*, infectious or pill-induced esophagitis). (*Courtesy of* Roy C. Orlando, MD.)

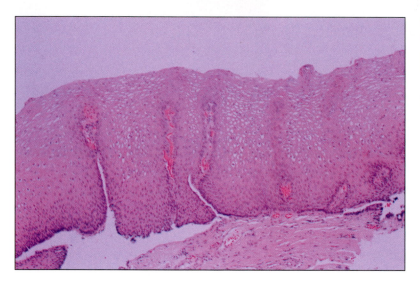

Figure 1-19. Histopathology of gastroesophageal reflux disease. Common alterations seen with early or mild reflux include hyperplasia of the basal zone and elongation of the lamina propria papillae beyond the normal 50% to 66% of the mucosal thickness. Although sensitive diagnostic features, these changes are not specific and may be found in the lower 2 to 3 cm of the esophagus in up to 20% of normal individuals. (*Courtesy of* Randall Lee, MD.)

Barrett's esophagus

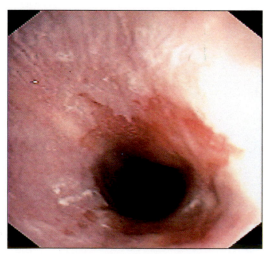

Figure 1-20. Barrett's esophagus: endoscopic pathology. The endoscopic appearance of a columnar-lined lower esophagus (*ie*, Barrett's) is shown for a patient with reflux esophagitis. The typical red coloration of the columnar epithelium is readily distinguished from the lighter pink or orange stratified squamous epithelium [2]. For a specific diagnosis, however, endoscopic biopsy is required for histologic confirmation of the nature of the epithelium lining the lower esophagus. (*Courtesy of* Roy C. Orlando, MD.)

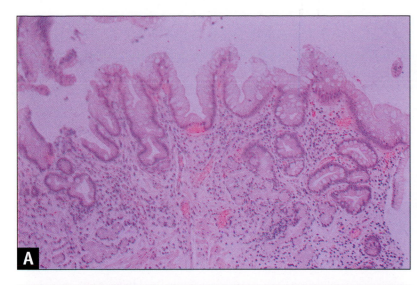

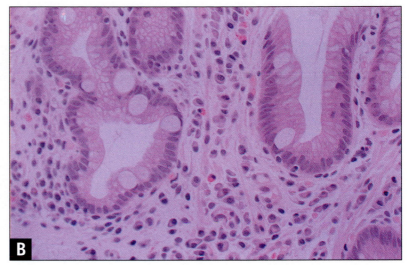

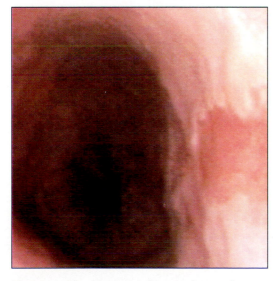

Figure 1-21. Histopathology of Barrett's esophagus. The distinctive metaplastic epithelium of Barrett's esophagus is the so-called specialized form characterized by goblet cells interspersed among tall columnar mucous cells (**A** and **B**). Less commonly noted are gastric cardia-type epithelium with mucous glands or gastric fundic-type epithelium with parietal and chief cells (**C**); the latter type is virtually confined to the distal 2 to 3 cm of Barrett's esophagus. (*Courtesy of* Randall Lee, MD.)

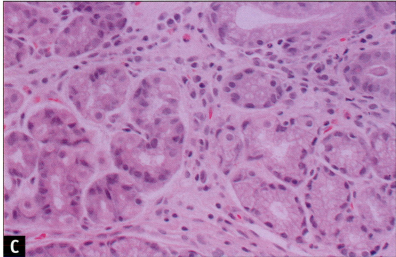

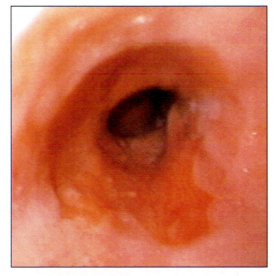

Figure 1-22. Tongue of Barrett's esophagus arising from the gastroesophageal junction into the proximal esophagus viewed endoscopically . (*Courtesy of* Harvey Young, MD.)

Figure 1-23. Endoscopic view of Barrett's esophagus arising circumferentially above the gastroesophageal junction into the distal esophagus. (*Courtesy of* Harvey Young, MD.)

Erosive esophagitis ....

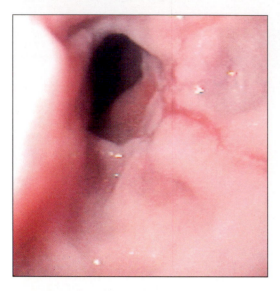

Figure 1-24. Mild erosive esophagitis with superficial linear ulcerations seen endoscopically . (*Courtesy of* Harvey Young, MD.)

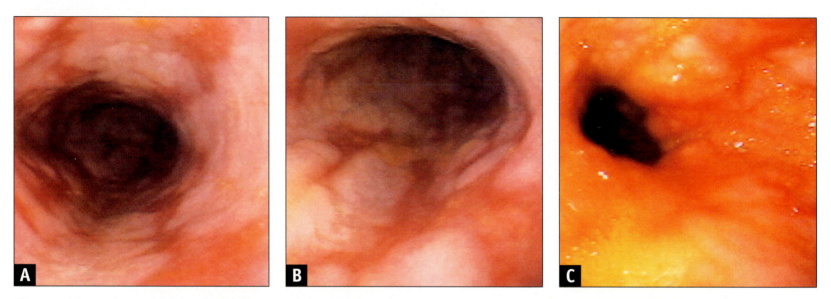

Figure 1-25. Endoscopic view of moderate erosive esophagitis of distal esophagus. (*Courtesy of* Harvey Young, MD.)

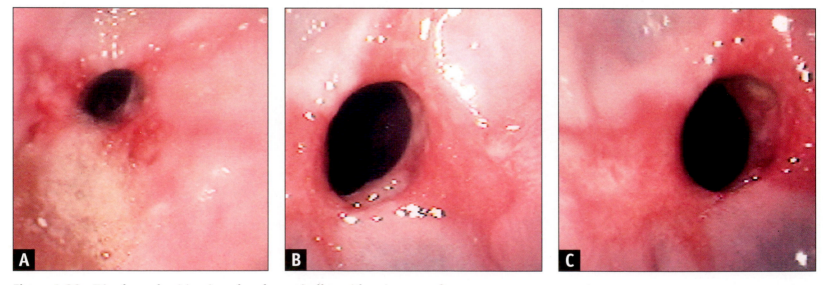

Figure 1-26. Distal esophagitis, viewed endoscopically, with stricture at the gastroesophageal junction. (*Courtesy of* Harvey Young, MD.)

Infectious Esophagitis

Human immunodeficiency virus–associated ulcer.

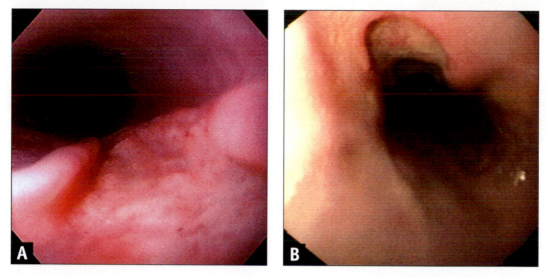

Figure 1-27. Endoscopic views of esophageal ulceration caused by human immunodeficiency virus. The endoscopic characteristics of an esophageal ulcer caused by human immunodeficiency virus (HIV) are variable, ranging from small, superficial shallow aphthous ulcers (0.5 to 1.0 cm) to large, deep ulcers with undermining borders (1 to 5 cm). To be considered as an ulcer caused by HIV other causes of esophageal ulceration must be excluded. These views demonstrate large 6-cm chronic ulcers with deep undermining edges and nodularity within the ulcer base. Idiopathic HIV-associated ulcers have been treated with intravenous corticosteroid therapy. In one study, 23 of 24 patients (95.8%) improved. Relapses were common after discontinuation of therapy. To maintain remission, long-term therapy was required. Trials of sucralfate four times daily mixed with dexamethasone (0.5) mg given as a slurry have been promising. These results must be tempered by the risk of additional long-term immunosuppressive therapy. (*Courtesy of* Matthew S.Z. Bachinski, MD, and Roy K.H. Wong, MD.)

Cytomegalovirus esophagitis.

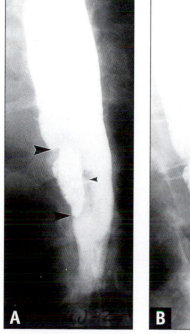 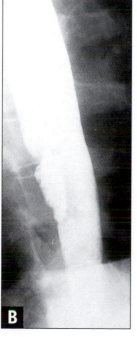

Figure 1-28. Esophagogram revealing a large, deep ulceration caused by cytomegalovirus. **A–B,** Esophagogram taken during the late phases of infection reveals large deep ulceration (*large arrowheads*) with raised borders secondary to edema. The small arrowhead identifies the edematous border.

Esophagogastroduodenoscopy with biopsy of the ulcer crater is required for diagnosis. Brushings of this area are not helpful. Findings early in the course include mucosal erythema and superficial erosions with geographic, serpiginous, nonraised borders. (*Courtesy of* Arunas E. Gasparitis, MD.)

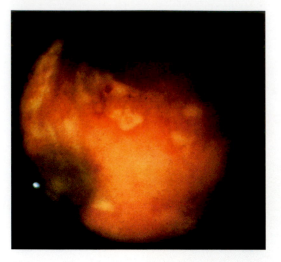

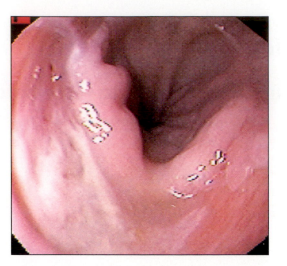

Figure 1-29. Shallow ulceration of the esophagus viewed endoscopically . This figure shows typical midcourse lesions with shallow ulcers 0.5 to 10 cm in which complete denudation of the esophagus is unusual. These ulcers may be indistinguishable from herpes simplex virus ulceration and biopsy is required. Cytomegalovirus infections of the esophagus is typically most prominent in the mid to distal esophagus. (*Courtesy of* Matthew S.Z. Bachinski, MD, and Roy K.H. Wong, MD.)

Figure 1-30. Endoscopic view of large ulcerations typical of the late course of infection caused by cytomegalovirus (CMV). These ovoid or elongated ulcers may extend for several centimeters. Herpes simplex virus ulcers are rarely more than several centimeters in length and the presence of one or more giant ulcers is suggestive of CMV esophagitis. Large ulcers may become hemorrhagic. (*Courtesy of* Matthew S.Z. Bachinski, MD, and Roy K.H. Wong, MD.)

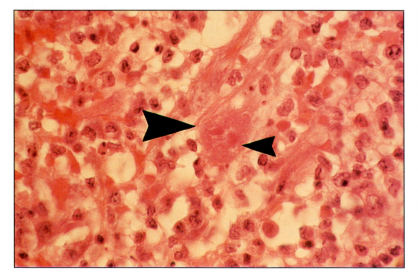

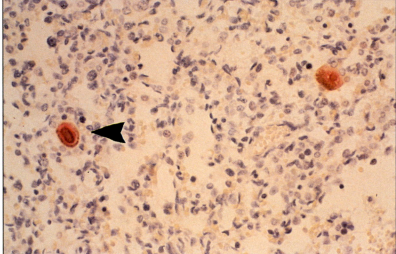

Figure 1-31. Viral culture revealing a CMV-infected cell. Viral culture for CMV can be sensitive if the biopsy is obtained from the correct location. Unfortunately, culturing technique requires long incubation periods (up to 3 weeks) and may not be clinically useful.

This figure shows a photomicrograph with hematoxylin and eosin staining showing typical changes associated with infection caused by cytomegalovirus (CMV). Cells have intranuclear inclusions, halos surrounding the nucleus, and intracytoplasmic inclusions. The large arrowhead identifies a CMV-infected cell whereas the small arrowhead shows the nuclear halo. (*Courtesy of* Matthew S.Z. Bachinski, MD, and Roy K.H. Wong, MD.)

Figure 1-32. An immunoperoxidase stain makes identification of cytomegalovirus (CMV)-infected tissue much easier. The peroxidase stain highlights CMV-infected cells (*arrowhead*), even at early stages of infection when classic cellular changes may not yet be evident. (*Courtesy of* Matthew S.Z. Bachinski, MD, and Roy K.H. Wong, MD.)

Herpes simplex virus esophagitis ································

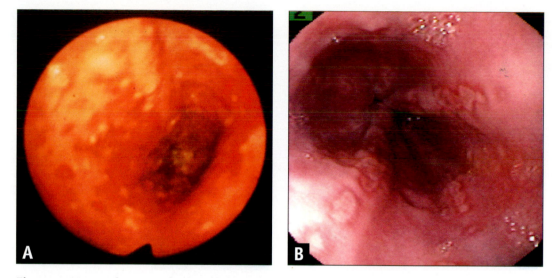

Figure 1-33. Endoscopic findings in esophagitis caused by herpes simplex virus (HSV). Endoscopic findings vary with the severity of the disease and the point at which endoscopy is performed. Early lesions are vesicular, occurring in the midesophagus, and are rarely seen because few endoscopies are performed at this stage, when the vesicles are fragile and easily ruptured. Midway in the course of the disease sharply demarcated small ulcers with raised margins are noted (**A**). The mucosa surrounding the ulcers is often erythematous and edematous. In the late necrotic phase of the disease process, diffuse esophagitis is noted with confluent esophageal ulcers (**B**).

The location of the biopsy site is essential to accurately diagnose esophagitis caused by HSV accurately. Because the virus is active only in epithelial cells, biopsies should be directed at the ulcer edge and not into the crater, which will only yield necrotic debris. (**A**, *Courtesy of* S. Kadakia, MD; **B**, *courtesy of* K. Yamamoto, MD.)

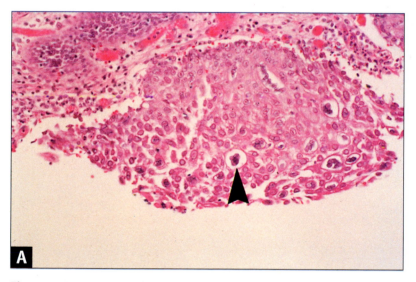

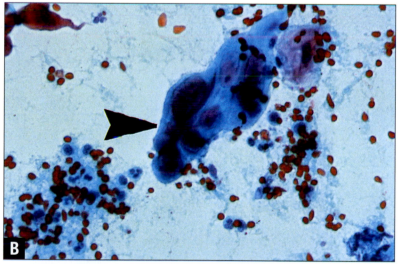

Figure 1-34. Histopathologic identification of esophagitis caused by HSV. Pathologists should be notified that esophagitis caused by herpes simplex virus (HSV) is suspected so that immunohistologic staining can be performed. **A**, HSV invades only the squamous epithelium, causing necrosis of the esophageal mucosa. Findings include multinucleated giant cells and ballooning degeneration of the squamous epithelial cells. Immunohistologic staining clearly identifies cells containing HSV. **B**, Characteristic findings of ballooning degeneration, ground glass nuclei, eosinophilic intranuclear inclusions, and herpetic giant cells (*arrowhead*). Special stains (Papanicolaou's stain) demonstrate multinucleated cells (*arrowhead*); this makes changes associated with HSV more evident.

Viral culture can be used to augment histopathology in diagnosing herpetic esophagitis. Viral culture is more sensitive than endoscopic inspection and microscopic examination. HSV can be rapidly grown in diploid fibroblasts or rabbit kidney cells. Cytopathic changes in culture occur rapidly and are evident within 24 to 96 hours after inoculation. (**A**, *Courtesy of* Matthew S.Z. Bachinski, MD, and Roy K.H. Wong, MD; **B**, *courtesy of* P. McNally, MD.)

Candida esophagitis . . . .

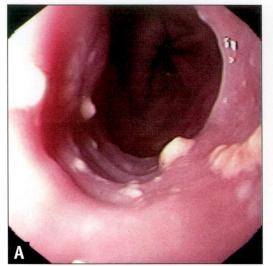
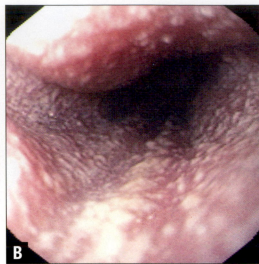

Figure 1-35. Endoscopic early findings of esophagitis caused by *Candida* with plaques not yet becoming confluent. As the infection worsens, there is associated hyperemia. Brushing and biopsy are diagnostic and help to rule out secondary causes of esophagitis. Generally plaques caused by *Candida* will not wash off. Biopsy should be obtained using hematoxylin and eosin stain as well as stains for fungus (silver and periodic acid-Schiff). **A**, Grade 1; **B**, grade 2. (**A**, *Courtesy of* A. Tsuchida, MD; **B**, *courtesy of* K. Yamamoto, MD.)

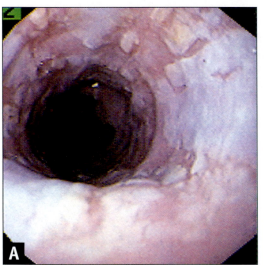
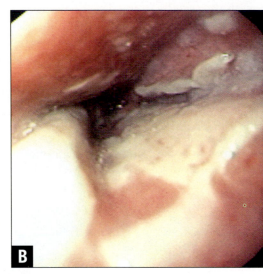

Figure 1-36. Panel A (grade 2-3,) and **panel B** (grade 3-4,) represent the progression of esophageal disease caused by candidiasis seen endoscopically. (**A**, *Courtesy of* Matthew S.Z. Bachinski, MD, and Roy K.H. Wong, MD; **B**, *courtesy of* M. Lyons, MD.)

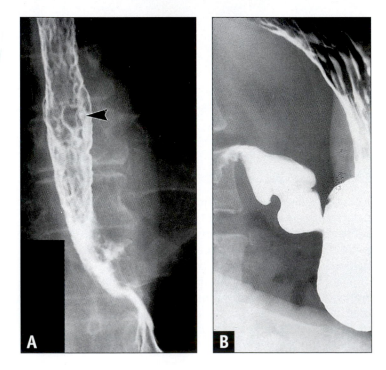

Figure 1-37. **A–B**, Esophagrams showing classic findings in acute esophagitis caused by *Candida*. Discrete plaque-like lesions, oriented longitudinally, producing linear or irregular filling defects with distinct margins (*arrowhead*). (*Courtesy of* Matthew S.Z. Bachinski, MD, and Roy K.H. Wong, MD.)

Pill-Induced Esophagitis

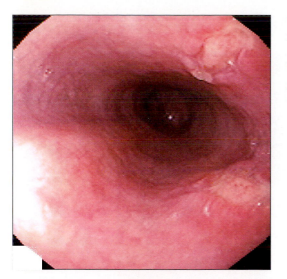

Figure 1-38. Endoscopic view of esophagitis caused by doxycycline pills. A 25-year-old female was prescribed doxycycline for treatment of acne. After she developed dysphagia and odynophagia acutely, she remembered that she had taken a dose of doxycycline just before she went to bed the night before. Endoscopy showed two ulcers in the midesophagus. The history and endoscopic appearance are perfectly compatible with the diagnosis of esophagitis caused by medication in pill form. (*Courtesy of* Wallace C. Wu, MB.)

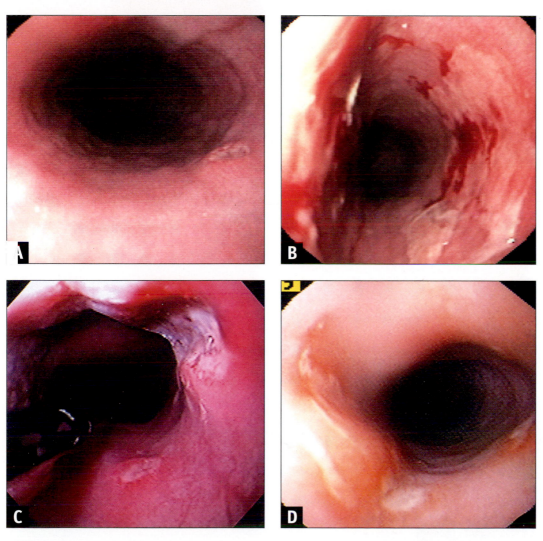

Patients with severe or persistent esophageal symptoms and an appropriate history of pill ingestion should have endoscopy. Findings, often including esophagitis, hiatal hernia, Schatzki's B-ring, or stricture, are all most commonly found in the distal esophagus. Most pill-induced lesions occur in the endoscopically normal esophagus, and are located between the junction of the proximal and middle esophagus. The lesions associated with pill-induced esophageal injury vary with the agent ingested and the duration of injury.

The type of pill and duration of esophageal contact may influence the injury. Punctate ulcers with well-circumscribed borders may be noted with antibiotics, such as doxycycline and erythromycin. A shallow plaque-like ulcer with a thin membrane can also be noted, resulting from lower toxic concentrations or shorter duration of injury. Raised, plaque-like membranes can be seen with quinidine-induced esophageal injury. Pill-induced lesions may be single or multiple, with remnants of pills sometimes noted within the ulcer crater.

A, A discrete tetracycline-induced ulcer with normal surrounding mucosa. **B,** Aggressive plaque-like, membranous ulceration, secondary to doxycycline with adjacent ulcers on each side of the esophagus. Friability and bleeding is noted following intubation of the endoscope. **C,** Large, deep ulcer and smaller more discrete ulceration secondary to erythromycin. **D,** Classic pill-induced "kissing ulcerations." (**A,** *Courtesy of* T. Peller, MD; **B,** *courtesy of* K. Yamamoto, MD; **C, D,** *courtesy of* Matthew S.Z. Brachinski, MD, and Roy K.H. Wong, MD.)

Figure 1-39. Pill induced esophagitis viewed endoscopically. Patients typically have no prior history of esophageal disease and present with sudden onset of retrosternal pain, exacerbated by swallowing. Pain may be mild or so severe that swallowing may be impossible. Typically, the pain increases over the first 72-hour pill ingestion and gradually subsides. Patients with preexisting esophageal problems, such as gastroesophageal reflux disease (GERD), frequently present with worsening symptoms of heartburn, regurgitation, and dysphagia. In more severe esophageal injury patients may present with odynophagia.

Bleeding Varices and Mallory-Weiss

Esophageal varices

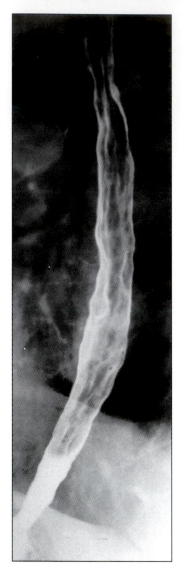

Figure 1-40. Esophageal varices as seen on barium swallow. Portal hypertension results in congestion and dilation with the deep intrinsic veins becoming grossly enlarged, thus displacing the more superficial venous systems. The deep veins eventually occupy a superficial subepithelial location and are identified radiographically and endoscopically as esophageal varices. (*Courtesy of* Frank Miller, MD.)

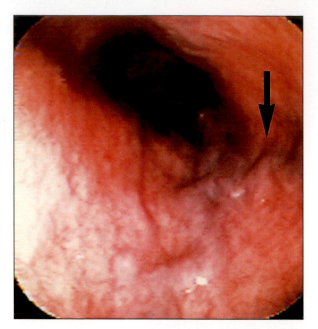

Figure 1-41. Esophageal varices seen endoscopically. The varices appear as slightly bluish dilated vessels (*arrow*). (*Courtesy of* Gulchin A. Ergun, MD, and Peter J. Kahrilas, MD.)

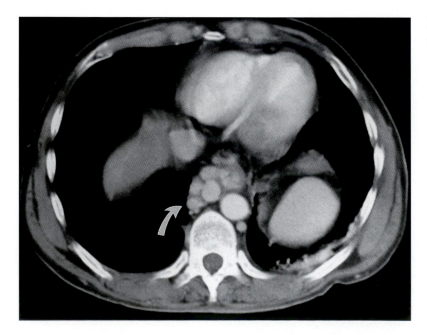

Figure 1-42. Gastroesophageal varices (*arrow*) demonstrated with computed tomography. (*Courtesy of* Frank Miller, MD.)

Squamous cell papilloma . . . .

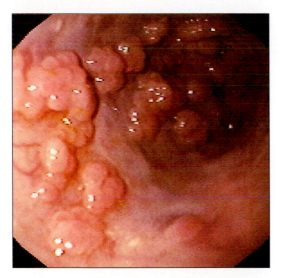

Figure 1-48. Endoscopic view of multiple squamous cell papilloma. Squamous cell papilloma of the esophagus is a rare benign tumor of the esophagus. It usually does not produce any symptoms and appears as a single or multiple wart-like lesion on the esophageal mucosa. This figure comes from a patient who was incidentally found to have multiple squamous cell papilloma. She had no esophageal symptoms, and because of the extent of the lesion endoscopic, excision was not contemplated. (*Courtesy of* Wallace C. Wu, MB.)

Squamous cell carcinoma . . . .

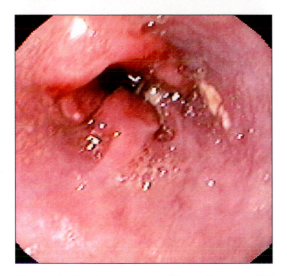

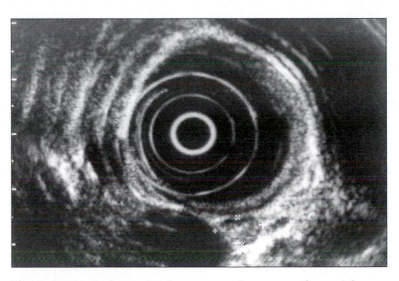

Figure 1-49. Squamous cell carcinoma of the esophagus seen endoscopically. A patient who experienced progressive solid-food dysphagia for several months and a 20-pound weight loss. Endoscopy of the patient confirmed the presence of an apparently malignant lesion in the esophagus. Biopsies showed a squamous cell carcinoma of the esophagus. (*Courtesy of* Wallace C. Wu, MB.)

Figure 1-50. Endoscopic ultrasonography was performed for staging. It clearly revealed lymph node metastasis. For this reason, the patient was not considered to be a candidate for primary surgical resection. Instead, he was treated with radiation and chemotherapy. (*Courtesy of* Wallace C. Wu, MB.)

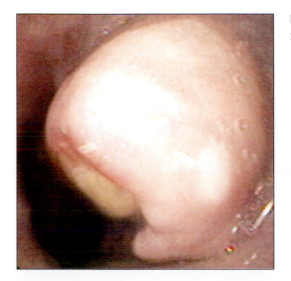

Figure 1-51. Endoscopic view of an 85-year-old Chinese man with squamous cell carcinoma of the esophagus from 26 to 30 cm. (*Courtesy of* Harvey Young, MD.)

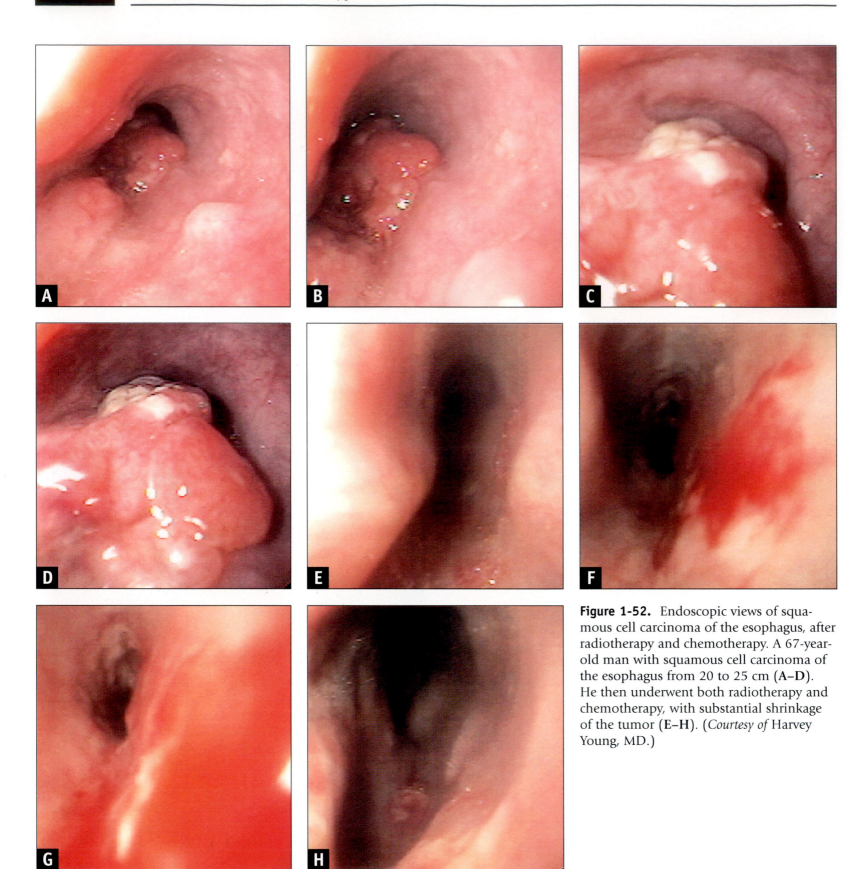

Figure 1-52. Endoscopic views of squamous cell carcinoma of the esophagus, after radiotherapy and chemotherapy. A 67-year-old man with squamous cell carcinoma of the esophagus from 20 to 25 cm (**A–D**). He then underwent both radiotherapy and chemotherapy, with substantial shrinkage of the tumor (**E–H**). (*Courtesy of* Harvey Young, MD.)

Expandable metal stent for cancer......................

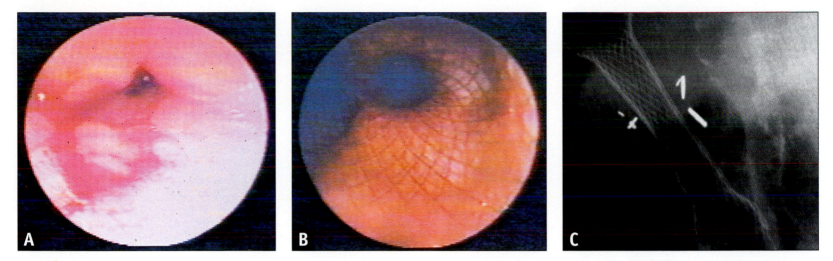

Figure 1-53. Techniques: expandable metallic stents. Self-expanding metallic stents are relatively new and may increase the use of stenting to palliate patients with esophageal cancer. They have several advantages over traditional stents. Their small pre-expansion diameter requires less dilation before stent placement and permits easier placement. Their post-expansion diameter is generally larger than rigid stents and, therefore, should provide more effective relief of dysphagia and longer stent patency. In the only prospective, randomized trial to date comparing expandable stents with rigid stents, the expandable metal stents were more cost-effective and had fewer complications [5]. In these models, tumor ingrowth through the mesh was a problem, although some more recent models are coated with synthetic membranes designed to prevent this. If tumor ingrowth or overgrowth at the margins occurs, then it is often treatable with laser or additional stent placement. Although metal stents are easier to place than traditional stents, initially after expansion, they are difficult to reposition, and, therefore, should only be placed by experienced physicians. **A–B**, Endoscopic views of an esophageal tumor before and after stent placement. **C**, a radiograph demonstrating the expanded stent in the esophagus. (*Courtesy of* R. Lee Meyers, MD, and Eugene M. Bozymski, MD.)

Laser treatment of cancer ....

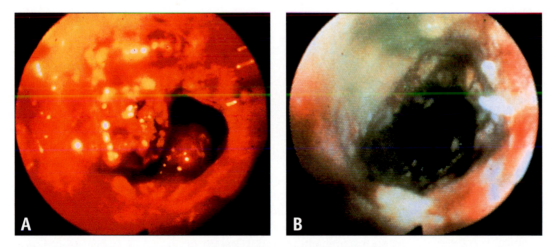

Figure 1-54. Endoscopic laser treatment of esophageal cancer: Technique. This procedure can generally be done with intravenous conscious sedation rather than general anesthesia. Two strategies for laser application exist. The initially developed method involves application of the laser beam with concentric destruction of tumor proceeding from the lumen to the wall, proximally to distally as much as possible during a single session. Progression to the distal portion of the tumor may be limited by the formation of edema with this method. The second, and more preferred, technique involves application of laser distal to proximal. If feasible, a guidewire is first placed distal to the lesion into the stomach; several Savary dilators are passed to facilitate maneuverability of the scope during the treatment. This latter method generally requires fewer treatment sessions. **Panel A** and **Panel B** demonstrate an exophytic tumor obstructing the esophagus and a patent lumen established after laser treatment. (*Courtesy of* R. Lee Meyers, MD, and Eugene M. Bozymski, MD.)

Malignant stricture ....

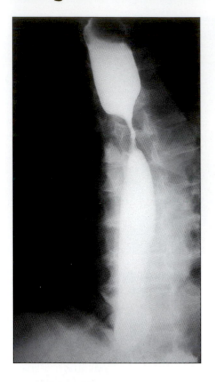

Figure 1-55. Esophagram demonstrating malignant stricture. (*Courtesy of* R. Lee Meyers, MD, and Eugene M. Bozymski, MD.)

Adenocarcinomas ....

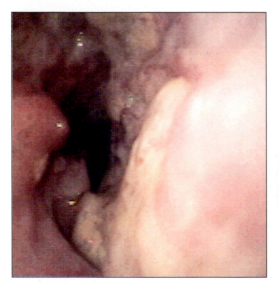

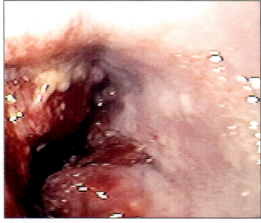

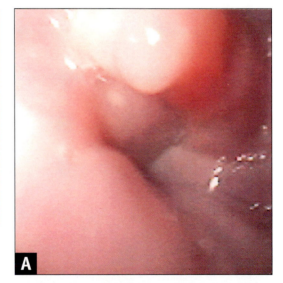

Figure 1-56. Adenocarcinoma of the esophagus viewed endoscopically. A 69-year-old man with adenocarcinoma of the esophagus extending from 33 to 40 cm; this lesion was T3N1 by endoscopic ultrasound. (*Courtesy of* Harvey Young, MD.)

Figure 1-57. Adenocarcinoma of the esophagus seen endoscopically. A 63-year-old man with adenocarcinoma of the esophagus extending from 32 to 37 cm and stage T3N1 by endoscopic ultrasound. (*Courtesy of* Harvey Young, MD.)

Figure 1-58. A–D, Endoscopic views of a 41-year-old man with adenocarcinoma arising from the gastroesophageal junction. (*Courtesy of* Harvey Young, MD.)

(*Continued on next page*)

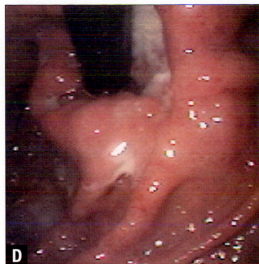
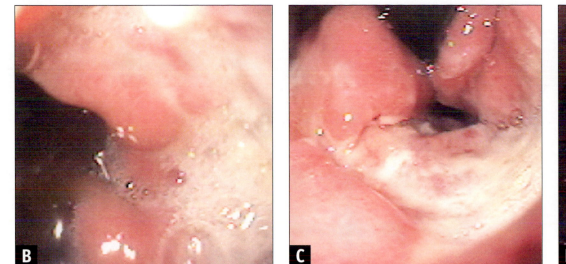

Figure 1-58. *(Continued)*

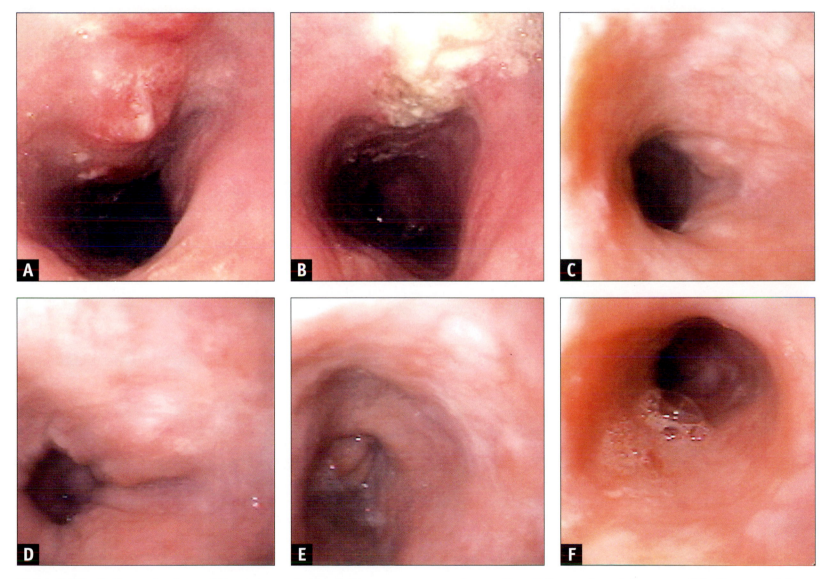

Figure 1-59. Endoscopic views of Barrett's esophagus. A 73-year-old man developed an adenocarcinoma of the esophagus arising in a Barrett's esophagus (**A**). He then underwent laser therapy, which caused necrosis and destruction of the tumor (**B**). One month later, esophagoscopy showed no evidence of the tumor (**C–F**). (*Courtesy of* Harvey Young, MD.)

Strictures

Peptic stricture

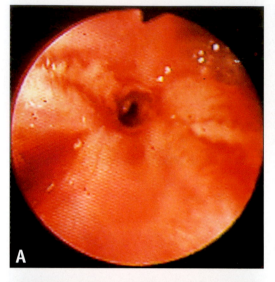

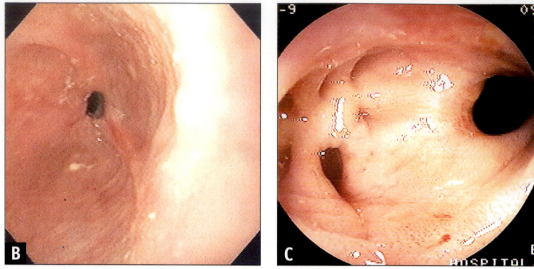

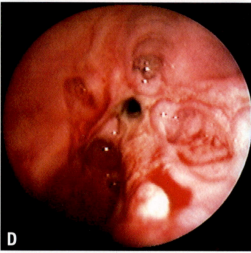

Figure 1-60. Endoscopic appearance of benign strictures. Acid-peptic strictures and Schatzki's rings are the most common strictures requiring dilation. Although in most instances endoscopic examination allows obvious distinction between the two, variation in air insufflation and the differences in magnification over short distances between the lower esophageal sphincter and the endoscope can make the assessment of the lower esophagus difficult in some patients. A subtle peptic stricture may be missed endoscopically, or, alternately, may be confused with a Schatzki's ring. Contrast radiology can be a more sensitive technique for demonstrating subtle rings and strictures and for calibrating the lumen more precisely. **A–D**, peptic strictures. Note the esophageal pseudodiverticula proximal to the septic stricture in *c* and *d*. Their presence increases the risk of unguided dilatation of the esophagus and mandates the use of a guidewire technique. (*Courtesy of* R. Lee Meyers, MD, and Eugene M. Bozymski, MD.)

Figure 1-61. Esophagram demonstrating Schatzki's ring. (*Courtesy of* R. Lee Meyers, MD, and Eugene M. Bozymski, MD.)

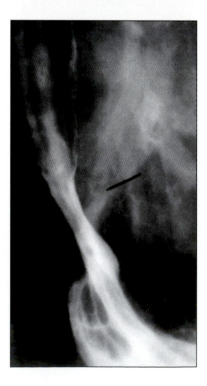

Radiation esophagitis and stricture . . . .

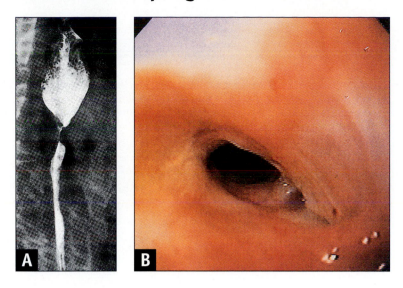

Figure 1-62. Esophageal strictures. At a radiation dose of less than 30 Gy patients have self-limited, asymptomatic esophagitis. At dosages above 30 Gy, there may be progression to fibrosis and scarring of the esophagus. Strictures are typically smooth and elongated with thickened walls. Neural elements of the esophageal wall are frequently damaged. Esophageal peristalsis may be absent proximal to the stricture. Other complications include ulceration, pseudopolyp formation, mucosal bridging, and fistulization to the tracheal or bronchia apparatus, mediastinum, or aorta. The findings noted at endoscopy vary with the duration of time that the patient has received radiation therapy. The series of endoscopic photos demonstrates a spectrum of injury from acute esophagitis to circumferential ulceration with stricture formation, as demonstrated both radiographically (**A**) and endoscopically (**B**). (*From* Wilcox [6]; with permission.)

Balloon dilators . . . .

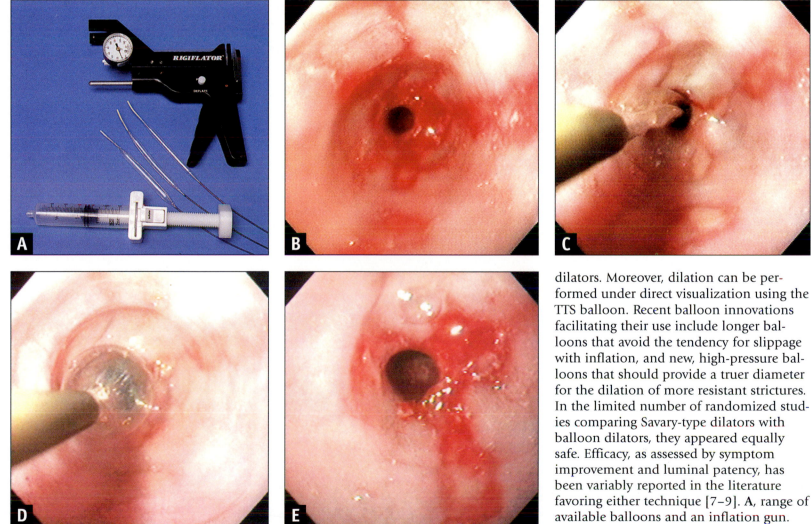

Figure 1-63. Types of dilators: balloons. Balloon dilators are an additional option for the endoscopist approaching an esophageal stricture. They may be placed over a guidewire or through the scope (TTS). Theoretically, balloons have the advantage of being safer because of the radial application of force and elimination of the shearing effect of rigid dilators. Moreover, dilation can be performed under direct visualization using the TTS balloon. Recent balloon innovations facilitating their use include longer balloons that avoid the tendency for slippage with inflation, and new, high-pressure balloons that should provide a truer diameter for the dilation of more resistant strictures. In the limited number of randomized studies comparing Savary-type dilators with balloon dilators, they appeared equally safe. Efficacy, as assessed by symptom improvement and luminal patency, has been variably reported in the literature favoring either technique [7–9]. **A,** range of available balloons and an inflation gun. **B–E,** a peptic stricture before and after balloon dilation, thus demonstrating the direct visualization that is possible with the TTS technique. (*Courtesy of* R. Lee Meyers, MD, and Eugene M. Bozymski, MD.)

References

1. McBride MA, Ergun GA: Role of upper endoscopy in the management of esophageal strictures. *Gastrointes Endosc Clin North Am* 1994, 4:595–621.

2. Tygat GNJ: Upper gastrointestinal endoscopy. In *Textbook of Gastroenterology*. Edited by Yamada T, Alpers DH, Owyang C, *et al*. Philadelphia: JB Lippincott; 1991:435–436.

3. Stiegman GV, Sun JH, Hammond WS: Results of experimental endoscopic esophageal varix ligation. *Am Surg* 1988, 54:105–108.

4. Cunningham ET Jr, Jones B, Donner MW: Normal anatiomy and techniques of examination of the pharynx. In *Alimentary Tract Radiology*. Edited by Freeny PC, Stevenson GW. St. Louis: Mosby–Year Book; 1994:94–130.

5. Knyrim K, Wagner HJ, Bethge N, *et al*.: A controlled trial of an expansile metal stent for palliation of esophageal obstruction due to inoperable cancer. *N Engl J Med* 1993, 329:1302–1307.

6. Wilcox CM: *Atlas of Clinical Gastrointestinal Endoscopy*. Philadelphia: WB Saunders; 1995.

7. Saeed ZA, Winchester CB, Feffo PA, *et al*.: Prospective randomized comparison of polyvinyl bougies and through-the-scope balloons for dilation of peptic strictures of the esophagus. *Gastrointest Endosc* 1995, 41:189–195.

8. Cox JGC, Winter RK, Maslin SC, *et al*.: Balloon or bougie for dilation of benign esophageal stricture? An interim report of a randomized controlled trial. *Gut* 1988, 29:1741–1747.

9. Shemesh E, Czemiak A: Comparison between Savary-Gilliard and balloon dilation of benign esophageal strictures. *World J Surg* 1990, 14:518–522.

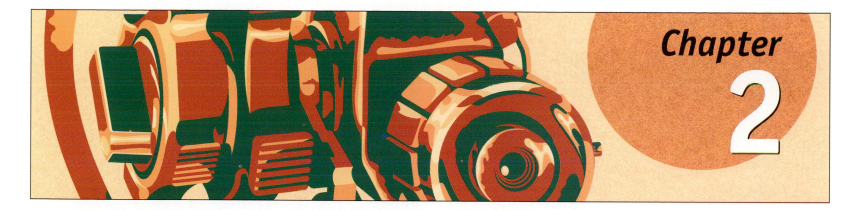

Chapter 2

Stomach

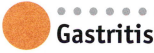

Gastritis

Erosive gastritis

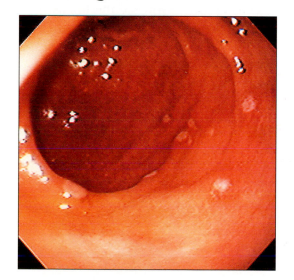

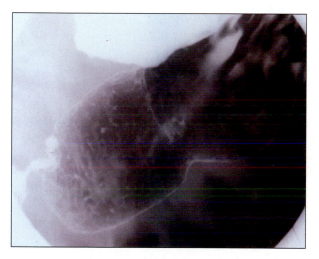

Figure 2-1. Endoscopic erosive gastritis. The observations of multiple erosive and hemorrhagic lesions may be defined endoscopically as gastritis. This figure is an example of endoscopic erosive gastritis. Common settings that may lead to endoscopic gastritis include use of nonsteroidal anti-inflammatory drugs, alcohol abuse, and the physiologic stress associated with serious illnesses (stress gastritis). Other less common causes include ingestion of corrosives, chemotherapeutic agents, or irradiation. There may also be no known demonstrable associated factor present (idiopathic). (*Courtesy of* W. Harford, MD.)

Figure 2-2. Erosive gastritis on upper gastrointestinal barium examination. Superficial gastric erosions appear radiographically as multiple tiny flecks of barium, which represent the erosions, surrounded by radiolucent halos, which represent surrounding mounds of edematous mucosa. Superficial gastric erosions can also appear as flat defects that coat with barium without surrounding reaction and are represented by reproducible linear streaks or dots of contrast. This barium study is an example of the radiographic appearance of erosive gastritis showing multiple tiny flecks, some surrounded by halos. It also shows areas of coalescence of lesions into linear streaks. (*Courtesy of* W. L. Peterson, MD.)

Gastritis associated with nonsteroidal anti-inflammatory drugs. . . . .

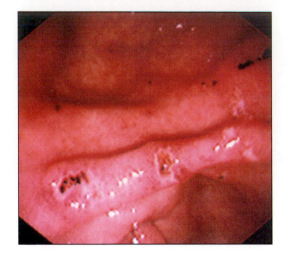

Figure 2-3. Endoscopic view of gastritis associated with aspirin and other nonsteroidal anti-inflammatory drug (NSAID) use. As shown in this figure, ingestion of aspirin and other NSAIDs can produce acute gastric mucosal erosions and subepithelial hemorrhages. Although found in all gastric locations, these NSAID–associated lesions have a predilection for the fundus and body. The constellation of multiple small erosions and multiple small submucosal hemorrhages throughout the stomach is very suggestive of NSAID use. On microscopic evaluation, the occurrence of a mucosal inflammatory infiltrate is not greater than that expected for age-matched controls who are not taking NSAIDs. Thus, NSAIDs do not actually cause a histologic gastritis. A more appropriate term for this condition is *NSAID gastropathy*. (*Courtesy of* Edward Lee, MD, and Byron Cryer, MD.)

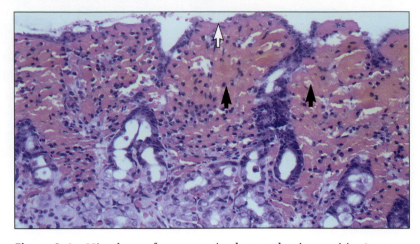

Figure 2-4. Histology of acute erosive hemorrhagic gastritis. As already mentioned, acute erosive hemorrhagic gastritis is the histologic correlate for the gross mucosal injury (erosions & hemorrhage) associated with agents such as nonsteroidal anti-inflammatory drugs. As shown here, the histologic features are erosions (*open arrow*) as evidenced by denuding of surface epithelium with necrosis of the glands involving the superficial third of the mucosa and hemorrhage (*closed arrows*) also involving the superficial portion of the gastric mucosa. It is this lack of penetration of the necrosis down to the muscularis layer that differentiates acute erosive gastritis from acute ulceration. (*Courtesy of* Edward Lee, MD, and Byron Cryer, MD.)

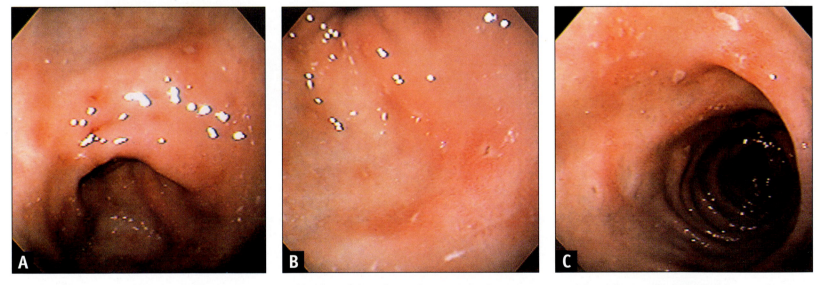

Figure 2-5. Nonsteroidal anti-inflammatory drug (NSAID)–induced disease seen endoscopically. Although NSAID–induced lesions may occur anywhere in the stomach or duodenum, the most common location is the antrum. In this patient, subepithelial hemorrhage, erosions and small ulcers are seen in the antrum (**A–B**).

(Continued on next page)

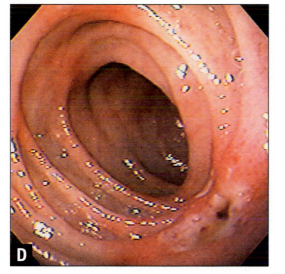

Figure 2-5. *(Continued)* Erosions in the duodenal bulb (**C**) and a posterior duodenal ulcer (**D**) are also present. (*Courtesy of* C. Mel Wilcox, MD.)

Alcoholic hemorrhagic gastritis. . . . .

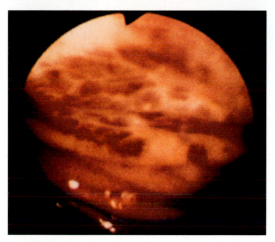

Figure 2-6. Endoscopic gastritis: alcohol. Alcohol consumption can result in endoscopic mucosal abnormalities termed *alcoholic hemorrhagic gastritis*. As shown in this figure, endoscopically such patients will have multiple subepithelial hemorrhages without any visible breaks in the mucosa. The appearance has been described as that of "blood under plastic wrap". These lesions are mainly confined to the body and fundus of the stomach and are infrequently seen in the antrum. (*From* Laine and Weinstein [1]; with permission.)

Pathologic features of gastritis. . . . .

A. Chronic gastritis: nonspecific gastritis- *Helicobacter pylori*

Classifications of chronic gastritis

Category	Nomenclature	Etiology
Nonspecific	Chronic active superficial gastritis	*H. pylori*, autoimmune and bile reflux
	or Chronic superficial gastritis	
	or Chronic atrophic gastritis	
Specific	Depends on etiology	Bacterial, viral, fungal, parasitic, granulomatous, eosinophilic, and hypertrophic

Figure 2-7. Chronic gastritis: nonspecific gastritis, *Helicobacter pylori*. As we move into the chronic gastritides, the classification of chronic gastritis is presented again for review. Nonspecific histologic gastritis is characterized by various patterns of gastric mucosal inflammation (as compared with the specific forms of gastritis that usually have a predictable pattern of mucosal inflammation). Nonspecific histologic gastritis is more precisely called *nonerosive nonspecific gastritis*, and since the discovery of *H. pylori*, it is almost always noted in association with this organism. Therefore, most cases of nonerosive nonspecific gastritis are said to be caused by *H. pylori*.

(Continued on next page)

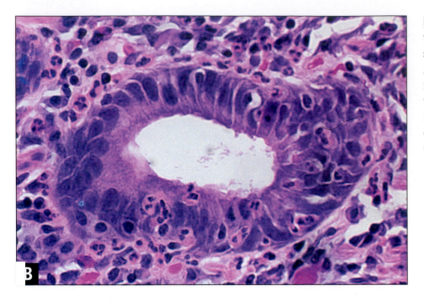

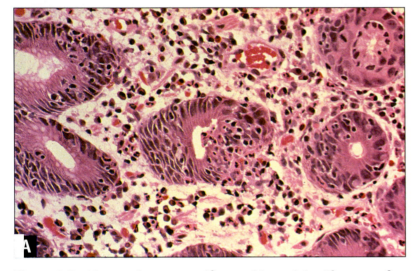

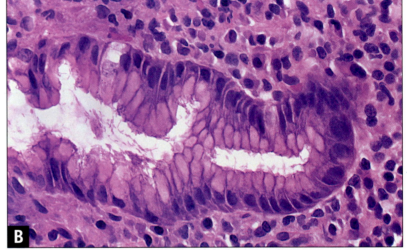

Figure 2-7. *(Continued)* *H. pylori* appear as small rods with a central bend or curve that are found beneath the mucus coat overlying surface epithelial cells. Although there are special stains to detect *H. pylori*, the organism can usually be easily seen on high-power microscopic examination of a hematoxylin and eosin–stained section as shown in this figure of a fundic mucosal biopsy with chronic active superficial gastritis; *H. pylori* is visible overlying the surface epithelium of the pits. (*Courtesy of* Edward Lee, MD, and Byron Cryer, MD.)

Figure 2-8. Nonerosive nonspecific gastritis: activity. The type of mucosal inflammatory infiltrate will determine the activity of the biopsy. **A**, Chronic active superficial gastritis is defined by an increase in both acute (neutrophils) and chronic (lymphocytes and plasma cells) inflammatory cells in the lamina propria. **B**, Chronic superficial gastritis is defined by an increase in only chronic inflammatory cells (lymphocytes and plasma cells) in the lamina propria. In this example of chronic superficial gastritis, note the markedly diminished number of neutrophils, the lack of neutrophil infiltration of the glands, and the numerous *Helicobacter pylori* present in the pits. (*Courtesy of* Edward Lee, MD, and Byron Cryer, MD.)

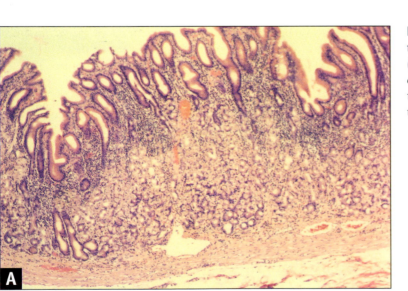

Figure 2-9. Nonerosive nonspecific gastritis: depth of inflammation. Nonerosive nonspecific gastritis is also defined by depth (severity) of mucosal inflammation. **A**, The least severe grade is chronic superficial gastritis in which the inflammation is confined to the gastric pit (foveolar) region. The glandular compartment is usually unaffected.

(Continued on next page)

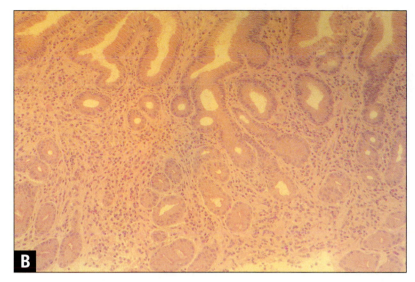

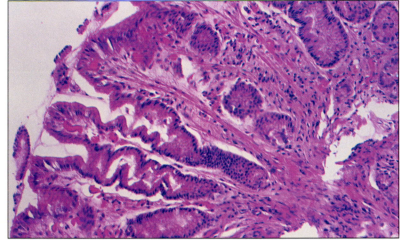

Figure 2-9. *(Continued)* **B**, In the higher grade, chronic atrophic gastritis, inflammation extends down into the mucosa to involve the glandular compartment and variable degrees of glandular atrophy may be present. Note in this example of chronic atrophic gastritis that a number of glands have been lost through destruction by inflammatory cells. (**A**, *Courtesy of* Edward Lee, MD, and Byron Cryer, MD; **B**, *courtesy of* Randall G. Lee, MD.)

Figure 2-10. Foveolar hyperplasia. Chronic inflammation of the gastric pits may lead to an increase in pit (foveolar) mitotic activity, ultimately resulting in pit elongation or foveolar hyperplasia. As shown, in addition to having become elongated, the gastric pits become more tortuous and develop a corkscrew appearance. Foveolar hyperplasia is the product of chronic inflammation associated with a number of conditions including gastropathy resulting from use of nonsteroidal anti-inflammatory drugs, Ménétrier's disease, hyperplastic polyps, and alkaline reflux gastritis in patients who have undergone partial gastric resections or gastrojejunostomies. (*Courtesy of* Edward Lee, MD, and Byron Cryer, MD.)

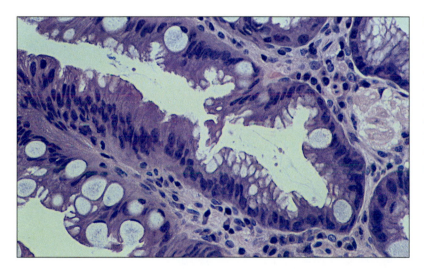

Figure 2-11. Intestinal metaplasia. The presence of intestinal metaplasia is characterized by a change of mucosal pattern from gastric type of epithelium to either a small intestinal type (paneth cells), colonic type (goblet cells), or both. In the stomach, intestinal metaplasia can occur in any gastric region and may arise in response to chronic injury such as in gastritis, especially chronic atrophic gastritis. Intestinal metaplasia is usually found in the pit region of the surface epithelium. This example demonstrates goblet cells lining many of the gastric pits. (*Courtesy of* Edward Lee, MD, and Byron Cryer, MD.)

Eosinophilic gastritis. . . . .

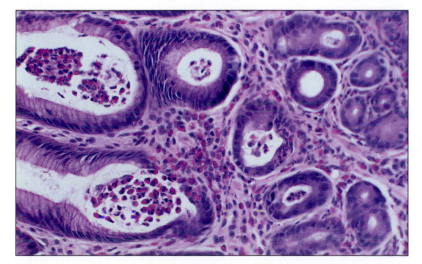

Figure 2-12. Histology of eosinophilic gastritis. The view of this condition represents the gastric component of the more generalized eosinophilic gastroenteritis. Endoscopically, usually no gross abnormality is present. Although all parts of the stomach may be involved, the eosinophilic infiltrate has a predilection for the antrum. This figure above demonstrates a gastric biopsy with numerous eosinophils most abundant in the superficial lamina propria and the lumen of the pits. On deeper sections the infiltrate may extend down into the muscularis mucosa. No ulceration, granulomas, or parasites were present. Such findings are consistent with a diagnosis of eosinophilic gastritis, a nonspecific diagnosis with a large differential that includes allergy, collagen vascular disorders such as Churg-Strauss syndrome or polyarteritis nodosa, parasitic infections such as schistosomiasis and strongyloidiasis, and lymphoma. (*Courtesy of* Edward Lee, MD, and Byron Cryer, MD.)

● ●

Ménétrier's Disease

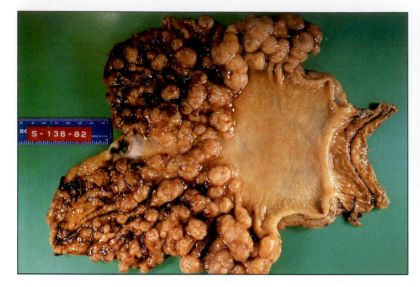

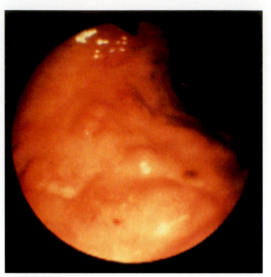

Figure 2-13. Ménétrier's disease: gross pathology. The clinical features diagnostic of Ménétrier's disease are giant folds, especially in the fundus and body of the stomach, protein-losing enteropathy with hypoalbuminemia, hypochlorhydria in advanced stages, and a marked increase in mucosal thickness overall. As shown in this figure, its gross pathological characteristics are enlarged gastric folds in the gastric body that typically spare the antrum. These folds have a nodular or polypoid configuration and may have associated erosions or ulcerations. (*Courtesy of* Edward Lee, MD, and Byron Cryer, MD.)

Figure 2-14. Ménétrier's disease: endoscopic characteristics. In common with the view shown in Figure 2-13, on endoscopy in Ménétrier's disease, large nodular gastric folds may also be appreciated. Shown is an endoscopic image of the gastric body taken from the retroflexed endoscopic angle of nodular and polypoid appearing gastric folds in a patient with Ménétrier's disease. (*Courtesy of* M. Feldman, MD.)

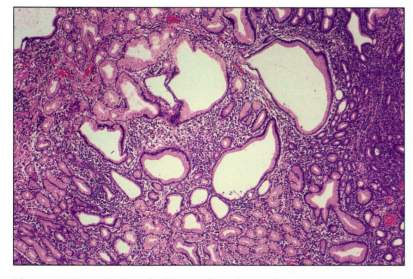

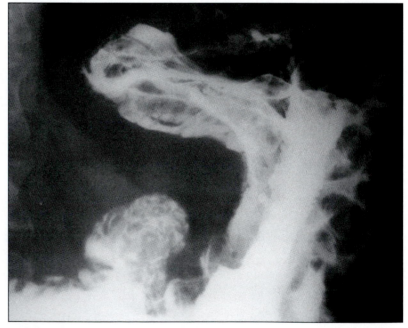

Figure 2-15. Ménétrier's disease: histologic characteristics. Histologically, Ménétrier's disease is characterized by marked elongation and cystic dilation of glands lined by foveolar epithelium and glandular atrophy. The lamina propria has a dense chronic (lymphocytic) inflammatory infiltrate. (*Courtesy of* Edward Lee, MD, and Byron Cryer, MD.)

Figure 2-16. Ménétrier's disease, upper GI series. Upper GI series demonstrating the giant folds in the fundus and body of the stomach. (*Courtesy of* Brooke Jeffrey, MD.)

Peptic Ulcer Disease

Gastric ulcer

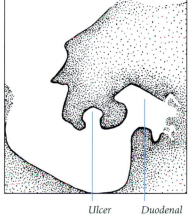
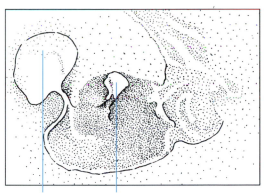
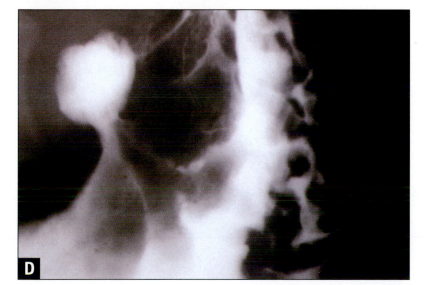
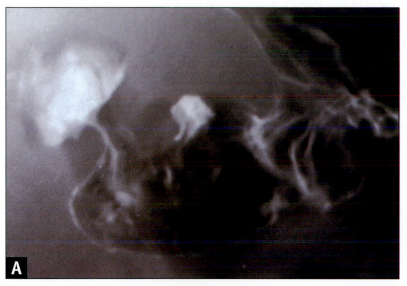
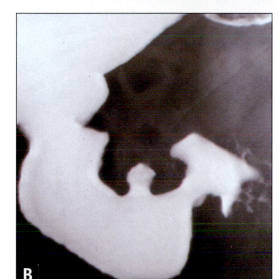
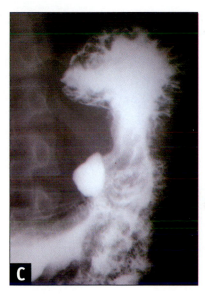
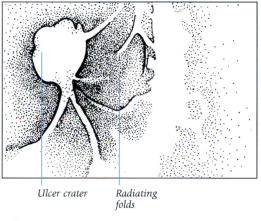

Figure 2-17. Typical radiographic features of a benign gastric ulcer. This ulcer on the distal lesser curvature in the antrum is well circumscribed (**A**) and lateral views (**B**) demonstrate projection of the crater away from the lumen. A large well-circumscribed ulcer is seen on the angularis (**C**). Rugal folds can be seen radiating to the crater (**D**).

(Continued on next page)

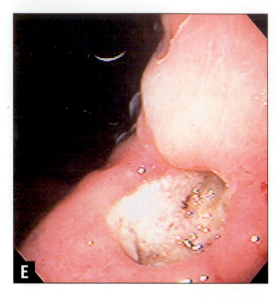

Figure 2-17. *(Continued)* The ulcer crater at endoscopy is shown in **E**. The lesion is large and well circumscribed with a symmetrical appearance. Multiple biopsies did not demonstrate carcinoma and the ulcer was demonstrated to heal on follow-up endoscopy. Radiographic features suggestive of a benign ulcer include projection of the ulcer away from the lumen, absence of mass effect or mucosal nodularity, and rugal folds of normal appearance, which extend to the ulcer crater. The sensitivity of barium radiography for the diagnosis of gastric ulcer is approximately 65% to 90%; the sensitivity increases with the size of the lesion. *(Courtesy of* C. Mel Wilcox, MD.)

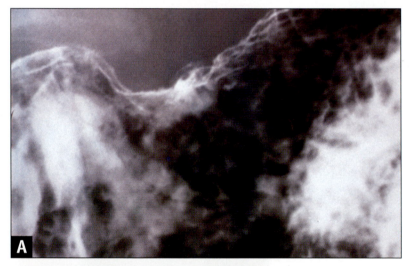

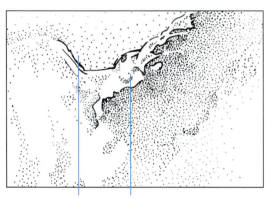

Retraction   Ulcer crater

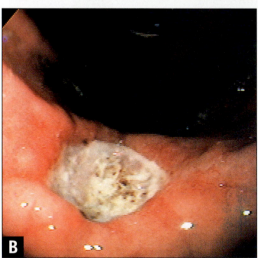

Figure 2-18. Benign gastric ulcer. **A,** Barium radiograph demonstrates a lesion on the angularis atypical for a benign lesion because the angularis is retracted. The ulcer margin is also not well demarcated. No abnormal rugal folds surround the lesion. Radiographically, a malignant lesion could not be excluded. **B,** Typical endoscopic appearance of a benign gastric ulcer. The ulcer is on the angularis—the most common location for a gastric ulcer—and is well circumscribed without any associated mass effect. The surrounding mucosa is mildly erythematous and without nodularity. *(Courtesy of* C. Mel Wilcox, MD.)

Gastric ulcer with adherent clot ....

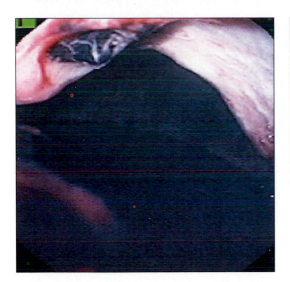

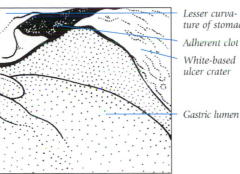

*Lesser curva-
ture of stomach*

Adherent clot

*White-based
ulcer crater*

Gastric lumen

Figure 2-19. Gastric ulcer with adherent clot seen endoscopically. This patient presented with massive upper gastrointestinal bleeding. This gastric ulcer lies on the lesser curvature in close proximity to the gastroesophageal junction (as evidenced by the endoscope seen on retroflexion view). Notice adherent clot within the ulcer crater—a diffuse, poorly organized collection of blood—that did not wash off the ulcer base with a jet of water from the endoscope. (*Courtesy of* Karl Fukunaga, MD, and Russell Yang, MD.)

Gastric ulcer with visible clot ....

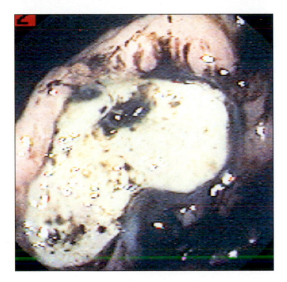

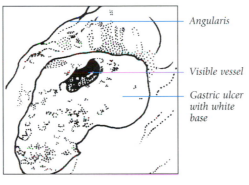

Angularis

Visible vessel

*Gastric ulcer
with white
base*

Figure 2-20. Endoscopic view of gastric ulcer with visible vessel. This gastric ulcer also lies along the lesser curvature and is so large that it occupies almost the entire angularis. Within the crater of the ulcer is a visible vessel—a well-circumscribed and glistening nodule. (*Courtesy of* Karl Fukunaga, MD, and Russell Yang, MD.)

Gastric ulcer with various stigmata of recent bleeding ....

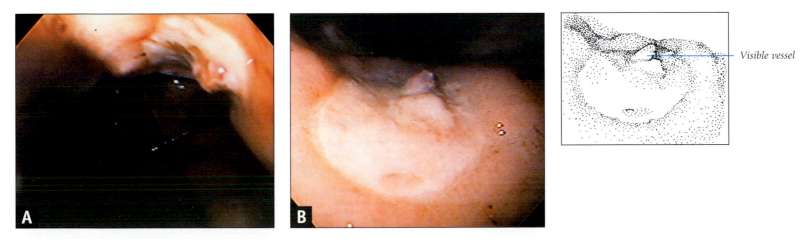

Visible vessel

Figure 2-21. Benign gastric ulcer. **A,** Close-up of the lesion demonstrates a visible vessel. **B,** A benign-appearing gastric ulcer located on the angularis has a protuberance in the center of the crater characteristic of a visible vessel (**B**) (*bottom* [**C, close up view**]).

(*Continued on next page*)

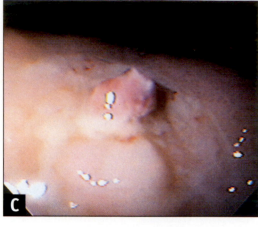

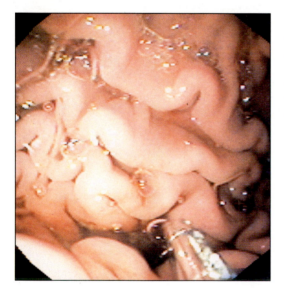

Adherent clot

Ulcer bed

Artery

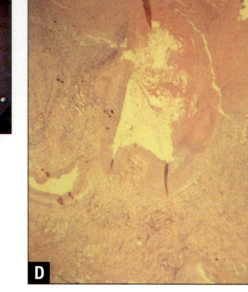

Figure 2-21. *(Continued)* This stigmata has approximately 50% chance of rebleeding. Certain colors of the visible vessel may increase the chance of rebleeding to 90%. (In this patient, hemorrhage recurred and gastric ulcer resection was performed.) **D,** The histopathologic equivalent of the visible vessel is shown. In this patient, a large artery is seen in the base of the ulcer with clot resulting in a nipplelike projection from the ulcer base. (*Courtesy of* C. Mel Wilcox, MD.)

Zollinger-Ellison Syndrome

Figure 2-22. Prominent gastric folds in a patient with Zollinger-Ellison syndrome (ZES) on gastroscopy. Gastrin has trophic effects on the gastric mucosa [2,3,4,5] resulting in prominent gastric folds, increased numbers of parietal cells, and increased numbers of enterochromaffin-like (ECL) cells. This figure shows the prominent gastric folds in a 17-year-old patient who presented with peptic ulcer disease (NIH #2663004), who was eventually diagnosed to have ZES. The presence of prominent folds such as this should lead to a possible suspicion of ZES in the patient. (*Courtesy of* Robert T. Jensen, MD.)

Miscellaneous Gastric Bleeding Lesions

Hemorrhagic gastritis

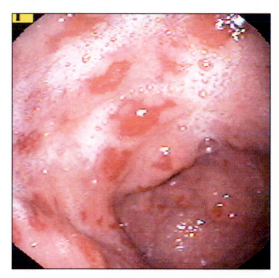

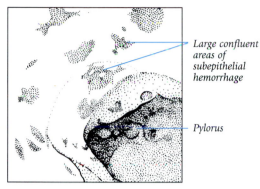

Large confluent areas of subepithelial hemorrhage

Pylorus

Figure 2-23. Hemorrhagic gastritis viewed endoscopically. *Gastritis* is a histologic term that does not necessarily correlate with the endoscopic appearance. Gastritis or more precisely, gastropathy, usually occurs in the setting of stress, alcohol abuse, or non-steroidal anti-inflammatory drug use. This figure is an extreme example of hemorrhagic gastritis. There are several areas of confluent subepithelial hemorrhage (with an appearance of blood under plastic wrap) separated by areas of eroded mucosa. (*Courtesy of* Karl Fukunaga, MD, and Russell Yang, MD.)

Osler-Weber-Rendu disease.

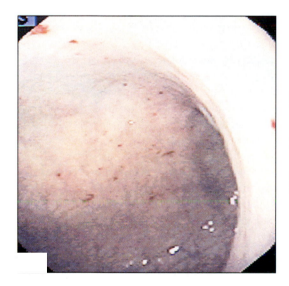

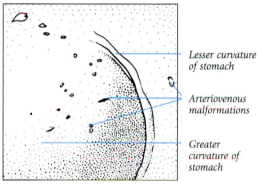

Lesser curvature of stomach

Arteriovenous malformations

Greater curvature of stomach

Figure 2-24. Endoscopic view of Osler-Weber-Rendu disease. Osler-Weber-Rendu disease (*ie*, hereditary hemorrhagic telangiectasia), an autosomal dominant disorder, may present with diffuse arteriovenous malformations throughout the gastrointestinal tract. If sufficiently localized, endoscopic ablation is the treatment of choice. If the lesions are diffuse, however, estrogen-progesterone therapy may be helpful [6]. Oral aminocaproic acid has also been reported to be of prophylactic benefit [7]. (*Courtesy of* Karl Fukunaga, MD, and Russell Yang, MD.)

Watermelon stomach

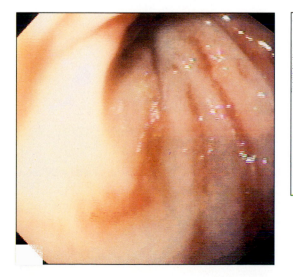

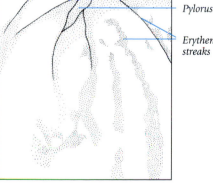

Pylorus

Erythematous streaks

Figure 2-25. Watermelon stomach [8] seen endoscopically. This lesion results from multiple antral vascular ectasias formed in a pattern of linear streaks radiating from the pylorus. Histologically, it consists of multiple dilated venules with focal thrombosis and fibromuscular hyperplasia. The cause of watermelon stomach is not known but it occurs primarily in older women. It presents with iron-deficient anemia, which is usually manageable with iron supplementation. In extreme cases, endoscopic thermal therapy or surgical antrectomy may be necessary. (*Courtesy of* Karl Fukunaga, MD, and Russell Yang, MD.)

Antral vascular ectasia . . . .

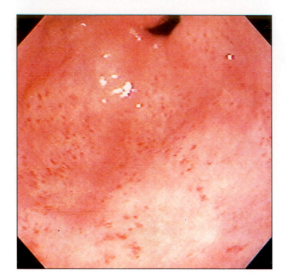

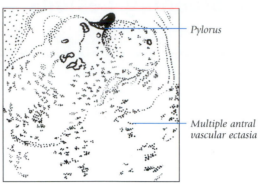

Pylorus

Multiple antral vascular ectasia

Figure 2-26. Antral vascular ectasia viewed endoscopically. Multiple antral vascular ectasia have been described in primary biliary cirrhosis usually when associated with the CREST (calcinosis, Raynaud's phenomenon, esophageal dysfunction, sclerodactyly, and telangiectasia) syndrome. The ectasia appears as multiple punctate areas of erythema on the antral mucosa. (*Courtesy of* Karl Fukunaga, MD, and Russell Yang, MD.)

Dieulafoy's lesion . . . .

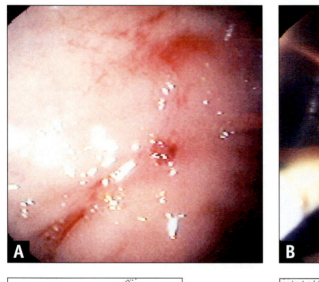

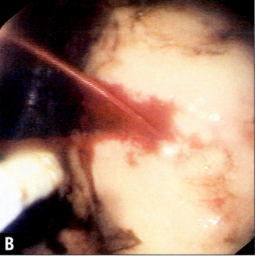

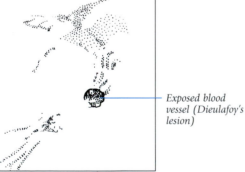

Exposed blood vessel (Dieulafoy's lesion)

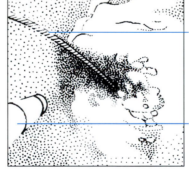

Spurting blood from Dieulafoy's lesion

Bipolar electro-coagulation probe

Figure 2-27. Endoscopic views of Dieulafoy's lesion. Dieulafoy's lesion is a rare cause of massive and recurrent upper gastrointestinal hemorrhage. The lesion is an extramural caliber artery present in the submucosa. Bleeding probably results from pressure exerted by such a blood vessel on the overlying mucosa so that it is ultimately exposed to the lumen. Dieulafoy's lesion is most common in the gastric cardia, 6 cm from the gastroesophageal junction. Mortality is high because the bleeding site is often difficult to identify. **A,** Rarely Dieulafoy's lesion may have the appearance of a visible blood vessel in the absence of an ulcer crater. **B,** When exposed to the lumen, the vessel's wall may actually break down and lead to dramatic bleeding [9]. (*Courtesy of* Karl Fukunaga, MD, and Russell Yang, MD.)

Gastric varices, fundus. . . . .

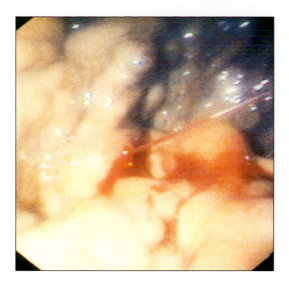

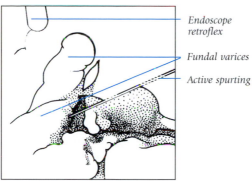

Endoscope retroflex

Fundal varices

Active spurting

Figure 2-28. Endoscopic view of fundal varices. Gastric varices usually occur in the fundus of the stomach. These fundal varices are best seen on retroflex view; they have the classic appearance of a submucosal *cluster of grapes*. These fundal varices, which are demonstrating active bleeding, occurred in a patient with hepatocellular carcinoma with sinistral portal hypertension secondary to tumor invasion of the portal vein. It is believed that up to 10% of variceal bleeds result from bleeding fundal varices [10]. Bleeding fundal varices are associated with a higher mortality rate than bleeding esophageal varices. In addition, conventional sclerotherapy has produced disappointing results with high rebleeding rates, often secondary to sclerotherapy-induced ulceration. There is some evidence that injection of fundal varices with a tissue adhesive, histoacryl, may be successful in controlling hemorrhage [11]. (*Courtesy of* Karl Fukunaga, MD, and Russell Yang, MD.)

Portal hypertensive gastropathy . . . .

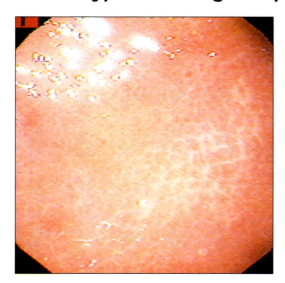

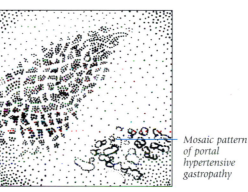

Mosaic pattern of portal hypertensive gastropathy

Figure 2-29. Portal hypertensive gastropathy. Typically portal hypertensive gastropathy has the appearance of a mucosal mosaic pattern with a speckling of subepithelial hemorrhages superimposed upon it. Histologically, it consists of vascular dilation and ectasia. Despite being very common in patients with portal hypertension, it is not clear if portal hypertensive gastropathy by itself is responsible for significant upper gastrointestinal hemorrhaging. (*Courtesy of* Karl Fukunaga, MD, and Russell Yang, MD.)

Gastric Tumors

Gastric carcinoma

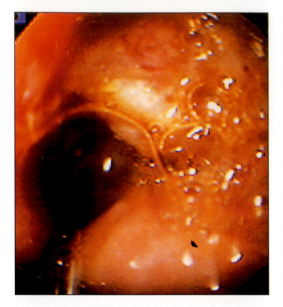

Figure 2-30. Endoscopic view of gastric carcinoma. The most common type of all malignant gastric neoplasms is the gastric adenocarcinoma. Squamous cell carcinomas of the stomach, as well as the hepatoid adenocarcinomas, are both very rare forms of gastric carcinomas. The 5-year survival rate for patients with gastric adenocarcinoma is 15%. It should be noted, however, that this percentage represents an average survival rate. Survival rates are thought to be considerably lower in younger patients than middle-aged and elderly patients. Treatment includes local resection for patients with "early gastric cancer", extensive resection and lymph node dissection for patients with advanced gastric cancer, and the addition of chemotherapeutic modalities for those patients in whom there is evidence of widespread metastatic disease. The possible role of adjuvant, neoadjuvant, hormonal, or radiographic therapy in the treatment of patients with advanced gastric cancer remains uncertain. Certain groups of patients are at significantly higher risk than others, including postpartial gastrectomy patients, patients with pernicious anemia, patients of lower socioeconomic status, and patients whose diet includes intake of large amounts of salted fish, starches, pickled vegetables, meat, smoked foods, nitrates, and nitrites. Even for such patients, routine endoscopic screening is not warranted. When a person from such a high-risk group develops symptoms, however, the patient should have upper gastrointestinal endoscopy. The possible endoscopic features seen can include such an ulcerated mass as shown in this figure. (*Courtesy of* Daniel C. DeMarco, MD.)

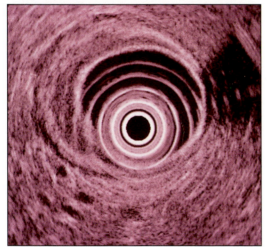

Figure 2-31. Use of endoscopic ultrasound confirms the depth of invasion of this lesion as seen in Figure 2-30. Involvement is to the fourth layer, which is composed of the muscularis mucosae. The serosa is not involved. No lymphadenopathy is seen. No adjacent organs are involved. This is classified as a $T_2 N_0 M_0$ lesion [12]. (*Courtesy of* Daniel C. DeMarco, MD.)

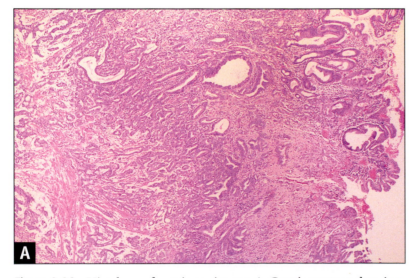

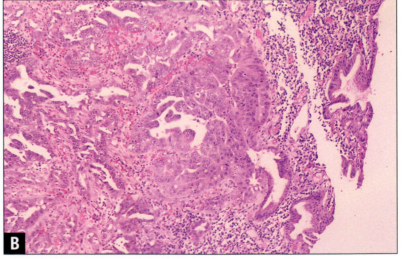

Figure 2-32. Histology of gastric carcinoma. **A,** Gastric mucosa showing infiltrating, moderately differentiated adenocarcinoma of the intestinal type. The tumor partially involves the surface and then infiltrates the underlying submucosa. Tumor cells form tubular glands of varying sizes and shapes with surrounding stromal desmoplasia (hematoxylin and eosin stain; original magnification × 40). **B,** Same view as *A,* although at different magnification (hematoxylin and eosin stain; original magnification × 100). (*Courtesy of* Daniel C. DeMarco, MD.)

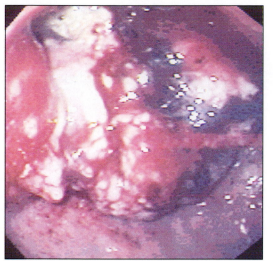

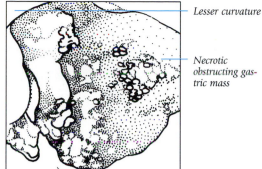

Lesser curvature

Necrotic obstructing gastric mass

Figure 2-33. Gastric carcinoma. Gastric adenocarcinoma accounts for more than 95% of the malignant tumors of the stomach. This lesion was discovered in a patient who presented with melenic stools and progressive anemia. This carcinoma is a fungating and friable mass, which could easily account for gastrointestinal bleeding. Unfortunately, most gastric carcinomas present as this one did and are not resectable at the time of diagnosis. (*Courtesy of* Karl Fukunaga, MD, and Russell Yang, MD.)

Ulcerative carcinoma ....

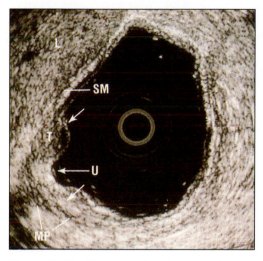

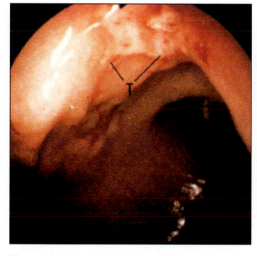

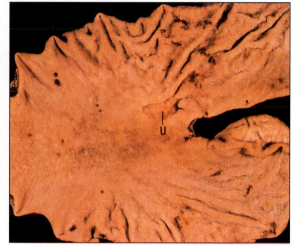

Figure 2-34. Endoscopic ultrasound of carcinoma in the body of the stomach. A 68-year-old man with a carcinoma in the body of the stomach was referred for preoperative staging. Endoscopic ultrasound shows an ulcer with nodular margins (*arrows*) containing an intrasubmucosal carcinoma (T). SM—submucosa. (*From* Tio [13]; with permission.)

Figure 2-35. In the same patient as shown in Figure 2-34, endoscopy shows an ulcerative carcinoma (T) located at the lesser curvature of the stomach. (*From* Tio [13]; with permission.)

Figure 2-36. Macroscopically, the resected specimen shows an ulcer (U) at the lesser curvature of the stomach. It was subsequently proven during additional analysis to be an early gastric carcinoma of submucosal type. (*From* Tio [13]; with permission.)

Carcinoma of the cardia . . . .

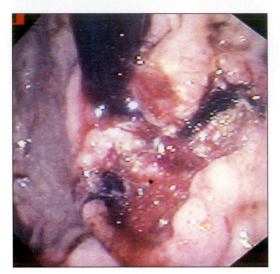

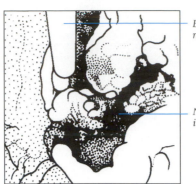

Endoscope on retroflex view

Necrotic tumor in cardia

Figure 2-37. Cardia carcinoma seen endoscopically. The gastric cardia is that portion of the stomach immediately adjoining the esophagus. Because of the proximity to the esophagus, carcinoma of the gastric cardia can result in dysphagia. This carcinoma is seen on retroflexion view and has a friable, necrotic appearance. Surgical resection of such a tumor is challenging because it may require an esophagectomy in addition to a partial gastrectomy. (*Courtesy of* Karl Fukunaga, MD, and Russell Yang, MD.)

Gastric carcinoid . . . .

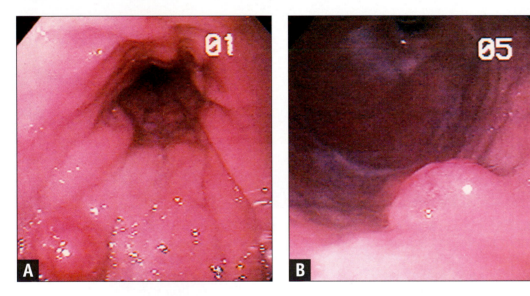

Figure 2-38. **A** and **B**, Carcinoid tumor: endoscopic view. Gastric carcinoids are rare tumors arising from enterochromaffin cells and are thought to be promoted by achlorhydria alone or combined with hypergastrinemia. They are rarely seen, even in persons on potent acid-inhibiting medication. This image shows multiple gastric carcinoids in a patient with chronic pernicious anemia. (*Courtesy of* Daniel C. DeMarco, MD.)

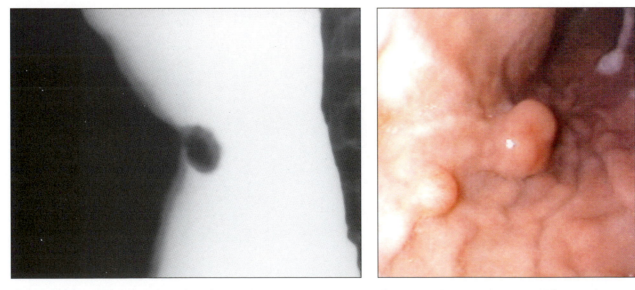

Figure 2-39. Gastric carcinoid: radiography. Upper GI series showing filling defect in the body of the stomach, later confirmed to be a carcinoid tumor. (*Courtesy of* Brooke Jeffrey, MD.)

Figure 2-40. Gastric carcinoid. Gastric carcinoid in mid body of the stomach. (*Courtesy of* Harvey Young, MD.)

Gastric carcinoid, pathology . . . .

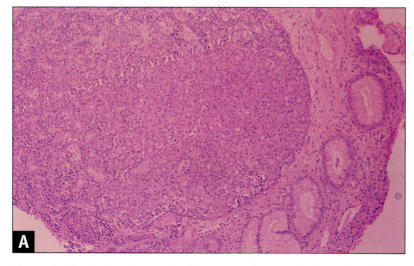

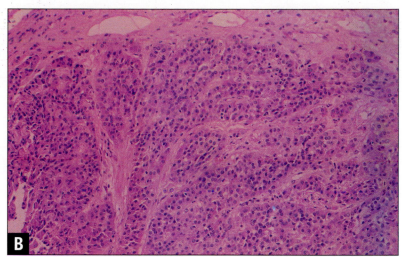

Figure 2-41. **A,** Gastric carcinoid tumor composed of small uniform cells arranged in nests. Tumor cells form irregular anastomosing ribbons as well as some acinar formation (hemotoxylin and eosin stain; original magnification × 40). **B,** Same view as in *A,* although at a different magnification (hematoxylin and eosin stain; original magnification × 100). (*Courtesy of* Daniel C. DeMarco, MD.)

Gastric lymphoma . . . .

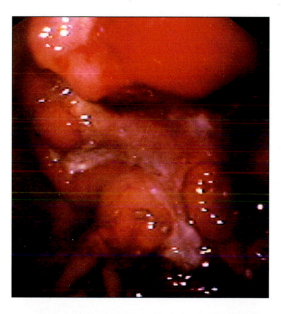

Figure 2-42. Endoscopic view of gastric lymphoma. Gastric lymphoma represents less than 5% of the gastric malignant neoplasms seen. The stomach remains the most common site of involvement for extranodal non-Hodgkin's lymphoma. Using only endoscopy and radiographic barium studies, lymphoma may be difficult to differentiate from gastric adenocarcinoma. Biopsies also are not particularly helpful in making the diagnosis. The 5-year survival rate for patients who have gastric lymphoma is approximately 50% when all combinations of patients and therapeutic modalities are considered. This endoscopic view reveals thickened folds. The differential diagnosis of thickened gastric folds includes many entities such as Zollinger-Ellison syndrome, Ménétrier's disease, varices lues, idiopathic hypertrophic gastrophy, eosinophilic gastritis, pseudolymphoma, and lymphoma. (*Courtesy of* Daniel C. DeMarco, MD.)

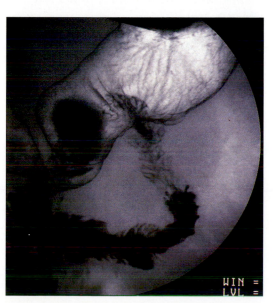

Figure 2-43. Radiography of gastric lymphoma. Thickened gastric folds and a mass noted involving the stomach. Often such deformities can extend into the duodenum. Such lesions are often difficult to distinguish from those present resulting from gastric adenocarcinoma. (*Courtesy of* Daniel C. DeMarco, MD.)

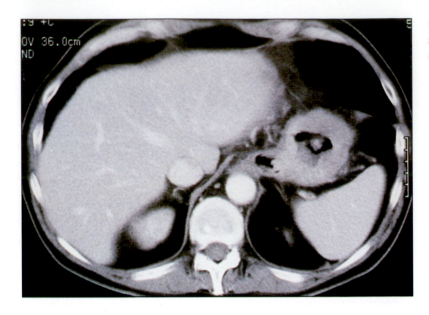

Figure 2-44. Image from a computed tomographic scan demonstrating gastric involvement with lymphoma. The duodenum, pancreas, liver, spleen, and retroperitoneum remain uninvolved. (*Courtesy of* Daniel C. DeMarco, MD.)

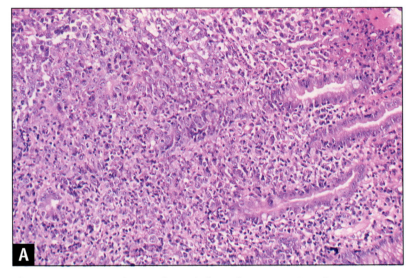

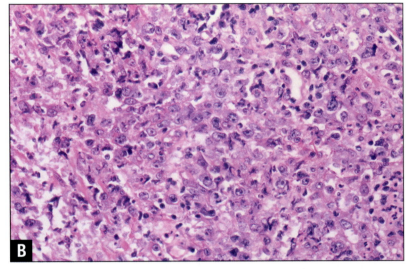

Figure 2-45. Histology of gastric lymphoma. **A**, Gastric mucosa with involvement by lymphoma. Infiltration of the lamina propria with destruction of glands by a diffuse infiltrate of large atypical lymphoid cells (hematoxylin and eosin stain; original magnification × 100). **B**, Same condition as shown in *A*, although at a different magnification (hematoxylin and eosin stain; original magnification × 200). (*Courtesy of* Daniel C. DeMarco, MD.)

Maltoma ·

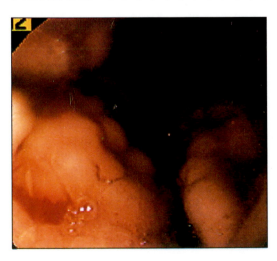

Figure 2-46. Maltoma. Endoscopic view of an edematous gastric mucosa with marked erythema and friability. (*Courtesy of* Daniel C. DeMarco, MD.)

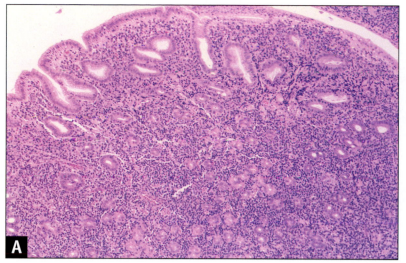

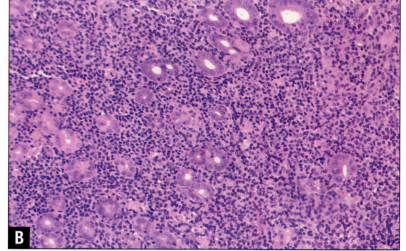

Figure 2-47. Histology of maltoma. **A**, View of gastric mucosa showing diffuse infiltration and expansion of the lamina propria of small atypical lymphocytes. Infiltration and destruction of gastric glands forming so-called lymphoepithelial lesions (hematoxylin and eosin stain; original magnification × 40). **B**, Same view as in *A*, although at a different magnification (hematoxylin and eosin stain; original magnification × 100). (*Courtesy of* Daniel C. DeMarco, MD.)

Gastric Kaposi's sarcoma ....

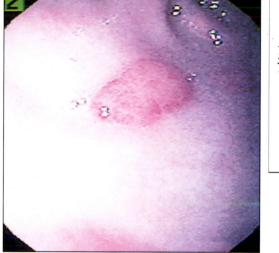

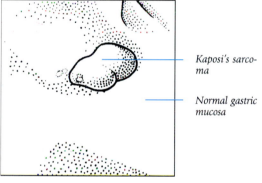

Kaposi's sarcoma

Normal gastric mucosa

Figure 2-48. Gastric Kaposi's sarcoma seen endoscopically. In the area of AIDS, a variety of bleeding gastrointestinal lesions have been noted. Kaposi's sarcoma is a spindle cell tumor that often has a submucosal location histologically; hence the yield of biopsy is low, 23%, despite a typical endoscopic appearance [14]. Although gastrointestinal Kaposi's sarcoma can occur in the absence of cutaneous lesions, increasing numbers of skin lesions predict a higher incidence of gastrointestinal lesions. The lesion is typically a well-circumscribed, submucosal, erythematous or violaceous mass lesion. Bleeding gastrointestinal Kaposi's sarcoma lesions are a reflection of advanced immunosuppression and poor long-term survival. Some authors have, however, reported good acute control of active bleeding with endoscopic sclerotherapy [15]. (*Courtesy of* Karl Fukunaga, MD, and Russell Yang, MD.)

Gastric leiomyosarcoma ....

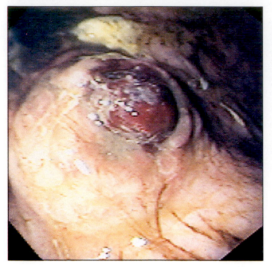

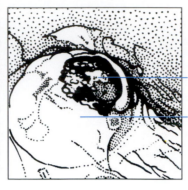

Overlying clot

Leiomyosarcoma

Figure 2-49. Endoscopic view of gastric leiomyosarcoma. Gastric leiomyosarcoma accounts for 1% of malignant tumors of the stomach. This leiomyosarcoma presented with hematemesis; notice that the tumor appears as a submucosal nodule within the gastric lumen. However, there is a clot overlying the lesion where the tumor had ulcerated and hemorrhaged. Although curative resection can be attempted, the 5-year survival rate is 25% to 30% [16]. (*Courtesy of* Karl Fukunaga, MD, and Russell Yang, MD.)

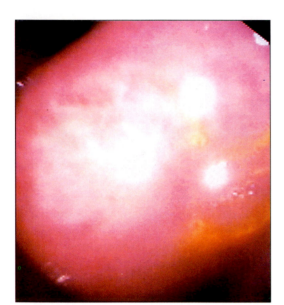

Figure 2-50. Leiomyoma. Leiomyomas and leiomyosarcomas are usually asymptomatic. Leiomyomas are the most common type of benign tumor of the stomach. Quite often, the benign leiomyoma and the malignant leiomyosarcoma are difficult to distinguish endoscopically, endosonographically, or even histologically. The leiomyosarcoma does, however, tend to be larger and more frequently ulcerated. Leiomyoma in a 62-year-old man with dyspepsia is depicted. Multiple, deep endoscopic biopsies were negative, however, because the lesion is submucosal and endoscopic biopsies are primarily biopsies of the mucosa. (*Courtesy of* Daniel C. DeMarco, MD.)

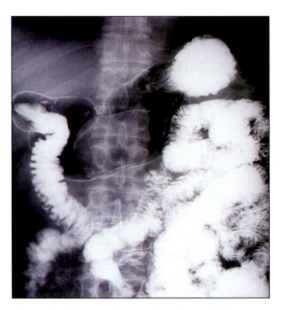

Figure 2-51. Radiographic view of leiomyoma. A series of tests of the upper gastrointestinal tract proved to be confirmative. Note the presence of a large submucosal, intramural mass and its effect on the gastric lumen. The existence of a hiatal hernia is noted, but the remainder of the study is unremarkable except for the evident mass. (*Courtesy of* Daniel C. DeMarco, MD.)

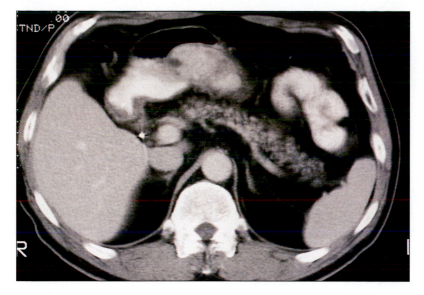

Figure 2-52. Leiomyoma. Computed tomographic scan shows no evidence of extragastric disease but very clearly demonstrates the presence of the tumor. The liver, pancreas, and biliary tree are free of involvement. (*Courtesy of* Daniel C. DeMarco, MD.)

Gastric polyp ·

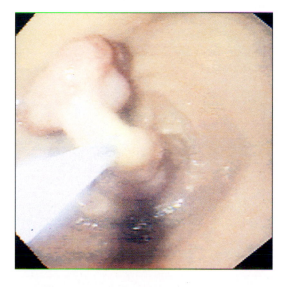

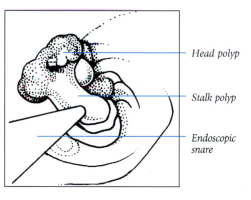

Head polyp

Stalk polyp

Endoscopic snare

Figure 2-53. Endoscopic view of gastric polyp. Gastric polyps have a prevalence of 0.4% in autopsy series [17]. The vast majority are symptomatic; however, when they are a large enough, surface ulceration and bleeding may occur. Polyps are most commonly hyperplastic, which are not premalignant; polyps are less commonly adenomatous, which are premalignant. This particular polyp was a 2-cm pedunculated polyp that was removed using an endoscopic coagulation snare. (*Courtesy of* Karl Fukunaga, MD, and Russell Yang, MD.)

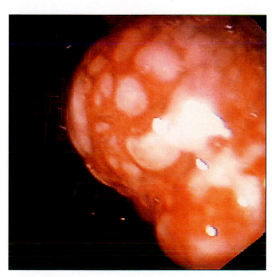

Figure 2-54. Hyperplastic gastric polyp. Gastric polyps are made up of hyperplastic or adenomatous tissues. Those formed by hyperplastic polyps are by far the most common, accounting for 75% to 90% of all gastric polyps. They have no potential for malignancy. Removal or resection is mandated only by symptoms or hemorrhage if present. Adenomatous polyps of the stomach are thought to have potential for malignant development and should be removed if the size of the polyp and condition of the patient permit such therapy. In this figure, an asymptomatic pedunculated benign gastric polyp as seen on upper gastrointestinal endoscopy is shown. Note the "malignant appearance." (*Courtesy of* Daniel C. DeMarco, MD.)

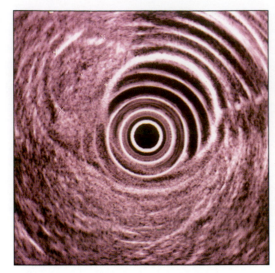

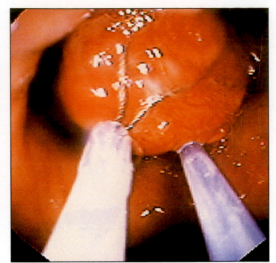

Figure 2-55. Hyperplastic gastric polyp seen on endoscopic ultrasound. View of the same lesion in Figure 2-54 imaged through use of endoscopic ultrasound. The muscularis propria (layer 4) is intact. No evidence of invasion is present. The neoplastic or hyperplastic tissue is hypoechoic. The sonographic appearance suggests that the polyp has multiple cystic areas. (*Courtesy of* Daniel C. DeMarco, MD.)

Figure 2-56. Snare removal of the polyp shown in Figure 2-54. A two-channel endoscope is used in combination with a basket and with snare electrocautery so that the polyp would not be lost should it migrate out of the stomach after polypectomy. The patient should be placed on antipeptic therapy after the polypectomy procedure. (*Courtesy of* Daniel C. DeMarco, MD.)

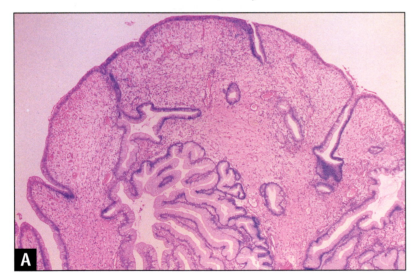

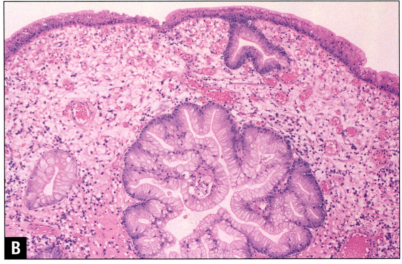

Figure 2-57. Histology of gastric polyp. **A,** Gastric hyperplastic polyp showing dilated, branching, hyperplastic glands. The surrounding stroma is edematous and inflamed (hematoxylin and eosin stain; original magnification × 40). **B,** Same view as seen in *A*, although at a different magnification (hematoxylin and eosin stain; original magnification × 100). (*Courtesy of* Daniel C. DeMarco, MD.)

Gastric lipoma ....

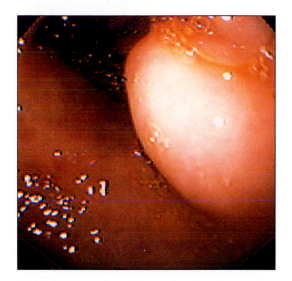

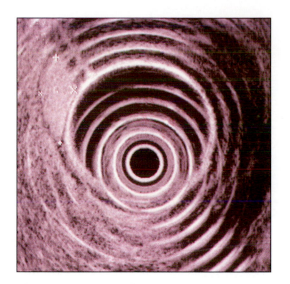

Figure 2-58. Gastric lipoma viewed endoscopically. Lipomas of the stomach tend to occur in the antrum, are rare, and are often distinguished endoscopically by a "cushion sign." (*Courtesy of* Daniel C. DeMarco, MD.)

Figure 2-59. Use of endoscopic ultrasound confirms the submucosal nature of the lesion. The lesion is confined to the third layer and is mildly hyperechoic. The experience with endoscopic ultrasound and the examination of liposarcomas are really limited because of the rare occurrence of the lesion. Thus far, it remains impossible to distinguish between lipomas and liposarcomas using endoscopic ultrasonography. (*Courtesy of* Daniel C. DeMarco, MD.)

Gastric Syphilis

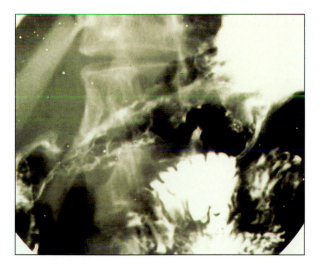

Figure 2-60. Gastric syphilis: upper gastrointestinal barium examination. Gastric syphilis is caused by infection with the organism *Treponema pallidum*. Gastric involvement usually presents in the secondary stage of the disease. On upper gastrointestinal system barium studies, gastric syphilis may be manifested as discrete, nodular gummalike lesions. Diffuse involvement of the stomach with a predominance of antral involvement is, however, more common. Swelling and thickening of the gastric wall can result in mural rigidity and narrowing of the lumen. As seen in this upper gastrointestinal barium study, diffuse thickening of the gastric wall resulted in narrowing of the antrum and scattered gummatous polyps. Luminal narrowing produces a tubular deformity or a funnel-shaped defect in which the apex of the funnel is at or near the pylorus. (*Courtesy of* Mark Feldman, MD.)

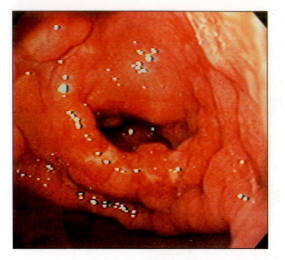

Figure 2-61. Gastric syphilis: endoscopic manifestations. Endoscopically gastric syphilis usually presents as thick gastric folds with submucosal infiltration and multiple erosions. The endoscopic picture is suggestive of gastric carcinoma. Shown in this figure is the gastric antrum of a patient with syphilis that endoscopically demonstrates massive submucosal infiltration and erosions. (*Courtesy of* Mark Feldman, MD.)

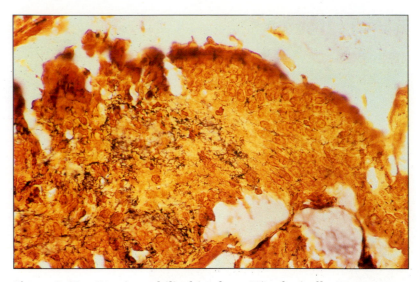

Figure 2-62. Gastric syphilis: histology. Histologically, *Treponema pallidum* is demonstrated in gastric biopsies either by silver staining or by fluorescent antibody staining. Histologic demonstration of the corkscrew appearance of the organisms in gastric biopsies is required for diagnosis. This figure shows a gastric body biopsy from the patient shown in Figure 2-61. It has been silver stained and demonstrates the organisms present. Granulomas would be another suggestive feature but not diagnostic for gastric syphilis. Other than the findings mentioned, the histology of gastric syphilis demonstrates a nonspecific inflammatory response. (*Courtesy of* Edward Lee, MD, and Byron Cryer, MD.)

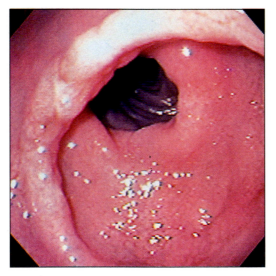

Figure 2-63. Gastric syphilis: posttherapy. Following appropriate antibiotic therapy for syphilis, the radiographic, endoscopic, and histologic abnormalities of gastric syphilis can be expected to resolve. This figure is an endoscopic photograph of the antrum of the gastric syphilis patient shown in Figure 2-61, 1 month after treatment with benzathine penicillin. As noted previously, the massive submucosal infiltration seen earlier has almost completely abated. (*Courtesy of* Mark Feldman, MD.)

Crohn's Disease

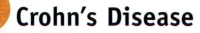

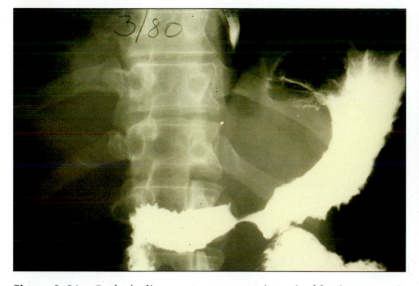

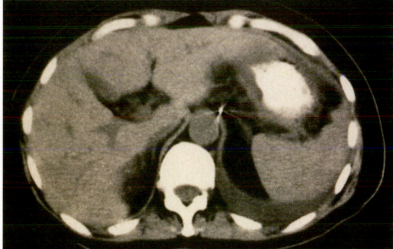

Figure 2-64. Crohn's disease: upper gastrointestinal barium examination. Although Crohn's disease can involve any portion of the gastrointestinal tract, clinically apparent isolated gastric Crohn's disease is a rare entity. Gastric Crohn's disease usually involves the antrum and pylorus. When gastric Crohn's disease is present, usually the proximal duodenum or other parts of the small and large intestines are involved as well. As in this figure, barium studies of the upper gastrointestinal tract may reveal gastric deformity with enlarged nodular folds, poor distensibility, and deformed pylorus. (*Courtesy of* Mark Feldman, MD.)

Figure 2-65. Crohn's disease seen using computed tomographic scan. Because transmural inflammation is seen in Crohn's disease, gastric wall thickening is a characteristic finding. In this computed tomographic scan of the abdomen with contrast, diffuse thickening of the wall of the stomach is seen. Endoscopy in such patients reveals aphthoid and serpiginous erosions, ulcerations, and mucosal irregularities. (*From* Cary *et al.* [18]; with permission.)

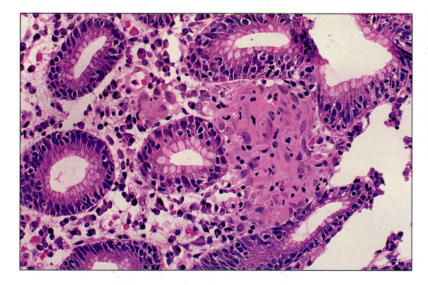

Figure 2-66. Crohn's disease: histology. Histologically, gastric Crohn's disease appears as an idiopathic granulomatous gastritis. Thus, in the absence of other clinical manifestations to suggest Crohn's disease, the diagnosis is difficult to make solely on the basis of histologic evidence. This figure shows two (one large and one small) granulomas (nodular collections of histiocytes) within the lamina propria. Acute and chronic inflammatory infiltrates involving the lamina propria are also present. (*Courtesy of* Edward Lee, MD, and Byron Cryer, MD.)

References

1. Laine L, Weinstein WM: Histology of hemorrhagic "gastritis": A prospective evaluation. *Gastroenterology* 1988, 94:1254–1262.

2. Crean GP, Marshall MW, Ramsey RD: Parietal cell hyperplasia induced by the administration of pentagastrin (ICI-50, 123) to rats. *Gastroenterology* 1969, 57:147–155.

3. Ekman L, Hansson E, Havu N, *et al.*: Toxicological studies on omeprazole. *Scand J Gastroenterol* 1985, 20(suppl 108):53–69.

4. Willems G: Trophic action of gastrin on specific target cells in the gut. In *Endocrine Tumors of the Pancreas: Recent Advances in Research and Management.* Edited by mignon M, Jensen RT. Basel: Karger; 1995:30–44.

5. Helander HF, Bordi C: Morphology of gastric mucosa during prolonged hypergastrinemia. In *Endocrine Tumors of the Pancreas: Recent Advances in Research and Management.* Edited by Mignon M, Jensen RT. Basel: Karger; 1995:372–384.

6. Van Custsem E, Rutgeerts P, Vantrappen G: Treatment of bleeding gastrointestinal vascular malformations with oestrogen-progesterone. *Lancet* 1990, 335:953–955.

7. Saba H, Morelli G, Logrono L: Treatment of bleeding in hereditary hemorrhagic telangiectasia with aminocaproic acid. *N Engl J Med* 1994, 330:1789–1790.

8. Jabbari J, Cherry R, Lough J, *et al.*: Gastric antral vascular ectasia: The watermelon stomach. *Gastroenterology* 1984, 87:1165–1170.

9. Eidus L, Rasuli P, Manion D, Heringer R: Caliber-persistent artery of the stomach. *Gastroenterology* 1990, 99:1507–1510.

10. Trudeau W, Prindiville T: Endoscopic injection sclerosis of bleeding gastric varices. *Gastrointest Endosc* 1986, 32:264–268.

11. Grimm H, Maydeo A, Noar M, Soehendra N: Bleeding esophagogastric varices: Is endoscopic treatment with cyanoacrylate the final answer? *Gastrointest Endosc* 1991, :A174.

12. Avuncluk C, Hampf F, Coughlin B: Endoscopic sonography of the stomach: Findings in benign and malignant lesions. *Am J Radiol* 1994, 163:591–595.

13. Tio TL: *Gastrointestinal TNM cancer staging by endosonography.* New York: Igaku-Shoin; 1995.

14. Friedman S, Wright T, Altman D: Gastrointestinal Kaposi's sarcoma in patients with acquired immunodeficiency syndrome: Endoscopic and autopsy findings. *Gastroenterology* 1985, 89:102–108.

15. Lew E, Dieterich D: Severe hemorrhage caused by gastrointestinal Kaposi's syndrome in patients with the acquired immunodeficiency syndrome. *Am J Gastroenterol* 1992, 87:1471–1474.

16. Bedikian A, Khankhanian N, Valdivieso M, *et al.*: Sarcoma of the stomach: Clinicopathologic study of 43 cases. *J Surg Oncol* 1980, 13:121–127.

17. Bentivenga S, Panagopoulos P: Adenomatous gastric polyps. *Am J Gastroenterol* 1965, 44:138–148.

18. Cary ER, Tremaine WJ, Banks PM, Nagorney DM: Case Report: Isolated Crohn's disease of the stomach. *Mayo Clin Proc* 1989, 64:776–779.

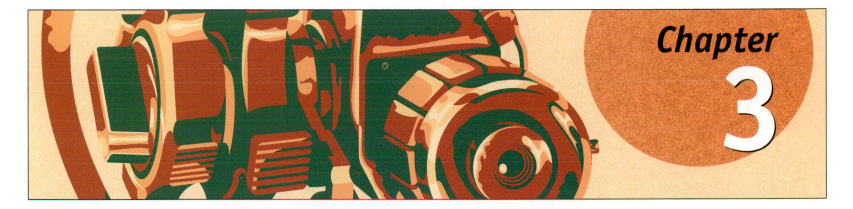

Chapter **3**

Duodenum and Small Bowel

 ## Duodenal Ulcer

Duodenal ulcer . . . .

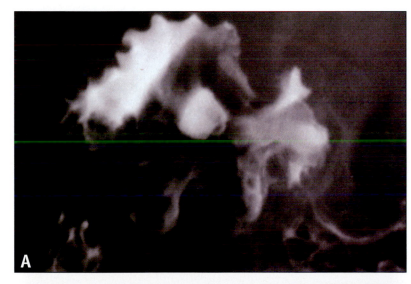

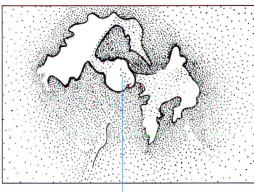

Ulcer crater

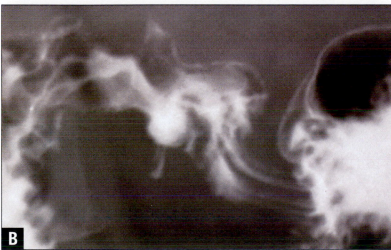

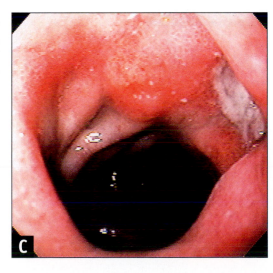

Figure 3-1. Typical radiographic features of duodenal ulcer. **A,** This duodenal bulb ulcer is associated with marked edema, resulting in the appearance of radiating folds to the ulcer crater. The bulb is also distored secondary to previously existing ulceration. **B,** A posterior bulbar ulcer is seen associated with distortion of the bulb. **C,** The duodenal ulcer as seen during endoscopy. The bulb is edematous and hemorrhagic with diffuse erosions. The sensitivity of barium studies for duodenal ulcer is 50% with the single-contrast technique but increases to between 80% and 90% when the double-contrast technique is performed. (*Courtesy of* C. Mel Wilcox, MD.)

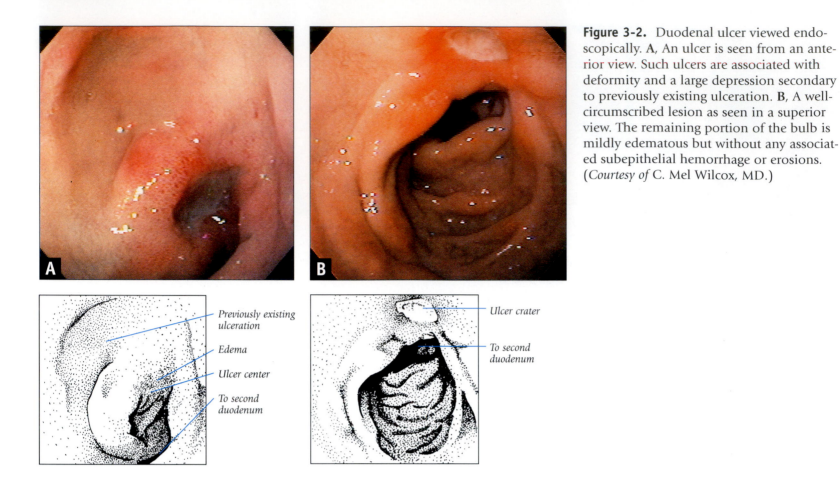

Figure 3-2. Duodenal ulcer viewed endoscopically. **A**, An ulcer is seen from an anterior view. Such ulcers are associated with deformity and a large depression secondary to previously existing ulceration. **B**, A well-circumscribed lesion as seen in a superior view. The remaining portion of the bulb is mildly edematous but without any associated subepithelial hemorrhage or erosions. (*Courtesy of* C. Mel Wilcox, MD.)

Previously existing ulceration
Edema
Ulcer center
To second duodenum

Ulcer crater
To second duodenum

Duodenal ulcer with clean base. . . . .

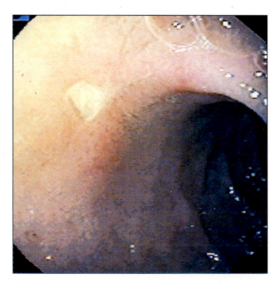

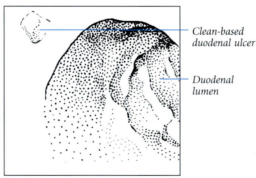

Clean-based duodenal ulcer
Duodenal lumen

Figure 3-3. Endoscopic view of duodenal ulcer with clean base. Approximately 50% of patients with upper gastrointestinal hemorrhage have experienced bleeding from a peptic ulcer. Bleeding duodenal ulcers are twice as common as gastric ulcers. Endoscopic appearance of an ulcer, that is, the presence or absence of stigmata predicting recurrent bleeding, is of value in assessing prognosis. A clean-based ulcer carries a 1% risk of recurrent hemorrhage. Some authors have advocated discharging from the hospital a patient with such a lesion immediately after replenishing intravascular volume. (*Courtesy of* Karl Fukunaga, MD, and Russell Yang, MD.)

Duodenal ulcer with flat pigmented spot . . . .

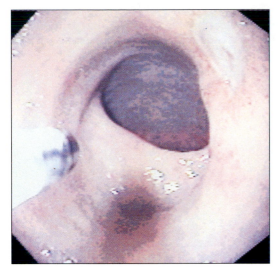

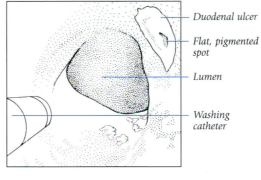

Figure 3-4.
Duodenal ulcer with flat pigmented spot, seen endoscopically. A flat, pigmented spot carries a 7% risk of recurrent bleeding. Notice that on tangential view there is no appearance of elevation in such a lesion. (*Courtesy of* Karl Fukunaga, MD, and Russell Yang, MD.)

Duodenal ulcer with visible vessel. . . . .

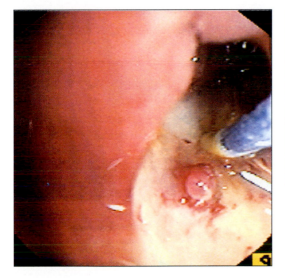

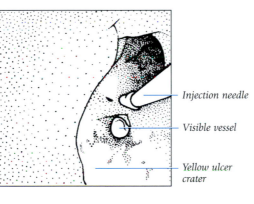

Figure 3-5. Endoscopic view of duodenal ulcer with visible vessel. This visible vessel was seen in an edematous duodenal bulb (hence the close-up view). It is actively oozing. A bipolar electrocoagulation probe is poised in the lower left corner before therapy. (*Courtesy of* Karl Fukunaga, MD, and Russell Yang, MD.)

Duodenal ulcer with various stigmata of recent bleeding. . . . .

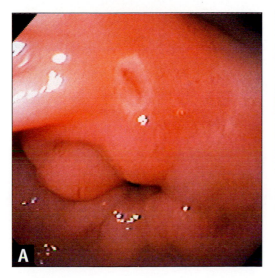

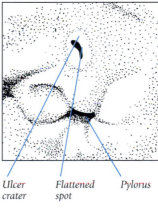

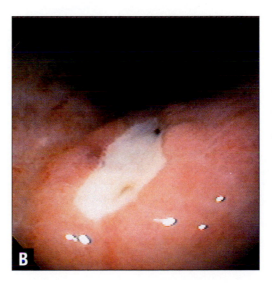

Figure 3-6.
Stigmata of recent hemorrhage seen endoscopically in patients with bleeding ulcer. **A,** A linear, flat, red spot in the base of a small peripyloric ulcer. **B,** Two flat black spots in the base of a benign-appearing ulcer on the angularis.

(Continued on next page)

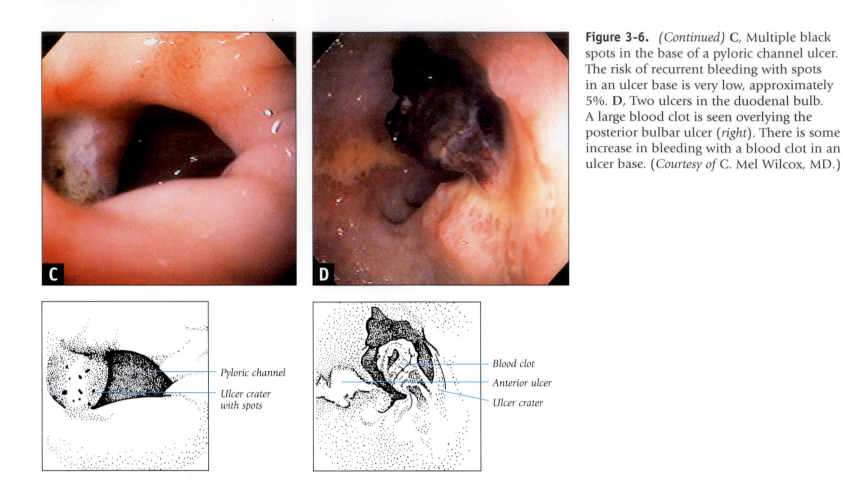

Figure 3-6. *(Continued)* **C,** Multiple black spots in the base of a pyloric channel ulcer. The risk of recurrent bleeding with spots in an ulcer base is very low, approximately 5%. **D,** Two ulcers in the duodenal bulb. A large blood clot is seen overlying the posterior bulbar ulcer *(right)*. There is some increase in bleeding with a blood clot in an ulcer base. *(Courtesy of C. Mel Wilcox, MD.)*

Pyloric ulcer with gastric outlet obstruction . . . .

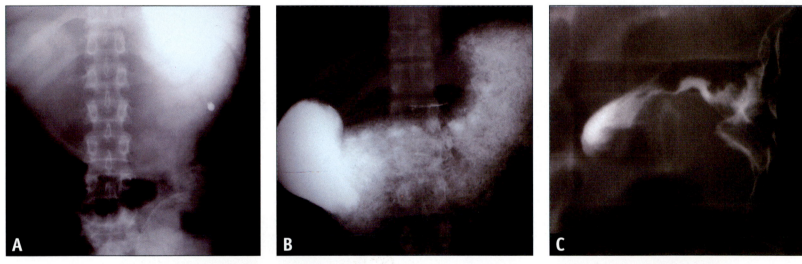

Figure 3-7. Pyloric outlet obstruction related to peripyloric ulcer disease is uncommon. Acutely, obstruction may result from edema. In some patients, however, chronic disease results in fixed fibrosis and outlet obstruction. **A,** Plain film of the abdomen in a patient presenting with nausea and vomiting and a succussion splash on physical examination demonstrates a massively enlarged stomach with inferior displacement of the transverse colon; a nasogastric tube is seen in the stomach. **B,** Barium upper gastrointestinal study demonstrates the size of the stomach. **C,** Edema, spasm, and a small ulcer crater are present in the pyloric channel area.

(Continued on next page)

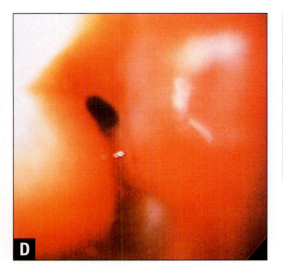

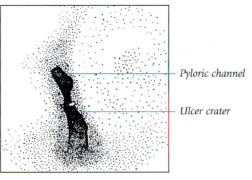

Pyloric channel

Ulcer crater

Figure 3-7. (*Continued*) **D,** Endoscopy demonstrates the pyloric obstruction with an active ulcer crater seen in the pyloric channel. Nasogastric suction and intravenous H_2-receptor antagonists resulted in a clinical cure. In some patients, surgery may be required. Endoscopic balloon dilation has been useful in some patients with fixed obstruction without active ulcer disease. (*Courtesy of* C. Mel Wilcox, MD.)

Duodenitis

Duodenitis, nodular

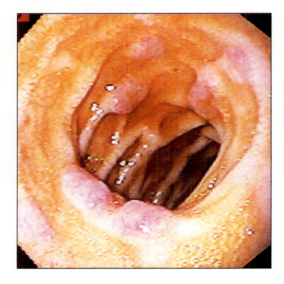

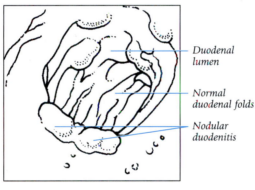

Duodenal lumen

Normal duodenal folds

Nodular duodenitis

Figure 3-8. Endoscopic view of nodular duodenitis. Esophagogastroduodenoscopy in stable hemodialysis patients reveals a mucosal abnormality as often as 50% of the time. Nodular duodenitis—raised areas of erythema and erosions in the duodenum— is commonly seen in patients with dialysis-dependent end-stage renal disease. These lesions appear to be reversible after renal transplantation [1]. (*Courtesy of* Karl Fukunaga, MD, and Russell Yang, MD.)

Duodenitis, erosive

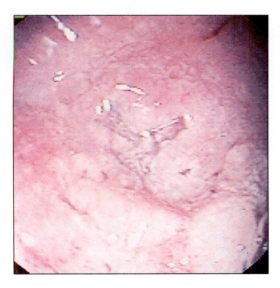

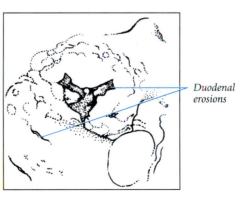

Duodenal erosions

Figure 3-9. Erosive duodenitis viewed endoscopically. Diffuse mucosal superficial defects, with or without subepithelial hemorrhages, may be associated with upper gastrointestinal bleeding. The subjective lack of depth in the mucosal defect distinguishes this lesion from an actual duodenal ulcer. This erosive duodenitis was present in a patient with Zollinger-Ellison syndrome; however, it can occur in patients without a hypersecretory state [2]. (*Courtesy of* Karl Fukunaga, MD, and Russell Yang, MD.)

Intestinal metaplasia. . . . .

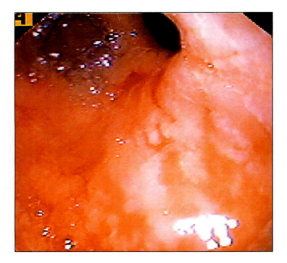

Figure 3-10. Intestinal metaplasia. This endoscopic view reveals multiple raised plaque-like areas. This can occur in any area of the stomach. It is thought to be a reaction to mucosal injury where epithelial cells develop the features of intestinal epithelia. (*Courtesy of* Daniel C. DeMarco, MD.)

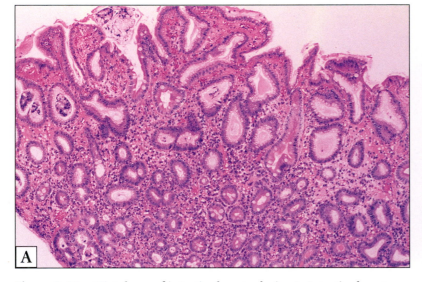

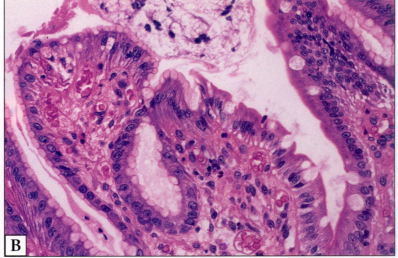

Figure 3-11. Histology of intestinal metaplasia. **A,** Intestinal metaplasia of the gastric mucosa. Intestinal type epithelium with columnar absorptive cells and goblet mucus cells replacing foveolar epithelium (hematoxylin and eosin stain; original magnification (× 100).

B, Same view as seen in *A,* although at a different magnification (hematoxylin and eosin stain; original magnification (× 200). (*Courtesy of* Daniel C. DeMarco, MD.)

Motility Disorders

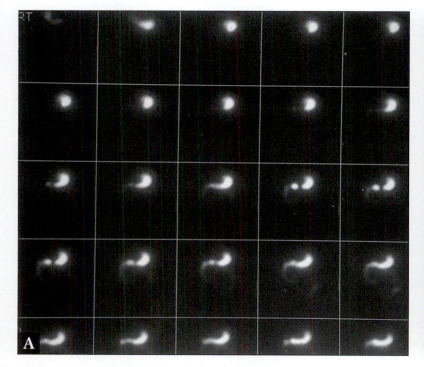

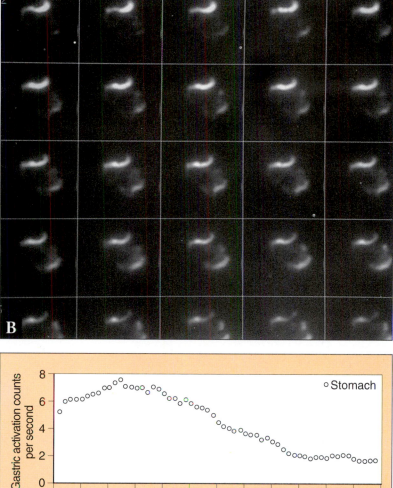

Figure 3-12. Scintigraphy is the most widely accepted technique for measuring gastric emptying. **A–B,** Sequential gamma camera images from a region of interest over the fundus following ingestion of a ^{99m}technetium-labeled scrambled egg meal. Note progression of the meal from the fundus through the corpus and antrum of the stomach, into the small intestine. **C,** The graph illustrates the disappearance of counts from the region of interest. The calculated half-emptying time was normal at 33 minutes. Scintigraphy is widely available, can separately or simultaneously measure liquid and solid emptying, and is relatively noninvasive, apart from radiation exposure. Furthermore, scintigraphy is quantifiable. Various liquid and solid meals can be radiolabeled. Indigestible solids are the most sensitive in detecting gastric motor dysfunction and liquids least. Most centers employ a semisolid meal, such as radiolabeled scrambled egg or chicken liver. Each center must define its own controls and interpret results accordingly. A limitation to gastric emptying studies is the inconsistent relationship between scintigraphic findings and symptoms. (*Courtesy of* Eamonn M.M. Quigley, MD.)

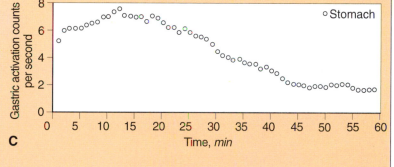

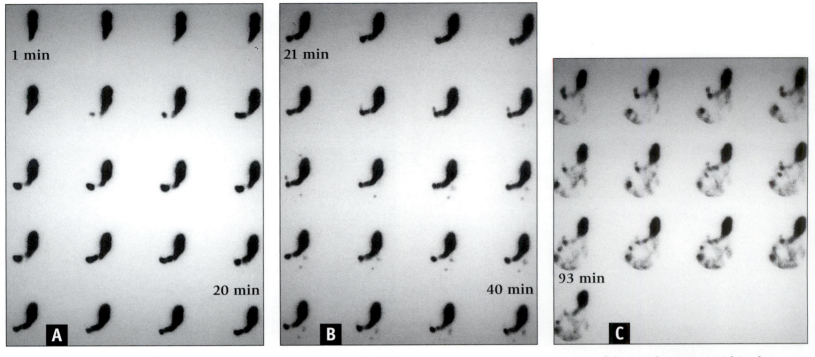

Figure 3-13. A–C, Delayed gastric emptying. A sequence of images from a patient with delayed gastric emptying. Note that even at 93 minutes the major portion of the meal remains within the stomach. (*Courtesy of* Eamonn M.M. Quigley, MD.)

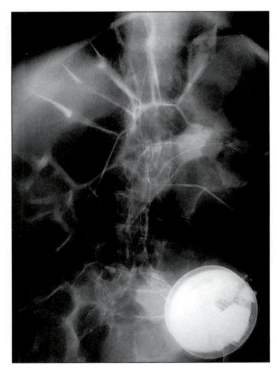

Figure 3-14. Radiographic view of acute intestinal pseudo-obstruction or ileus. Although ileus is an expected consequence of abdominal and other surgical procedures, it may also occur in other nonsurgical situations, such as in patients with pneumonia, pancreatitis, cholecystitis, myocardial infarction, and a variety of neurological conditions. Occasionally, ileus may occur without an obvious cause—idiopathic ileus. This figure illustrates marked dilatation of small and large intestine, a finding consistent with ileus, in a patient with multiple sclerosis. Note patient also had an implanted pump to deliver the muscle relaxant baclofen. (*Courtesy of* Eamonn M.M. Quigley, MD.)

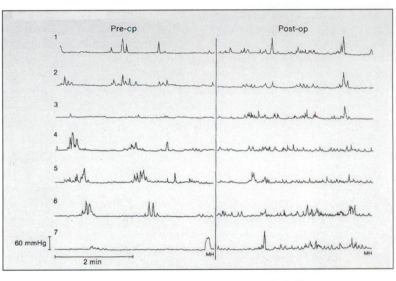

Figure 3-15. Intestinal obstruction. Figure on left illustrates manometric features of intestinal obstruction. Note repetitive, propagated clusters of phasic contractions and rapidly propagated high-amplitude waves in the postprandial period. On right, note return of normal fed pattern in the same patient following successful operative relief of obstruction. (*Adapted from* Summers *et al.* [3].)

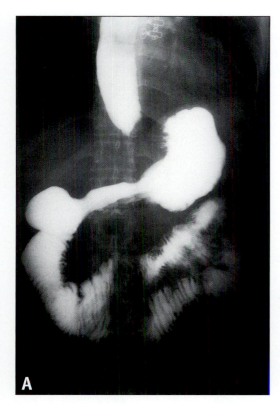

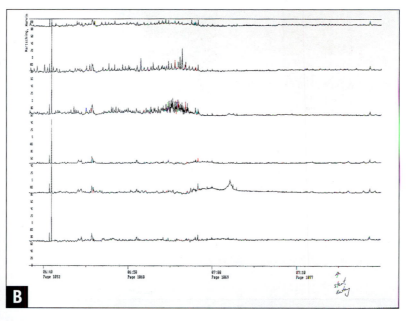

A

B

Figure 3-16. Chronic intestinal pseudo-obstruction. **A,** Upper gastrointestinal barium radiography demonstrates the typical features of scleroderma involving the small intestine. Note the dilated jejunal loops with prominent valvulae conniventes, giving a "stacked coin" or "coiled spring" appearance. **B,** Simultaneous recordings of antral (top two traces) and duodenal (bottom three traces) motility from a patient with advanced scleroderma. Fasting recording demonstrates virtually complete absence of motor activity; during phase III of the migrating motor complex, a very low-amplitude phase III is evident in the antrum and duodenum. (**A,** *Courtesy of* Eamonn M.M. Quigley, MD; **B,** *adapted from* Quigley [4].)

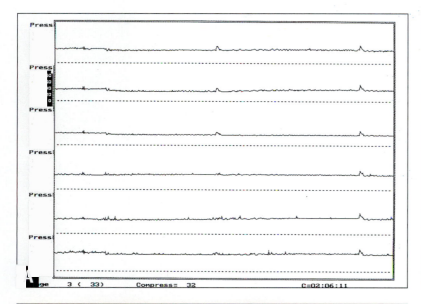

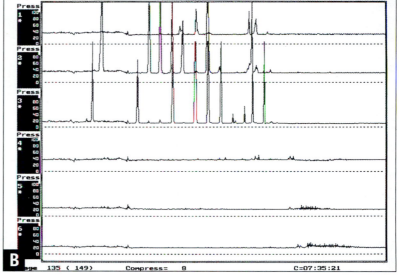

A

B

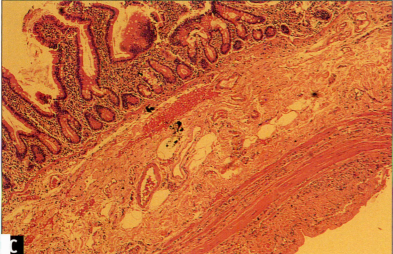

C

Figure 3-17. Intestinal myopathy. **A,** Simultaneous recording of antral (top three traces) and duodenal (lower three traces) motor activity from a patient with an intestinal myopathy and idiopathic megaduodenum. Note marked suppression of motor activity.

B, Figure demonstrating duodenal hypomotility in a patient with an intestinal myopathy. Normal phase III of the migrating motor complex in the antrum (upper three traces), but marked suppression of the amplitude of phasic contractions during phase III in the duodenal recording sites (bottom three traces) are seen.

Pathologic features of intestinal myopathy. **C,** Full-thickness intestinal biopsy from a patient with an intestinal myopathy demonstrating essentially complete replacement of the circular muscle layer by fibrosis. Note relative preservation of longitudinal muscle layer.

(Continued on next page)

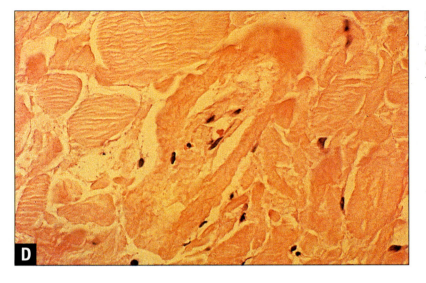

Figure 3-17. *(Continued)* **D**, Amyloidosis of the small intestine. Duodenal biopsy demonstrating extensive infiltration by amyloid, seen as homogenous pink hyaline substance. (**A**, **B**, and **D**, *Courtesy of* Eamonn M.M. Quigley, MD; **C**, *from* Quigley [4]; with permission.)

Malabsorption

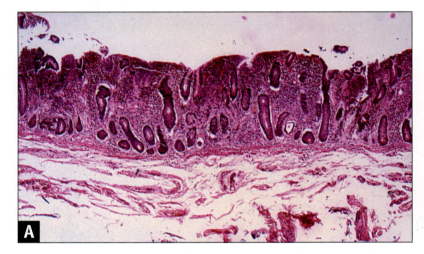

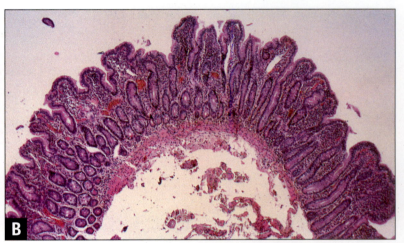

Figure 3-18. Jejunal mucosal biopsy from a patient with celiac sprue before (**panel A**) and 3 months after (**panel B**) treatment with a gluten-free diet. Celiac sprue is characterized by small intestinal mucosal damage and nutrient malabsorption in susceptible persons after ingesting gluten, the water-insoluble protein component of certain grains. **Panel A** illustrates the flat mucosal surface, absence of villi, hyperplastic crypts, and increased lamina propria cellularity that are characteristic of the disease. After 3 months of treatment (**panel B**) the mucosa is markedly improved and recognizable villi are present. The villi are short, however, and crypt hyperplasia and lamina propria hypercellularity persist.

The severity of malabsorption and clinical symptoms can vary markedly in patients with celiac sprue, and are directly correlated with the length of the intestinal lesion. Usually, the proximal intestine is most involved and disease severity decreases distally along the length of small bowel. Patients with severe disease have flatulence, progressive weight loss, and multiple nutrient deficiencies. The diarrhea is often voluminous and may float on water because of increased air and fat content. However, some patients have increased fecal mass without loose stools and complain of constipation. Removal of dietary gluten, present in wheat, rye, barely, oats, food additives, emulsifiers, and stabilizers, is essential for successful management. Patients who do not respond to a strict gluten-free diet may have refractory sprue or lymphoma. (*Courtesy of* Samuel Klein, MD.)

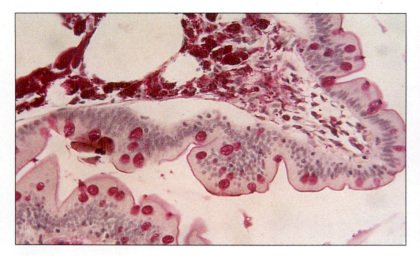

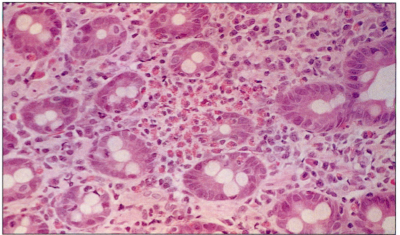

Figure 3-19. Jejunal biopsy from a patient with Whipple's disease. The histologic appearance of biopsies obtained from involved small intestine is diagnostic for Whipple's disease. In this patient, the villi are flat and widened. There is also extensive infiltration of the lamina propria with large periodic acid-Schiff–positive macrophages. Whipple's disease is caused by a bacterial infection with a gram-positive bacillus. The gastrointestinal tract, musculoskeletal system, cardiovascular system, central nervous system, pulmonary system, skin, and lymph nodes may be involved, causing a broad range of symptoms. Treatment with appropriate antibiotics usually results in dramatic clinical improvement within 2 weeks. Antibiotic therapy should be continued for 1 year to decrease the risk of relapse. Short-term nutritional therapy to correct protein-calorie malnutrition and specific nutrient deficiencies, such as vitamin C deficiency, is often necessary until absorptive function improves. (*Courtesy of* Samuel Klein, MD.)

Figure 3-20. Jejunal biopsy from a patient with eosinophilic gastroenteritis. A dense inflammatory cell infiltrate, composed almost entirely of eosinophils, is present in the mucosa and submucosa. Specific clinical symptoms depend on which layer of the intestinal wall is predominantly involved. Clinical manifestations of mucosal and submucosal disease include abdominal pain, nausea, vomiting, diarrhea, and weight loss. Approximately 25% of patients have steatorrhea. (*Courtesy of* Samuel Klein, MD.)

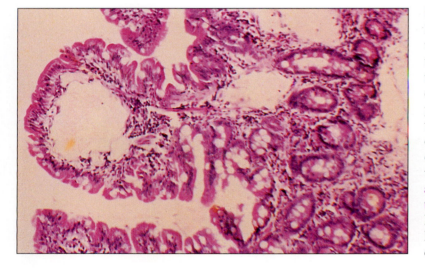

Figure 3-21. Jejunal biopsy demonstrating dilated submucosal lacteals in a patient with lymphangiectasia. Congenital malformation or secondary obstruction of the lymphatic system causes dilatation of intestinal lacteals and rupture of intestinal lymphatics through the mucosa. The leakage of lymph, containing chylomicrons, protein, and lymphocytes, into the intestinal lumen causes protein, fat, and lymphocyte losses. Therefore, the clinical manifestations of intestinal lymphangiectasia include peripheral edema, chylous ascites, hypoproteinemia, lymphopenia, and impaired delayed cutaneous hypersensitivity. Treatment involves therapy of the underlying disease in patients with secondary lymphangiectasia and careful monitoring of dermatologic complications. Resection of the involved intestine can be beneficial in patients with a localized lymphatic lesion. The goal of diet therapy is to decrease intestinal lymph flow by having the patient consume a low-fat (reduced long-chain triglyceride) diet [5]. (*Courtesy of* Samuel Klein, MD.)

Small Bowel Bleeding

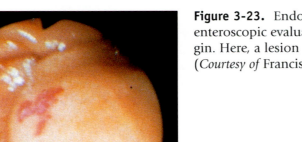

Figure 3-22. Enteroscopic equipment. **A**, Push enteroscope with overtube (Olympus SIF-10L [Olympus America, Inc, Lake Success, NY]). **B**, Sonde-type enteroscope (Olympus SIF-SW). **C**, SIF-SW sonde-type enteroscope with its inflated balloon tip is seen advancing in the small bowel. (*Courtesy of* Francisco C. Ramirez, MD.)

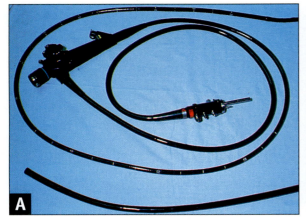

Figure 3-23. Endoscopic view of small-bowel arteriovenous malformation found during enteroscopic evaluations in two patients with gastrointestinal hemorrhage of obscure origin. Here, a lesion is found in the proximal jejunum using the push-type enteroscope. (*Courtesy of* Francisco C. Ramirez, MD.)

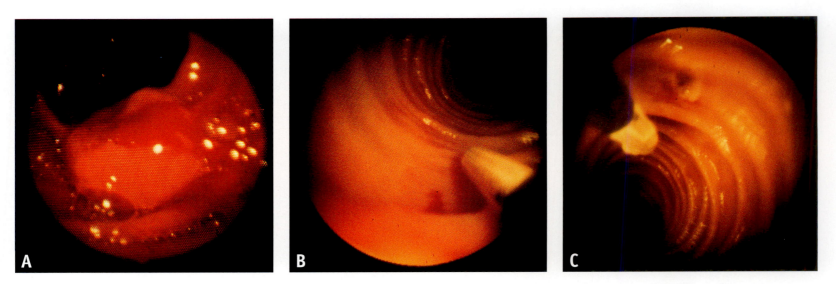

Figure 3-24. Endoscopic views of a malignant-appearing tumor (**panel A**), a bleeding leiomyoma (**panel B**), and villous adenoma with adenocarcinoma (**panel C**) in three patients presenting with gastrointestinal bleeding of obscure origin. These diagnoses were made possible by enteroscopy. (*Courtesy of* Francisco C. Ramirez, MD.)

Mesenteric Vascular Insufficiency

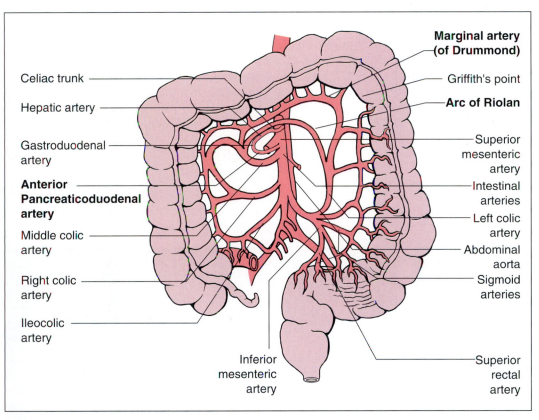

Celiac trunk

Hepatic artery

Gastroduodenal artery

Anterior Pancreaticoduodenal artery

Middle colic artery

Right colic artery

Ileocolic artery

Marginal artery (of Drummond)

Griffith's point

Arc of Riolan

Superior mesenteric artery

Intestinal arteries

Left colic artery

Abdominal aorta

Sigmoid arteries

Inferior mesenteric artery

Superior rectal artery

Figure 3-25. Mesenteric arterial anatomy. Three unpaired arterial branches of the aorta provide the small and large intestines with arterial blood. Direct arterial flow to the small intestine depends on patent celiac and superior mesenteric arteries (SMA). Potential exists for the development of collateral (anastomotic) channels between celiac arteries and SMA, as well as between superior and inferior mesenteric arteries when gradual occlusion of the primary vascular trunks occurs.

In most instances, veins parallel arteries in the mesenteric circulation. The superior mesenteric vein joins the splenic vein to form the portal vein, which enters the liver at its hilum. The inferior mesenteric vein anastomoses with the splenic vein near the point at which the superior mesenteric and splenic veins join to form the portal vein [6]. (*Adapted from* Rogers and David [6].)

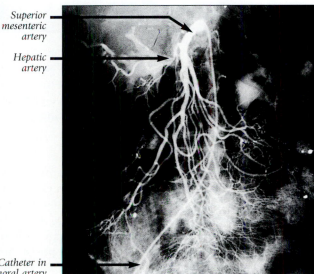

Superior mesenteric artery

Hepatic artery

Catheter in femoral artery

Figure 3-26. Superior mesenteric artery anatomy seen arteriographically. This arteriogram was performed by selective injection of the superior mesenteric artery (SMA). The catheter is shown ascending from its entrance site in the right femoral artery, traversing the abdominal aorta, with the catheter tip in the SMA (obscured by the contrast medium). The hepatic artery is the first major branch, as seen in this patient; an anatomic variant occurs in approximately 25% of normal individuals [7]. (*From* American Gastroenterological Association [7]; with permission.)

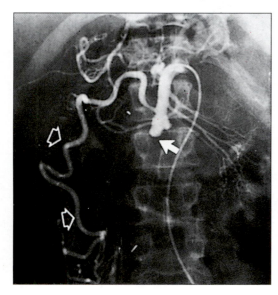

Figure 3-27. Embolic occlusion of the superior mesenteric artery (SMA). The usual origin of a mesenteric arterial embolus is a mural thrombus from the left atrium or ventricle. Predisposing conditions include atrial fibrillation, rheumatic heart disease, prosthetic heart valves, myocardial infarction, ventricular aneurysms, and invasive angiographic procedures. The clinician should be alert to the possibility of embolism to a major mesenteric artery when severe periumbilical abdominal pain, vomiting, diarrhea, and leukocytosis arise acutely in the appropriate clinical setting. Emboli to the SMA most often lodge in the middle colic branch, but can affect any of its four branches. Emboli tend to lodge within 3 to 8 cm of the origin of the SMA, usually where the vessel narrows. This angiogram reveals occlusion of the SMA by a thrombus. The solid arrow points to complete occlusion distal to the origin of the middle colic artery. The open arrows reveal some collateral flow through the middle colic–right colic anastomosis [6]. (*From* Rogers and David [6]; *courtesy of* Stanley Baum, MD.)

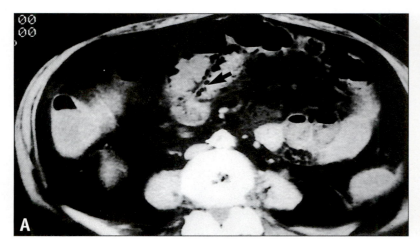

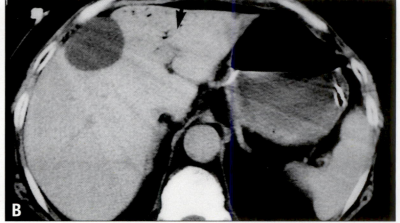

Figure 3-28. Pneumatosis intestinalis with hepatic portal venous gas demonstrated by computed tomography. **A,** Gas collections within the intestinal wall, termed *pneumatosis intestinalis* (PI) in (*arrow*), can be a manifestation of a variety of disorders. **B,** The additional finding of hepatic portal venous gas (HPVG) (*arrow*) dramatically shortens the list of potential disorders. Portal venous gas is virtually always associated with bowel necrosis, bacteremia, or both. It generally represents a grave prognostic sign. Mesenteric vascular occlusion, as in this case, rapidly progresses to intestinal infarction and necrosis of long segments of small bowel, commonly associated with PI. HPVG is often present in this setting [8]. (*Courtesy of* J. Casillas, MD.)

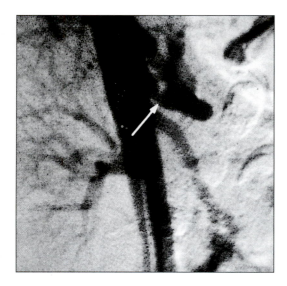

Figure 3-29. Chronic intestinal ischemia. This can be encountered in patients with severe atherosclerotic disease of the splanchnic circulation. These patients present with postprandial abdominal pain, sitophobia (fear of eating), and weight loss. The site of arterial narrowing is often seen near the origin of the feeding artery from the aorta. Shown here is an oblique view of the abdominal aorta during digital subtraction angiography in an individual with chronic upper abdominal pain. There is stenosis of the celiac axis with poststenotic dilation (*arrow*). Although surgical reconstruction may be attempted, the results are often suboptimal. (*From* Pounder *et al.* [9]; with permission.)

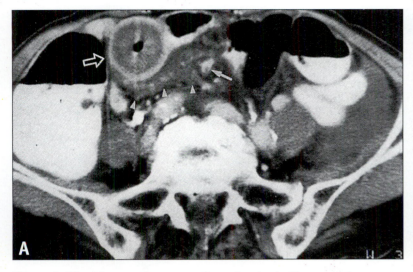

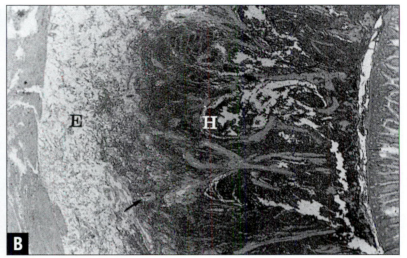

Figure 3-30. Mesenteric venous thrombosis. **A,** Computed tomography with intravenous contrast exhibits marked thickening of the jejunal wall with alternating layers of high and low density and peripheral enhancement. The branches of the superior mesenteric vein have thrombus (*closed arrow*); mesenteric edema is present (*arrowheads*). **B,** The histology of the resected specimen reveals hemorrhage (H), edema (E), and thrombus in submucosal veins (*arrow*). (*From* Kim *et al.* [10]; with permission.)

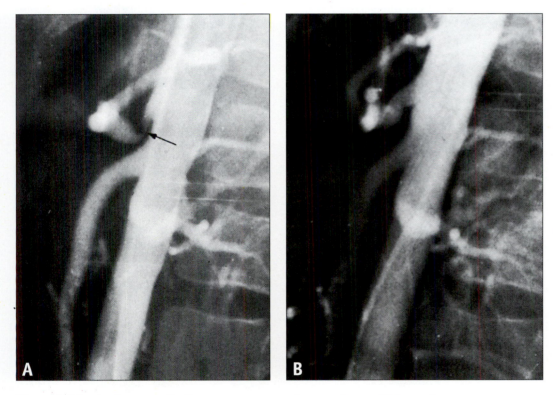

Figure 3-31. Angiogram of celiac artery compression syndrome. This syndrome presents as chronic recurring upper abdominal pain, which can be attributed to compression of the celiac axis (CA) by surrounding structures. Structures that may contribute to compression of the proximal CA include the inferior portion of the median arcuate ligament of the diaphragmatic crura and the celiac plexus. Patients with this syndrome are generally young and otherwise in good health. They are usually young women with complaints of abdominal discomfort, which is not consistently related to meals and is frequently associated with other symptoms, such as nausea, vomiting, and weight loss. A high-midline systolic bruit that decreases with inspiration may be the only helpful physical finding. The angiogram shown exhibits a smooth tapered compression of the CA in a 12-year-old boy with epigastric pain. A bruit could be heard over the epigastrium. **A,** The lateral abdominal aortogram shows compression of the CA by the median arcuate ligament (*arrow*). **B,** A repeat aortogram after surgical division of the constricting ligament reveals patency of the CA lumen. The child became asymptomatic after the surgery. Considerable forethought must be exercised before recommending surgery; this remains a poorly defined syndrome with an unproven pathogenesis [6]. (*From* Rogers and David [6]; *courtesy of* Stanley Baum, MD.)

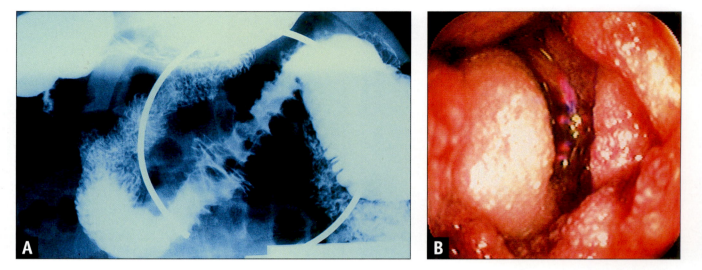

Figure 3-32. Polyarteritis nodosa (PAN). PAN results in a necrotizing vasculitis of medium and small arteries. The presentation of a vasculitis affecting small intestinal arteries can be the first or only manifestation of the patient's disease. The vessel involvement in PAN is classically segmental, as in **panel A**. Note the mucosal effacement and thumbprinting (*arrow*) caused by submucosal edema on this barium contrast study of the upper gastrointestinal tract. **B**, An endoscopic picture of the acute stage of intestinal ischemia characterized by hyperemia and edema [11]. Endoscopy is an important adjunct for the clinician in diagnosis of ischemic diseases of the gastrointestinal tract. It enables a direct inspection of the intestinal mucosa and permits access to perform biopsies, if necessary [12]. (*Courtesy of* Tony DeMondesert, MD.)

Crohn's Disease

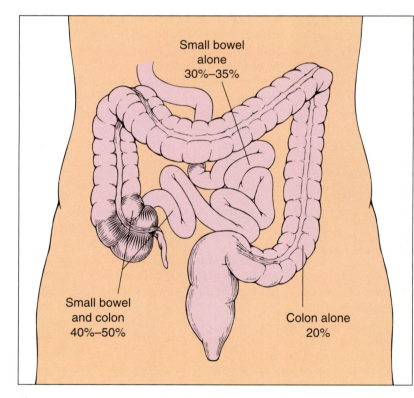

Figure 3-33. Anatomic distribution in Crohn's disease. Crohn's disease affects the small bowel alone in approximately 33% of cases and the colon alone in approximately 20%; nearly 50% of the cases involve both the small and large bowels (ileocolitis). (*Courtesy of* Ellen J. Scherl, MD, and David B. Sachar, MD.)

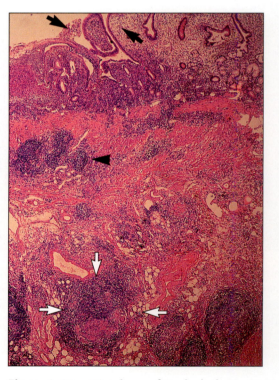

Figure 3-34. Histology of Crohn's ileitis. Mucosal edema and ulceration (*closed arrows*) are early pathologic findings in Crohn's disease. Lymphoid aggregates (*arrowhead*) organize into discrete, noncaseating granulomas (*open arrows*), shown here in the deep submucosa. Although granulomas seem to be a pathognomonic feature of Crohn's disease, the absence of granulomas does not rule out the diagnosis. (*Courtesy of* Ellen J. Scherl, MD, and David B. Sachar, MD.)

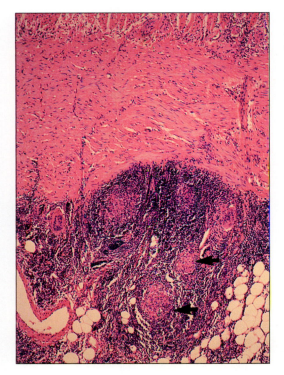

Figure 3-35. Chronic subserositis. The inflammatory process spreads transmurally. Note lymphoid aggregates and granulomas in the background of chronic subserositis (*arrows*). (*Courtesy of* Ellen J. Scherl, MD, and David B. Sachar, MD.)

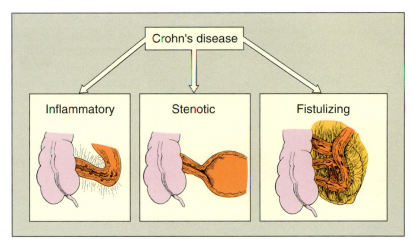

Figure 3-36. Behavioral patterns of Crohn's disease. It has proven useful, both for defining natural history and for selecting therapy, to think of the heterogeneous entity of Crohn's disease as comprising at least three different patterns of clinical and pathologic behavior: inflammatory, fibrostenotic, and fistulizing. (*Courtesy of* Ellen J. Scherl, MD, and David B. Sachar, MD.)

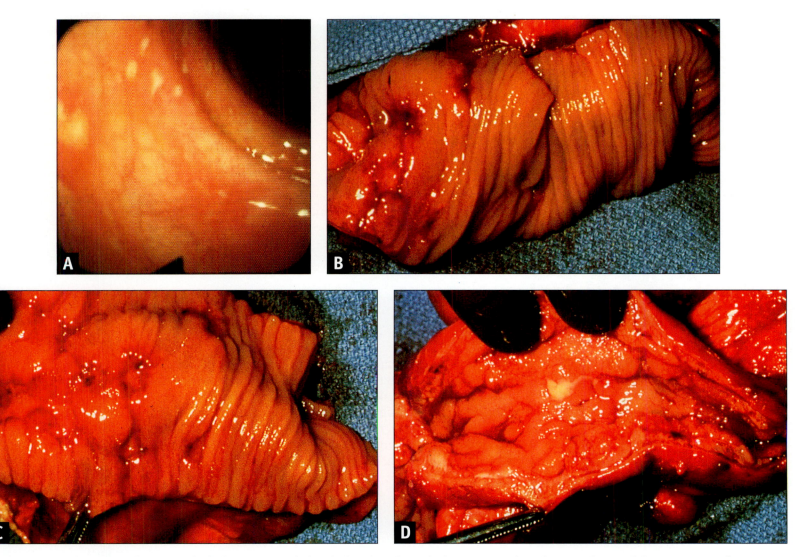

Figure 3-37. Ulcerations due to Crohn's disease. A. Aphthoid ulcerations are the earliest visible mucosal lesions of Crohn's disease. Discrete patchy ulcerations in the areas with submucosal edema (**panel B**) progressively enlarge and spread, becoming confluent (**panel C**), until they obliterate normal mucosa entirely (**panel D**). (*Courtesy of* Ellen J. Scherl, MD, and David B. Sachar, MD.)

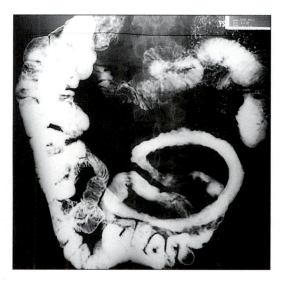

Figure 3-38. Radiographic appearance of Crohn's disease of the terminal ileum. Nodularity, ulceration, narrowing, and irregularity of the lumen, characteristically affecting the terminal ileum, may result from transmural inflammation and lymphoid proliferation. Separation of involved loops of intestine from adjacent segments of bowel reflects luminal narrowing, thickening of bowel wall, and mesenteric hypertrophy. (*Courtesy of* Ellen J. Scherl, MD, and David B. Sachar, MD.)

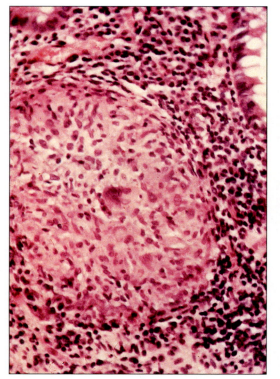

Figure 3-39. Granuloma. The typical granuloma of Crohn's disease consists of one or more Langhans' giant cells and epithelioid cells surrounded by a rim of T lymphocytes. (*Courtesy of* Ellen J. Scherl, MD, and David B. Sachar, MD.)

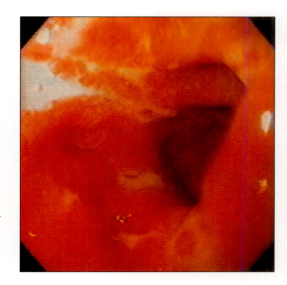

Figure 3-40. Endoscopic view of ileal Crohn's disease. Edema, hyperemia, and confluent linear ulcerations are classic endoscopic findings of inflammatory Crohn's disease. (*Courtesy of* Ellen J. Scherl, MD, and David B. Sachar, MD.)

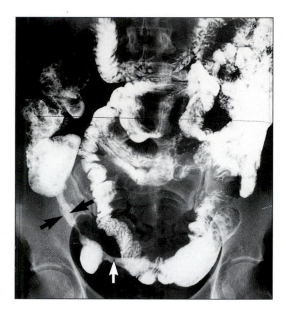

Figure 3-41. Radiographic "string sign" of Crohn's disease. In the early stages of stenosing Crohn's disease, edema and spasm produce intermittent obstructive symptoms, such as increasing postprandial pain. The spasm and edema are also responsible for the classic radiographic "string sign" (*open arrow*). Over several years the persistent inflammation progresses to scarring, narrowing, and finally, to stricture. Narrowing may be associated with asymmetric outpouchings or "pseudodiverticulae" (*closed arrows*). (*Courtesy of* Ellen J. Scherl, MD, and David B. Sachar, MD.)

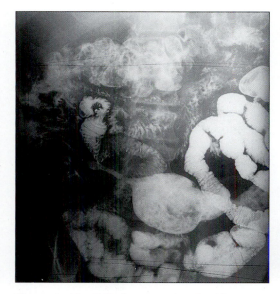

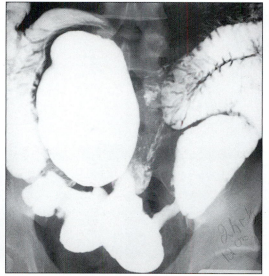

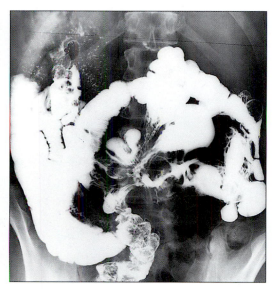

Figure 3-42. Dilation associated with Crohn's disease. Over the years, dilation proximal to fixed stenotic strictures becomes increasingly prominent. (*Courtesy of* Ellen J. Scherl, MD, and David B. Sachar, MD.)

Figure 3-43. When multiple strictures produce multiple areas of massively dilated proximal bowel over periods of many years, huge sacs, or "saddlebags," may develop. This saccular pattern is often accompanied by clinical sequelae of malnutrition due to impaired intake, bacterial overgrowth, and malabsorption. (*Courtesy of* Ellen J. Scherl, MD, and David B. Sachar, MD.)

Figure 3-44. Radiographic view of enteroenteric fistulas. Fistulization is the process in which transmural sinus tracts burrow all the way through to the serosa. These tracts often penetrate into adjacent loops of bowel to form ileoileal, ileocecal, or ileosigmoid fistulas. This figure shows complex ileal fistulas extending into adjacent ileal loops and cecum. (*Courtesy of* Ellen J. Scherl, MD, and David B. Sachar, MD.)

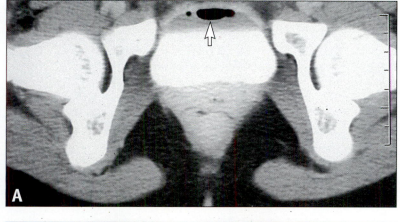

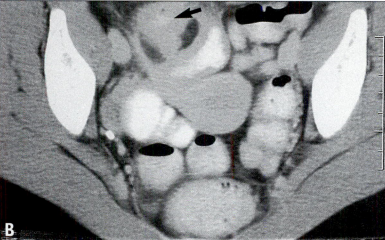

Figure 3-45.
Radiographic view of enterovesical fistulas. Enterovesical fistulization is a common complication of Crohn's disease as the distal ileum traverses the dome of the bladder. These figures show air in the bladder (**panel A**) and contrast in an ileal loop (*open arrow*) with a fistulous tract into the bladder (*closed arrow*) (**panel B**). (*Courtesy of* Ellen J. Scherl, MD, and David B. Sachar, MD.)

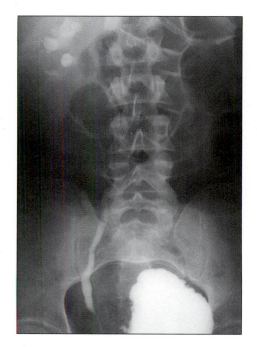

Figure 3-46. Retroperitoneal fistulas. When a sinus tract penetrates posteriorly from the ileum to the retroperitoneum, the resulting phlegmon may entrap the right ureter and compress it against the psoas muscle, resulting in noncalculous hydroureter and hydronephrosis. (*From* Sachar *et al.* [13]; with permission.)

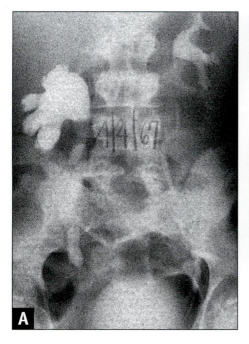

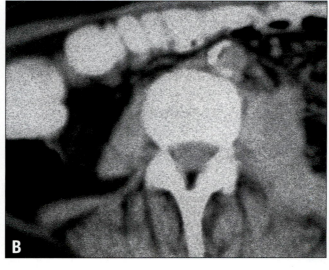

Figure 3-47. Frank psoas abscess. A–B, More advanced cases of retroperitoneal fistulization may produce a frank psoas abscess. The computed tomographic scan shows an abscess in the psoas muscle, which is nearly three times its normal thickness and contains an area of central liquefaction. (*From* Sachar *et al.* [13]; with permission.)

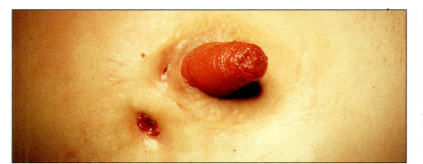

Figure 3-48. Enterocutaneous fistulas. Enterocutaneous fistulas follow the path of least resistance. Therefore, in a patient who has undergone previous surgery, an enterocutaneous fistula invariably emerges through the surgical scar, as shown here. In the absence of earlier surgery, it may dissect along a persistent urachal segment and drain through the relatively thin fascia layer at the umbilicus. Alternatively, it may track along the psoas muscle and present in the groin or extend directly to the anterior abdominal wall in the right lower quadrant. (*Courtesy of* Adrian Greenstein, MD.)

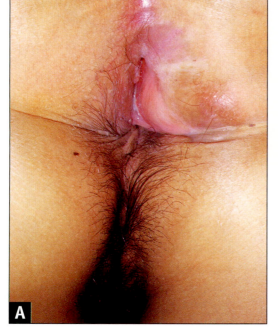

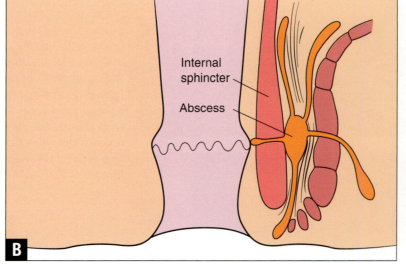

Figure 3-49. Perianal fistulas. A, Perianal lesions occur in as many as one third of all patients with Crohn's disease. Although perianal complications are more prevalent in patients with colonic disease, they are also seen in up to one quarter of patients with small-bowel disease alone. B, Perianal fistulas develop from the extension of intersphincteric abscesses. The lesions generally follow a course independent of the intra-abdominal disease. (**A**, *Courtesy of* Daniel Present, MD. **B**, *Adapted from* Wexner [14].)

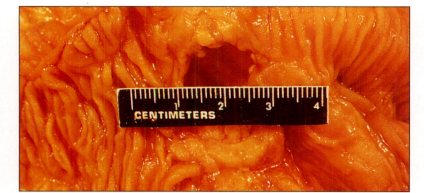

Figure 3-50. Gastointestinal carcinoma. There is an increased incidence of gastrointestinal (GI) carcinoma in Crohn's disease. Most of the GI malignancies in Crohn's disease occur in grossly diseased bowel, but as many as one third may arise in clinically uninvolved areas of the GI tract. This figure shows a small ileal carcinoma in an inactive ileum. The predominant risk factor for small-bowel carcinoma in Crohn's disease is a very long duration of disease, usually 20 years or more, applying equally to bypassed loops and to bowel in continuity with the rest of the intestine. In extensive Crohn's disease of the colon, the risk for colorectal cancer is as high as that for ulcerative colitis of comparable extent and duration (*Courtesy of* Adrian Greenstein, MD.).

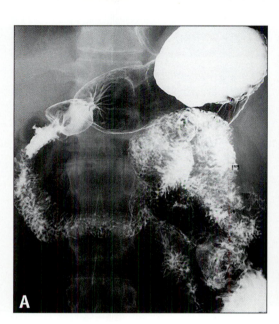

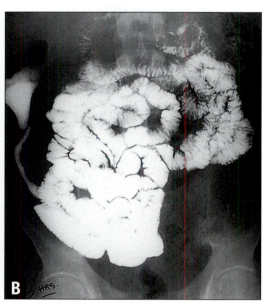

Figure 3-51. Upper gastrointestinal and small-bowel series. When the history, physical examination, and laboratory testing suggest Crohn's disease, an upper gastrointestinal (**panel A**) and small-bowel series (**panel B**) is generally the best first diagnostic test. If only an upper gastrointestinal series is performed, however, without thorough small-bowel follow-through and visualization of the terminal ileum, even the most obvious diagnosis of Crohn's disease may be completely missed. (*Courtesy of* Ellen J. Scherl, MD, and David B. Sachar, MD.)

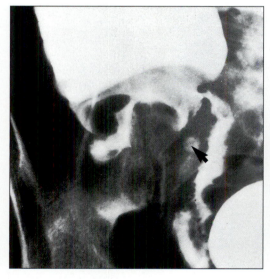

Figure 3-52. Appendiceal abscess. The distal 8 cm of terminal ileum are spastic, irritable, and markedly contracted in association with deformity and narrowing of the cecum. A 1-cm appendicolith is present (*arrow*). In this case, the inflammatory changes in the terminal ileum are secondary to the adjacent appendiceal abscess. (*Courtesy of* Daniel Maklansky, MD.)

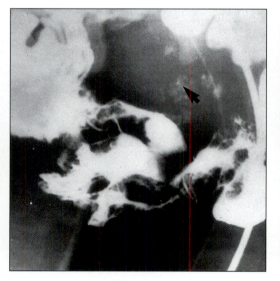

Figure 3-53. Carcinoma of cecum invading the ileocecal valve and terminal ileum. Superficially, this case mimics ileocolitis. The distal 6 cm of terminal ileum are markedly narrowed in association with several short fistulous tracts extending from the ileum to the cecum, which is also markedly contracted. These findings are secondary to an infiltrating mass from a cecal carcinoma. Note the psammoma bodies representing calcifications (*arrow*) in the carcinoma. (*Courtesy of* Daniel Maklansky, MD.)

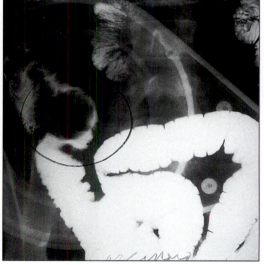

Figure 3-54. Carcinoid. Distal ileum. There is a golf-ball-sized submucosal mass fixing and indenting the distal ileum with minimal pleating of the adjacent folds. (*Courtesy of* Daniel Maklansky, MD.)

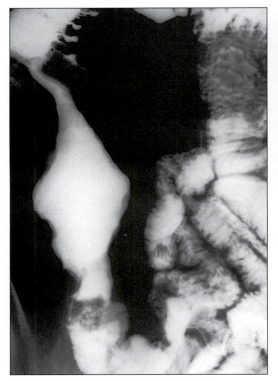

Figure 3-55. Lymphoma dilatation. The distal 15 cm of ileum are dilated in association with scalloped margins indicating mass. These findings represent a large ulcerating neoplasm. The term *aneurysmal* derives from the fact that the ulcerating mass is wider than the normal dimension of the bowel at this site. (*Courtesy of* Daniel Maklansky, MD.)

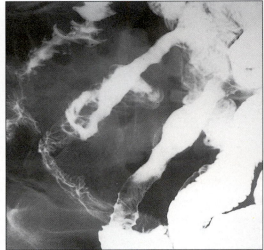

Figure 3-56. Lymphoma (separation of the loops). The loops of the distal ileum are rigid, fixed, and separated by lymphoma infiltrating the walls and the mesentery. Note that the margins are scalloped, indicating the presence of submucosal nodules. There is no ulceration. (*Courtesy of* Daniel Maklansky, MD.)

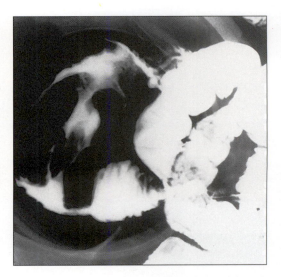

Figure 3-57. Lymphoma (mid-ileum). There is an irregular ulceration which traverses the center of the mass and divides in two, simulating a fistulous tract. The findings actually represent irregular necrotic changes within the lymphoma mass. (*Courtesy of* Ellen J. Scherl, MD, and David B. Sachar, MD.)

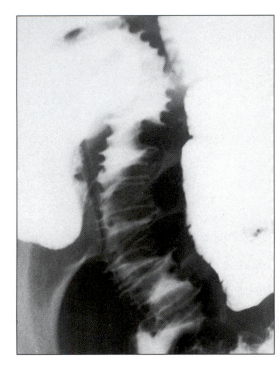

Figure 3-58. Vasculitis and edema of the terminal ileum. The patient is a 29-year-old female on birth control pills presenting with acute right lower quadrant pain. The "stack of coins" appearance indicates edema of the lamina propria and submucosa. (*Courtesy of* Daniel Maklansky, MD.)

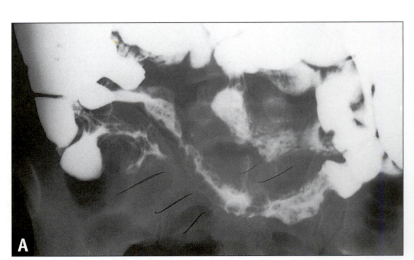

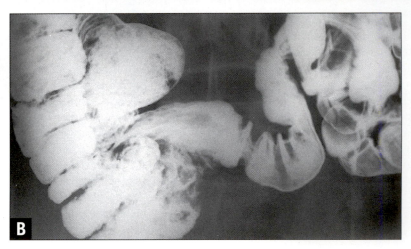

Figure 3-59. A, Tuberculosis A. The distal 15 to 20 cm of ileum are involved with an inflammatory mass characterized by extensive linear ulceration, slight transverse ulceration, and separation of the loops. There are no fistulae. From the roentgen findings alone, this cannot be differentiated from Crohn's disease. B, Tuberculosis B. Same patient as in **panel A** after 5 months of treatment with appropriate therapy. (*Courtesy of* Daniel Maklansky, MD.)

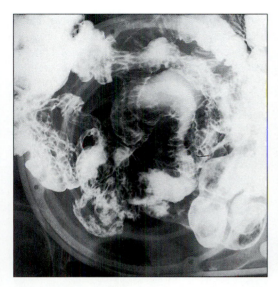

Figure 3-60. Radiation enteritis. The loops of the distal ileum are fixed and angulated in position with slight separation. The mucosal folds are thickened, and in some sites, nodular. There are no fistulas or sinus tracts. (*Courtesy of* Daniel Maklansky, MD.)

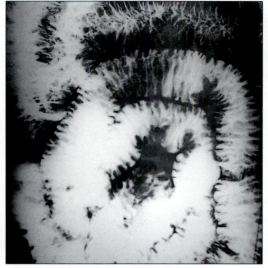

Figure 3-61. Amyloid. There is marked thickening and slight rigidity of the valvulae of the jejunum and ileum. Note that the folds in the distal ileum have the appearance of those in the jejunum, termed *jejunization* of the ileum. (*Courtesy of* Henry Janowitz, MD.)

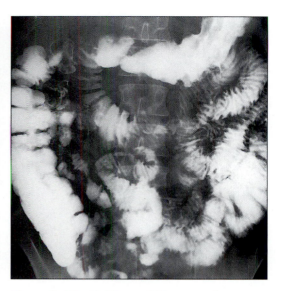

Figure 3-62. Zollinger-Ellison syndrome. There is moderate thickening of the folds of the jejunum and proximal ileum associated with marked increased secretions simulating jejunitis. Markedly thickened gastric folds are also present. (*Courtesy of* Daniel Maklansky, MD.)

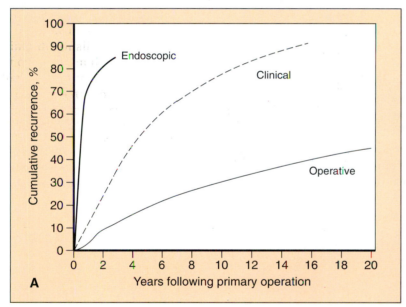

Figure 3-63. Postoperative recurrence of Crohn's disease. **A,** Although surgery is frequently necessary and highly effective in managing complications, achieving rehabilitation, and restoring a healthier quality of life in patients with Crohn's disease, postoperative recurrence is almost inevitable. The magnitude of this problem of postoperative recurrence depends largely on the definition of *recurrence*—whether endoscopic, clinical, or surgical. **B,** Postoperative recurrent ileitis is characterized by edema, ulcerations, and narrowing in the neoterminal ileum.

(Continued on next page)

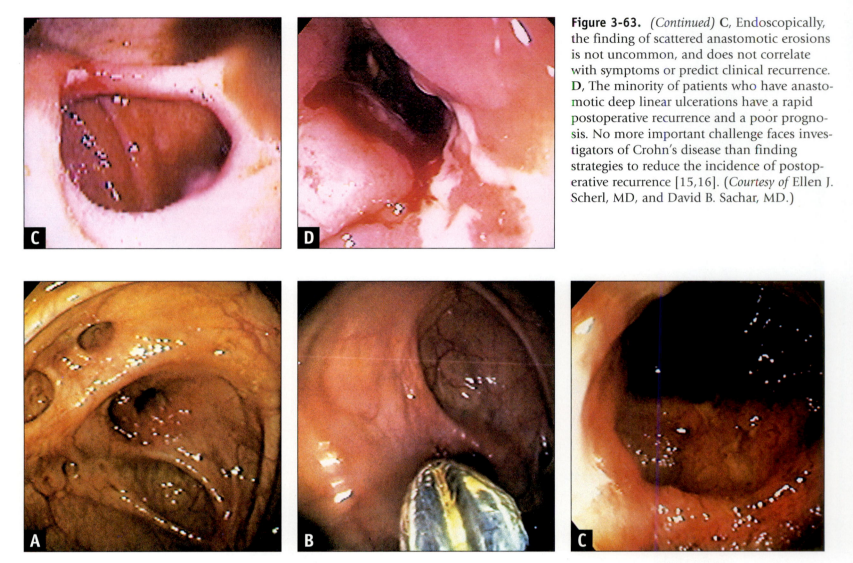

Figure 3-63. *(Continued)* **C**, Endoscopically, the finding of scattered anastomotic erosions is not uncommon, and does not correlate with symptoms or predict clinical recurrence. **D**, The minority of patients who have anastomotic deep linear ulcerations have a rapid postoperative recurrence and a poor prognosis. No more important challenge faces investigators of Crohn's disease than finding strategies to reduce the incidence of postoperative recurrence [15,16]. (*Courtesy of* Ellen J. Scherl, MD, and David B. Sachar, MD.)

Figure 3-64. **A–C**, Endoscopic balloon dilation of short postoperative stricture. An alternative strategy for short, inactive ("burnt-out") postoperative strictures is balloon dilation. No controlled trials are currently ongoing to assess this approach, but it offers an intriguing alternative in the management of postoperative recurrence [17,18]. (*Courtesy of* Ellen J. Scherl, MD, and David B. Sachar, MD.)

Neoplastic Diseases

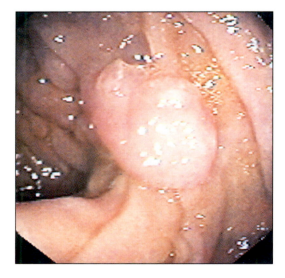

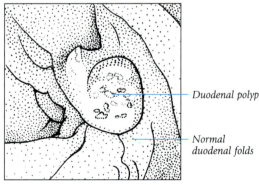

Duodenal polyp

Normal duodenal folds

Figure 3-65. Duodenal polyp viewed endoscopically. Duodenal polyps may occur sporadically as they did in this patient. They also occur in patients with colonic polyposis syndromes. If they are located near the ampulla of Vater, they may present a challenge during endoscopic polypectomy. (*Courtesy of* Karl Fukunaga, MD, and Russell Yang, MD.)

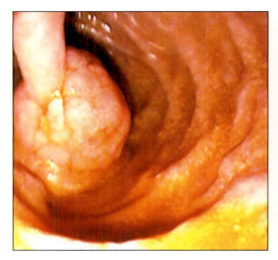

Figure 3-66. Endoscopic view of pedunculated adenomatous polyp. This polyp was found in the second portion of the duodenum in a patient with nausea and epigastric discomfort. Although this patient did not carry a diagnosis of familial adenomatous polyposis (FAP), polyps in FAP patients have a similar appearance [19–21]. (*Courtesy of* Gordon D. Luk, MD, Herbert J. Smith, MD, and Edward L. Lee, MD.)

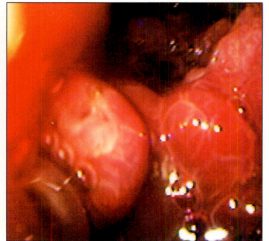

Figure 3-67. Multiple adenomatous polyps. Multiple sessile adenomatous polyps were seen in the second portion of the duodenum in a patient with familial adenomatous polyposis. The surface of the polyps have the slightly lobulated appearance suggestive of adenomas [20,21]. (*Courtesy of* Gordon D. Luk, MD, Herbert J. Smith, MD, and Edward L. Lee, MD.)

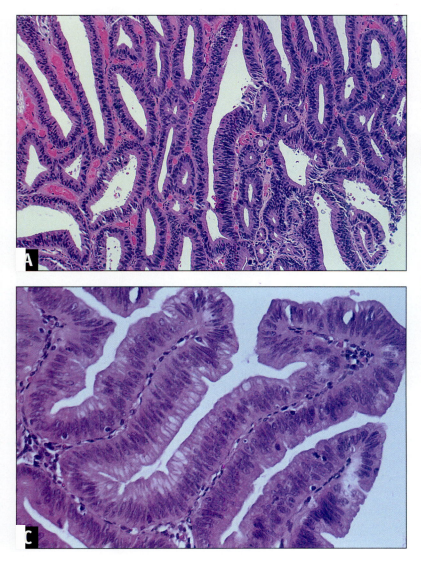

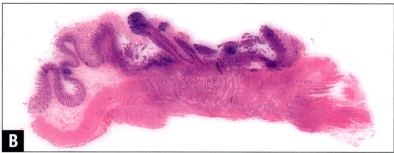

Figure 3-68. Histology of adenomatous polyps. **A**, Adenoma with severe atypia. Note the predominant villous pattern, the tightly packed glands and cells, the elongated hyperchromatic nuclei with loss of basal polarity, and the markedly increased nuclear:cytoplasmic ratio. **B**, Adenoma with mild atypia. Note the well-preserved villus architecture, with closely packed epithelial glands. The nuclei are hyperchromatic but still retain a predominant basal orientation, with only mildly increased nuclear:cytoplasmic ratio. **C**, Adenocarcinoma. This adenocarcinoma apparently arose from preexisting adenomatous epithelium. Note the transition from relatively normal-appearing mucosa to adenomatous epithelium and to adenocarcinoma. (*Courtesy of* Gordon D. Luk, MD, Herbert J. Smith, MD, and Edward L. Lee, MD.)

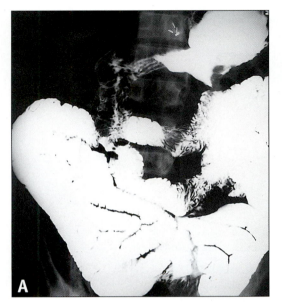

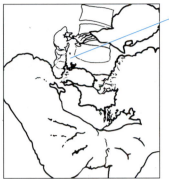

Napkin-ring lesion and displacement of adjacent tissues by mass effect

Figure 3-69. Adenocarcinoma. Although many duodenal and proximal jejunal tumors may be seen by endoscopy or enteroscopy, most are beyond the reach of even the longest instruments. Such tumors require either conventional small-bowel follow-through radiograms or enteroclysis for their detection. **A–B,** In this patient, the annular napkin-ringlike lesion was seen to best advantage at enteroclysis. **C,** The marked narrowing of the lumen by the circumferentially growing adenocarcinoma was seen in the resection specimen. **D,** The bulkiness of the tumor was also evident on histologic examination [19,22,23]. (*Courtesy of* Gordon D. Luk, MD, Herbert J. Smith, MD, and Edward L. Lee, MD.)

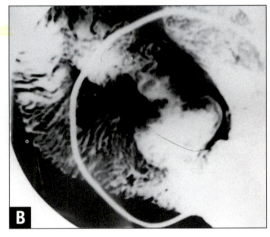

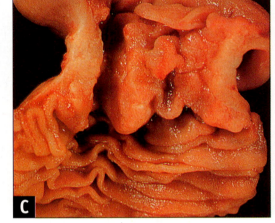

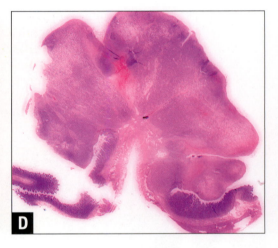

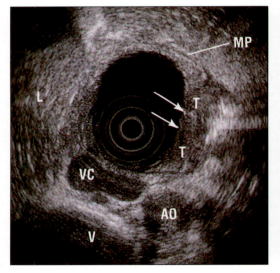

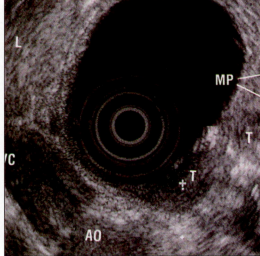

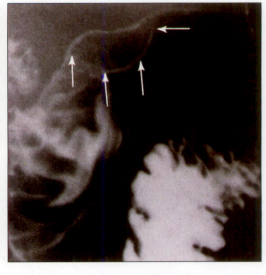

Figure 3-70. Ultrasound revealing a diffuse, hypoechoic tumor. A 40-year-old man with a primary duodenal carcinoma found endoscopically was referred for staging. Endoscopic ultrasound reveals a diffuse, hypoechoic tumor (T) with exophytic margins (*arrows*). AO—aorta; L—right lobe of the liver; MP—muscularis propria; V—vertebral body; VC—vena cava. (*From* Tio [24]; with permission.)

Figure 3-71. Another transverse section shows a deeply penetrating carcinoma (T) with minimal penetration into the subserosa. AO—aorta; L—right lobe of the liver; MP—muscularis propria, VC—vena cava. (*From* Tio [24]; with permission.)

Figure 3-72. Barium swallow shows a polypoid tumor (arrows) positioned in the distal part of the second portion of the duodenum. (*From* Tio [24]; with permission.)

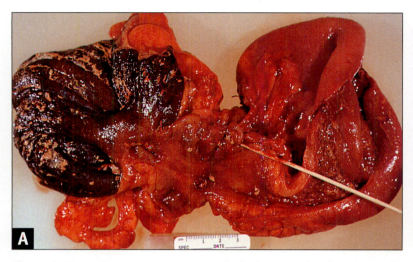

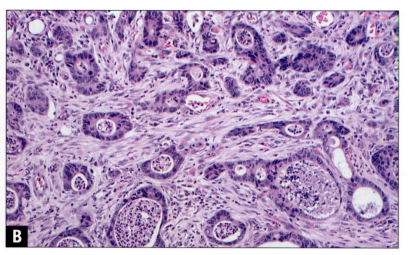

Figure 3-73. Adenocarcinoma in Crohn's disease. The diagnosis of adenocarcinoma in patients with longstanding active Crohn's disease may be extremely difficult. There are strictures, mucosal thickening, and inflammatory changes that may be difficult to differentiate from adenocarcinoma. A high index of suspicion is necessary, and all accessible strictures and masses should undergo biopsy or brushing. This patient with Crohn's disease of 22 years' duration developed worsening abdominal cramping pain and intestinal obstruction. Biopsies of the terminal ileum were highly suspicious for adenocarcinoma. The surgical specimen showed the tumor mass (*white pointer*). **A,** The cecum and proximal colon with melanosis coli are seen on the left side of the specimen. **B,** Histologic examination found moderately well-differentiated adenocarcinoma and active Crohn's disease [22,25]. (*Courtesy of* Gordon D. Luk, MD, Herbert J. Smith, MD, and Edward L. Lee, MD.)

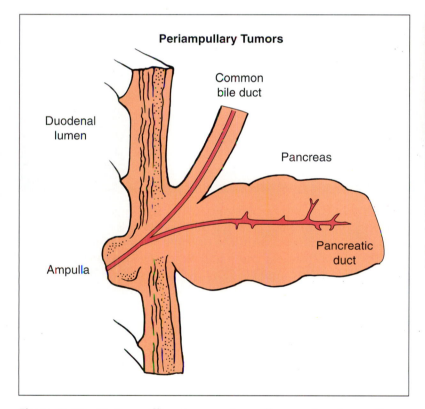

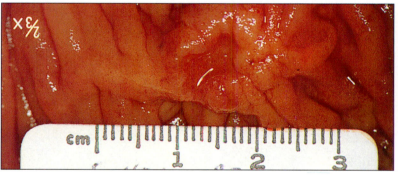

Figure 3-75. Ampullary carcinoma (pancreatic). This ampulla had invasive adenocarcinoma that was found to be pancreatic in origin. The patient underwent a pancreaticoduodenectomy (Whipple's procedure) [27]. (*Courtesy of* Gordon D. Luk, MD, Herbert J. Smith, MD, and Edward L. Lee, MD.)

Figure 3-74. Periampullary tumors. Ampullary and periampullary tumors most commonly arise from the pancreatic duct, but may also arise from the ampulla itself or the periampullary duodenal mucosa (commonly in familial adenomatous polyposis), the common bile duct, and even the gallbladder, liver, and other adjacent organs [22,26,27]. (*Courtesy of* Gordon D. Luk, MD, Herbert J. Smith, MD, and Edward L. Lee, MD.)

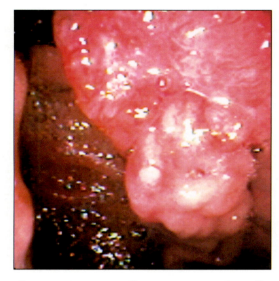

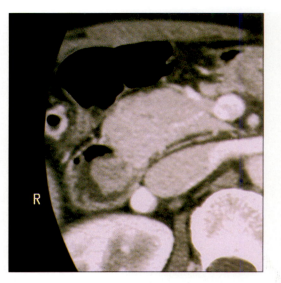

Figure 3-76. Ampullary carcinoma (papilla of Vater). This patient has a large ampullary carcinoma that protrudes from the papilla of Vater at the time of ERCP (*Courtesy of* Harvey Young, MD.)

Figure 3-77. Ampullary carcinoma. A CT scan from the same patient in Fig. 3-76 shows a mass in the lumen of the duodenum extending from the medial wall (*Courtesy of* Brooke Jeffrey, MD.)

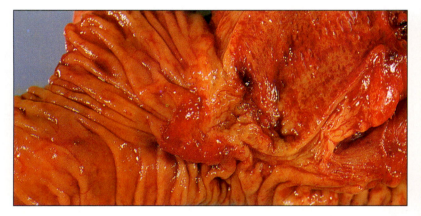

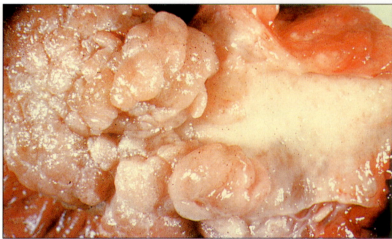

Figure 3-78. Ampullary carcinoma. This ampullary carcinoma was found to arise within the ampulla itself. The common bile duct has been opened lengthwise; no tumor involvement was seen and no evidence of pancreatic involvement was present [27]. (*Courtesy of* Gordon D. Luk, MD, Herbert J. Smith, MD, and Edward L. Lee, MD.)

Figure 3-79. Ampullary carcinoma. This was a large tumor mass, virtually obliterating the ampulla. In cases like this, macroscopic dissection to determine the tissue of origin is very difficult. In this case, the tumor histology was highly suggestive of a carcinoma originating from the ampulla [22,27]. (*Courtesy of* Gordon D. Luk, MD, Herbert J. Smith, MD, and Edward L. Lee, MD.)

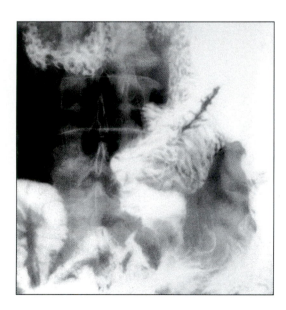

Figure 3-80. Carcinoid. This tumor was visualized as a well-circumscribed intraluminal mass in the midileum by enteroclysis. Without histologic examination, the exact etiology of this polypoid mass cannot be ascertained, although its distal location is suggestive of a carcinoid [28,29]. (*Courtesy of* Gordon D. Luk, MD, Herbert J. Smith, MD, and Edward L. Lee, MD.)

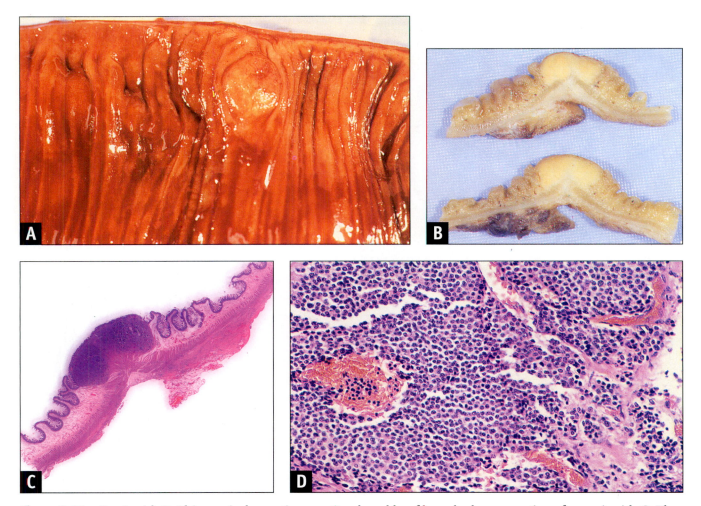

Figure 3-81.   Carcinoid. **A,** This surgical resection specimen shows a well-circumscribed intraluminal mass with apparently normal overlying mucosa and a central umbilication. **B,** On cut section, the tumor showed a pale-yellow meaty appearance, suggestive of a carcinoid; the muscular layer and serosa have undergone retractile changes that resulted in the formation of a knuckle of bowel, also suggestive of a carcinoid. **C,** The histology shows normal mucosa overlying the submucosal tumor, which consists of a monotonous array of bland tumor cells (**panel D**), which are characteristic of carcinoid [30,31]. (*Courtesy of* Gordon D. Luk, MD, Herbert J. Smith, MD, and Edward L. Lee, MD.)

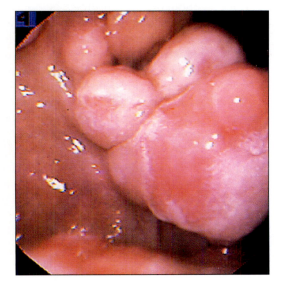

Figure 3-82.   Endoscopic image of multiple duodenal carcinoids in a 48-year-old woman who presented with gastrointestinal bleeding. These lesions may originate from anywhere in the gastrointestinal tract or in the bronchopulmonary tree. After they have a metastatic effect to the liver, these tumors can cause symptoms of the carcinoid syndrome [32]. (*Courtesy of* Daniel C. DeMarco, MD.)

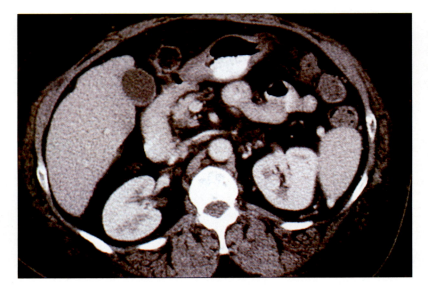

Figure 3-83. Computed tomographic scan of duodenal carcinoid tumors. Image from computed tomographic scan surprisingly shows a normal duodenum and no evidence of metastatic disease in this patient with the duodenal carcinoid tumors as already noted in Fig. 3-82. (*Courtesy of* Daniel C. DeMarco, MD.)

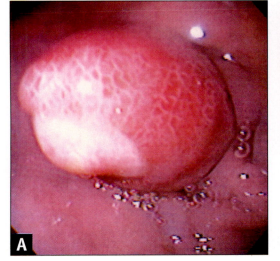

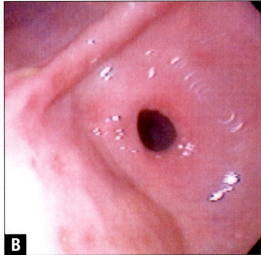

Figure 3-84. Endoscopic view of pedunculated duodenal carcinoid. This pedunculated 2-cm duodenal polyp had a long pliable stalk and moved freely through the pylorus into the gastric lumen (**panel A**) and retracted totally into the duodenal bulb (**panel B**) with peristalsis or attempted endoscopic maneuvers. (*Courtesy of* Gordon D. Luk, MD, Herbert J. Smith, MD, and Edward L. Lee, MD.)

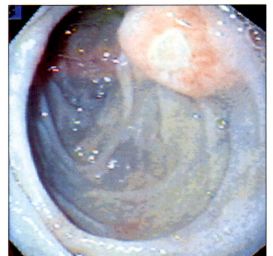

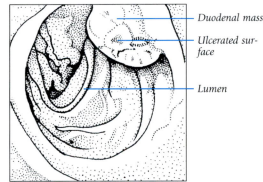

Duodenal mass

Ulcerated surface

Lumen

Figure 3-85. Duodenal mass seen endoscopically. The differential diagnosis for a duodenal mass is broad. Neoplastic causes include both benign and malignant types. Of the benign tumors, one must consider benign adenomatous polyp, villous adenoma, leiomyoma, carcinoid tumor, and benign inflammatory masses. Malignant causes include primary adenocarcinoma, metastatic tumor, leiomyosarcoma, carcinoid tumor, or lymphoma. This patient, who carried a diagnosis of AIDS, had a duodenal lymphoma. Notice that the surface of the tumor is ulcerated. (*Courtesy of* Karl Fukunaga, MD, and Russell Yang, MD.)

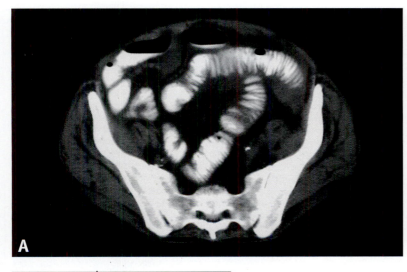

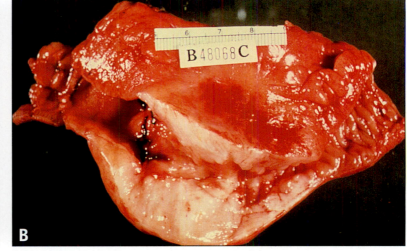

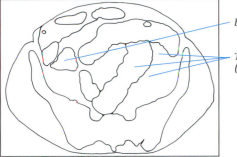

Bowel lumen (contrast)

Thickened bowel well (tissue density)

Figure 3-86. Primary small-bowel lymphoma. Lymphomas may present as diffuse infiltration, ulcerations, circumferential masses, or polypoid masses. **A**, This case of lymphoma with diffuse thickening of the small-bowel wall was visualized by CT scan. **B**, The surgical specimen confirmed the diffuse wall thickening. The cut surface shows the typical fish-flesh appearance [29,33,34]. (*Courtesy of* Gordon D. Luk, MD, Herbet J. Smith, MD, and Edward L. Lee, MD.)

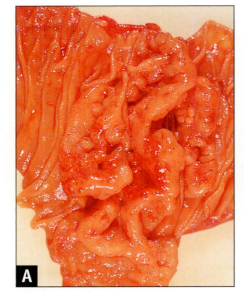

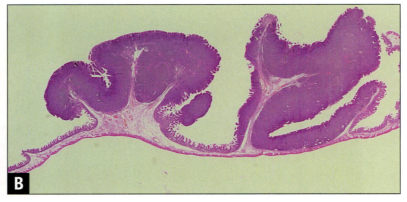

Figure 3-87. Polypoid lymphoma. **A**, This surgical specimen showed the diffuse polypoid involvement of the small-bowel wall by an infiltrative process. **B**, Histology confirmed the diagnosis of lymphoma, with the presence of lymphomatous polyps [33,34]. (*Courtesy of* Gordon D. Luk, MD, Herbert J. Smith, MD, and Edward L. Lee, MD.)

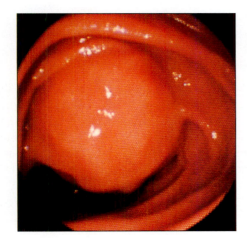

Figure 3-88. Leiomyoma viewed endoscopically. Leiomyomas and leiomyosarcomas are characteristically spherical submucosal masses with intact overlying mucosa. Large tumors may develop a central ulceration, which can lead to gastrointestinal bleeding or perforation. Size is an important prognostic factor, and tumors that are 5 cm or larger are generally classified as malignant, although most authors depend on histology (*see* Fig. 3-90). This 3-cm proximal jejunal tumor was visualized by enteroscopy and was histologically a benign leiomyoma. However, surgical resection is almost always indicated and was performed in this patient [35–37]. (*Courtesy of* Gordon D. Luk, MD, Herbert J. Smith, MD, and Edward L. Lee, MD.)

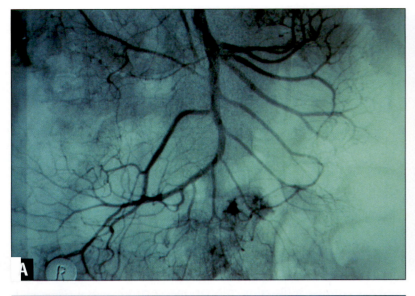

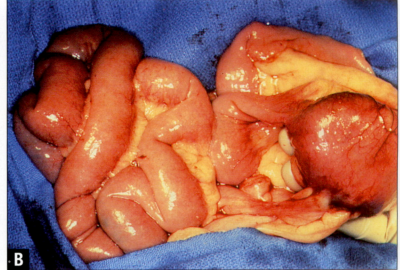

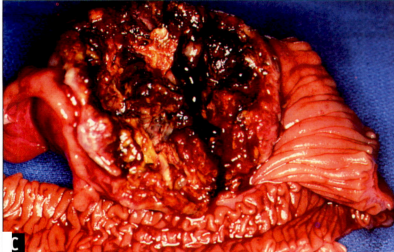

Figure 3-89. Leiomyosarcoma. Most leiomyosarcomas are beyond the reach of even the longest enteroscope. **A,** Arteriography may sometimes be helpful because leiomyosarcomas (and leiomyomas) are hypervascular and have a dense, well-circumscribed blush [38]. **B,** After arteriographic visualization, this patient underwent surgery; the tumor was identified and resected. **C,** The surgical specimen was opened longitudinally and revealed the large bulky hypervascular tumor. This tumor was 6 cm in diameter, and subsequently found to be a leiomyosarcoma by using histology [36,37]. (*Courtesy of* Gordon D. Luk, MD, Herbert J. Smith, MD, and Edward L. Lee, MD.)

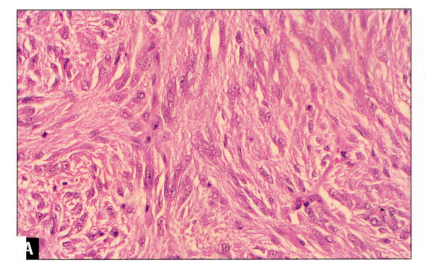

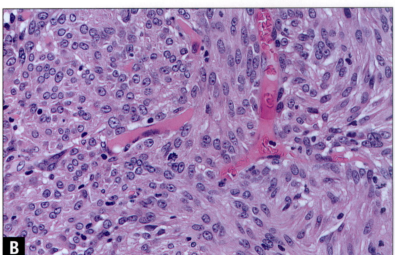

Figure 3-90. Histology of leiomyoma versus leiomyosarcoma. Although size is predictive of the nature of a stromal tumor, with tumors larger than 5 cm tending to be aggressive and malignant, smaller tumors may also be malignant. A reasonable index of malignancy is the level of mitotic activity. Tumors with more than five mitoses per 10 high-power fields tend to be malignant, although even tumors with lower mitotic indices may be or become malignant. Thus, surgical resection is almost always indicated for symptomatic tumors. **A,** No mitoses, a finding suggestive of a benign leiomyoma. **B,** Five mitoses within a single high-power field, a finding strongly suggestive of a malignant leiomyosarcoma [36,37]. (*Courtesy of* Gordon D. Luk, MD, Herbert J. Smith, MD, and Edward L. Lee, MD.)

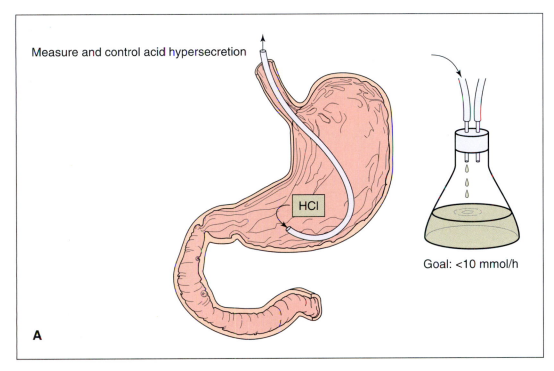

Measure and control acid hypersecretion

HCl

Goal: <10 mmol/h

A

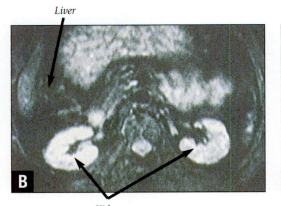

Liver

Kidneys

B

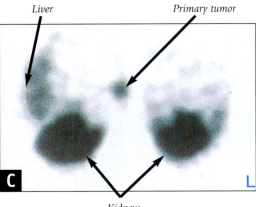

Liver   *Primary tumor*

Kidneys

C   L

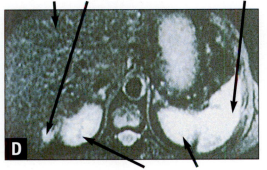

Liver   *Right lobe liver metastasis*   *Spleen*

Kidney

D

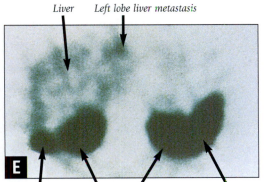

Liver   *Left lobe liver metastasis*

Right lobe liver metastasis   *Kidney*   *Spleen*

E

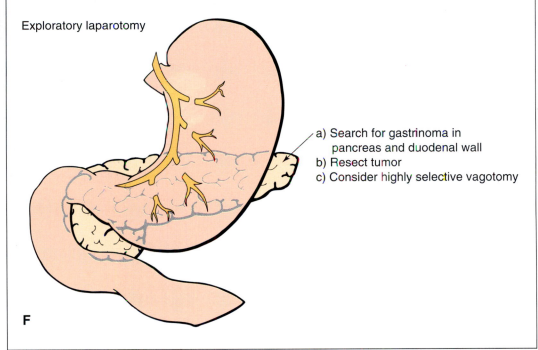

Exploratory laparotomy

a) Search for gastrinoma in pancreas and duodenal wall
b) Resect tumor
c) Consider highly selective vagotomy

F

Figure 3-91. Treatment of Zollinger-Ellison syndrome (ZES) involves both medical and surgical therapies [39]. Acid secretion can be effectively controlled in most patients by histamine$_2$-receptor antagonists or proton-pump inhibitors. It is essential that basal acid secretion be reduced to less than 10 mmol/hr if symptoms are to be controlled. The effectiveness of therapy needs to be measured with gastric analysis (**panel A**). After acid secretion is controlled, evidence for the resectability of tumor should be sought; computerized tomography, upper gastrointestinal endoscopy, endoscopic ultrasound, and radiolabeled octreotide scanning can be powerful tools for this purpose. B–E, These figures contrast findings of MR imaging (**panels B and D**) with findings of radiolabeled octreotide scanning (SRS) at the same anatomic levels (**panels C and E**) in detection of the primary tumor in one patient (**panels B and C**) and metastatic disease in another patient (**panels D and E**) with gastrinoma. The octreotide scans are clearly positive whereas the MR images do not always show the tumor [40]. If there is no evidence for metastasis, surgical exploration should be considered to identify and resect tumor (**panel F**). This is reasonable because now that acid secretion can be controlled, patients with ZES die from tumor metastasis and not acid-related complications, such as perforation. Vagotomy can be considered at the time of surgery to minimize the need for antisecretory drugs. (**B–E,** *Courtesy of* Robert T. Jensen, MD.)

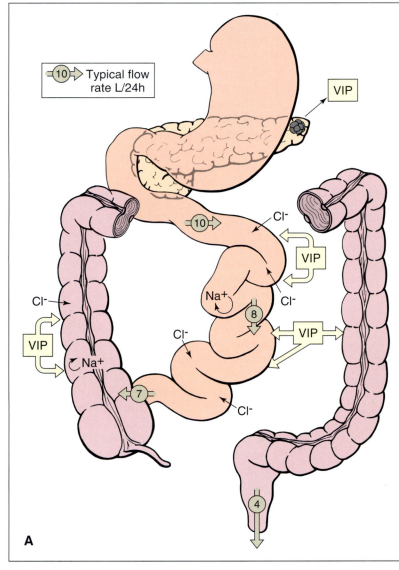

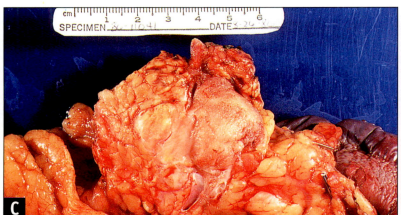

A

Figure 3-92. VIPomas. **A,** Vasoactive intestinal polypeptide (VIP)–secreting tumors produce the Verner-Morrison syndrome, also known as *pancreatic cholera syndrome,* or watery diarrhea, hypokalemia, and achlorhydria syndrome. VIP produces a secretory state in the intestine by raising enterocyte cyclic AMP levels, causing chloride secretion and inhibiting sodium absorption. Stool outputs of up to 5 L per day can be observed. The tumors typically are located in the pancreas, but tumors in other locations (ganglioneuromas, pheochromocytomas) can also produce this neuropeptide. Treatment with resection is ideal, but injection of octreotide, the somatostatin analogue, has allowed good control of symptoms in many patients. **B,** A bulky VIPoma (*arrow*) in the tail of the pancreas as shown by computerized tomography. **C,** Resected tumor in the same patient. **D,** Histology of this tumor showing nest of enteroendocrine cells.

The somatostatin analogue, octreotide, often produces dramatic decreases of serum VIP levels and daily stool weights in patients with pancreatic cholera syndrome. **E–F,** These figures are from an early report and show the results of starting octreotide on day 7 on serum VIP concentration (**panel E**) and stool weight (**panel F**). (**A–D,** *Courtesy of* Lawrence R. Schiller, MD; **E–F,** *adapted from* Maton *et al.* [41].)

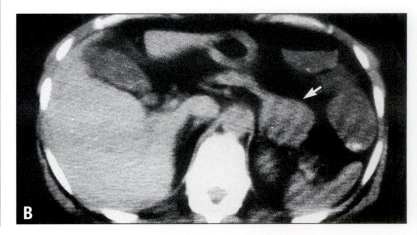

B

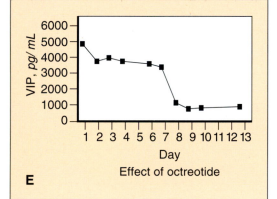

C

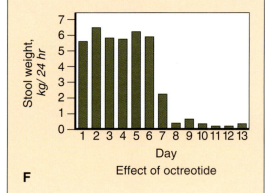

D

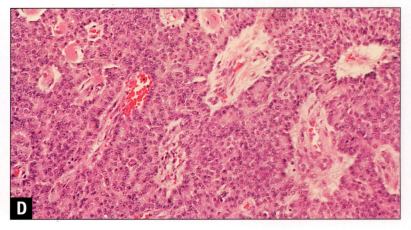

E

F

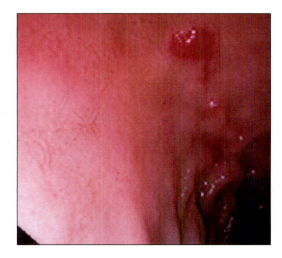

Figure 3-93. Kaposi's sarcoma. Kaposi's sarcoma in patients with AIDS might be considered a systemic disease, and has been found to arise throughout the entire gastrointestinal tract. In this patient there are multiple flat and raised reddish submucosal lesions, with only a thin layer of overlying mucosa in the distal duodenum. Although patients with AIDS are often found to harbor Kaposi's sarcoma on endoscopic examination, it is unclear whether these small lesions cause symptoms. Biopsy will often yield the diagnosis [42]. (*Courtesy of* Gordon D. Luk, MD, Herbert J. Smith, MD, and Edward L. Lee, MD.)

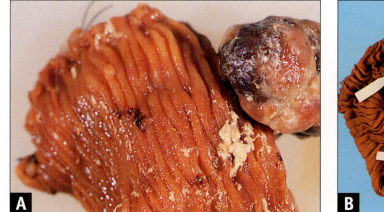

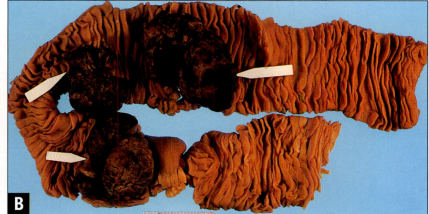

Figure 3-94. Metastatic melanoma. Melanoma is the most common tumor metastatic to the small bowel and is found in about half of patients dying with metastatic melanoma. The metastases may appear as a single mass (**panel A**) or multiple masses (**panel B**). Most melanoma metastases are pigmented. Because tumors tend to be bulky, patients often develop obstruction or intussusception [43]. (*Courtesy of* Gordon D. Luk, MD, Herbert J. Smith, MD, and Edward L. Lee, MD.)

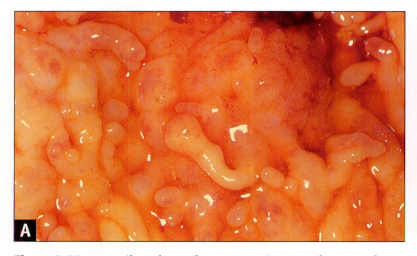

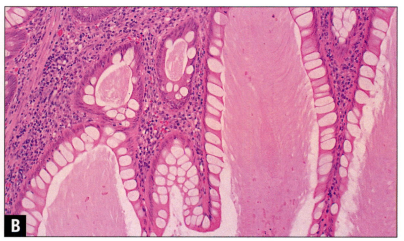

Figure 3-95. Juvenile polyps. These serpentine, translucent polyps were seen in the proximal jejunum of a patient who was complaining of dyspepsia, but who was otherwise healthy. **A**, This surgical specimen shows their characteristic translucent appearance. **B**, Histology revealed the hamartomatous nature of the polyp with distended mucus-filled glands and edematous lamina propria. Except in familial juvenile polyposis syndromes, these juvenile polyps are considered benign [44]. (*Courtesy of* Gordon D. Luk, MD, Herbert J. Smith, MD, and Edward L. Lee, MD.)

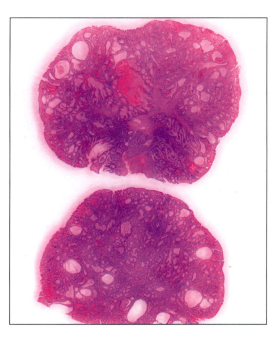

Figure 3-96. Peutz-Jeghers polyp. This 2-cm surgical specimen was found in the midjejunum of a patient with Peutz-Jeghers syndrome who had intermittent intestinal obstruction. The histology reveals the characteristic arborization of smooth muscle and epithelial elements, along with cystic dilation and edematous lamina propria containing abundant vasculature. Although the syndrome has been associated with an increased risk of carcinoma, primarily outside the gastrointestinal tract, the polyps themselves are not considered premalignant [44]. (*Courtesy of* Gordon D. Luk, MD, Herbert J. Smith, MD, and Edward L. Lee, MD.)

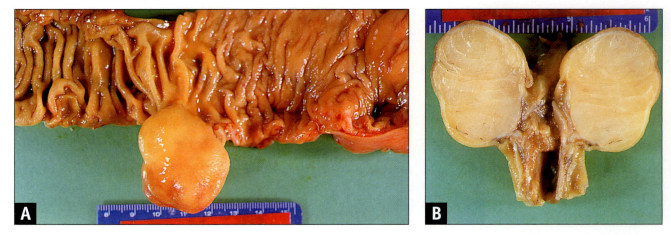

Figure 3-97. Lipoma. This 3-cm polyp was found in the distal ileum of a patient with intermittent intestinal obstruction. **A,** The surgical specimen had the characteristic glistening, yellowish appearance of a lipoma. **B,** The cut surface revealed the characteristic color and texture of fat. (*Courtesy of* Gordon D. Luk, MD, Herbert J. Smith, MD, and Edward L. Lee, MD.)

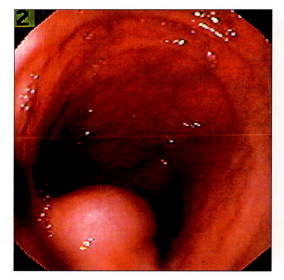

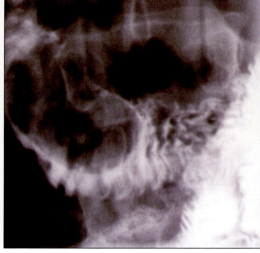

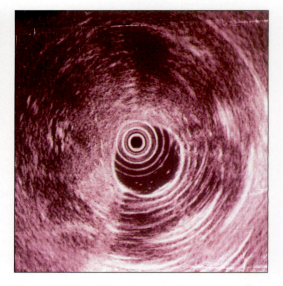

Figure 3-98. Duodenal lipoma. Endoscopic view of a submucosal mass in the duodenum of a patient who presented with refractory nausea. (*Courtesy of* Daniel C. DeMarco, MD.)

Figure 3-99. Upper gastrointestinal series shows a lesion to be located in the third portion of the duodenum. (*Courtesy of* Daniel C. DeMarco, MD.)

Figure 3-100. Ultrasonography cannot reliably demonstrate or differentiate lipoma from liposarcoma. However, there is no evidence of metastatic disease in this patient. Furthermore, liposarcomas remain exceedingly rare. (*Courtesy of* Daniel C. DeMarco, MD.)

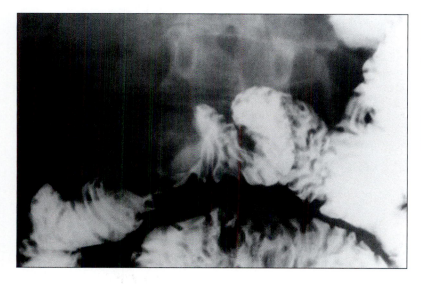

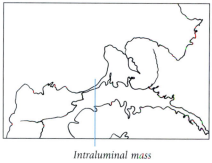

Intraluminal mass

Figure 3-101. Neurofibroma. This large intraluminal mass with a smooth domed surface was visualized by enteroclysis. Subsequently, the mass was found to be a neurofibroma. (*Courtesy of* Gordon D. Luk, MD, Herbert J. Smith, MD, and Edward L. Lee, MD.)

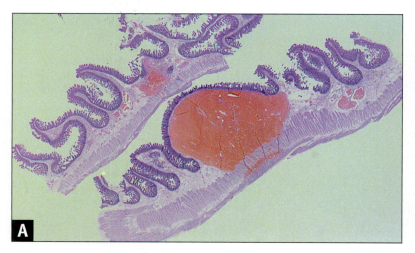

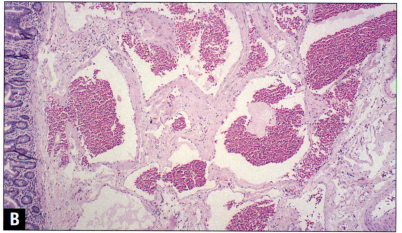

Figure 3-102. Hemangioma. **A,** The low-power view of this hemangioma specimen showed cavernous dilation of the vascular structures. **B,** Higher magnification revealed that almost all vascular structures are dilated. (*Courtesy of* Gordon D. Luk, MD, Herbert J. Smith, MD, and Edward L. Lee, MD.)

Small Bowel Transplantation

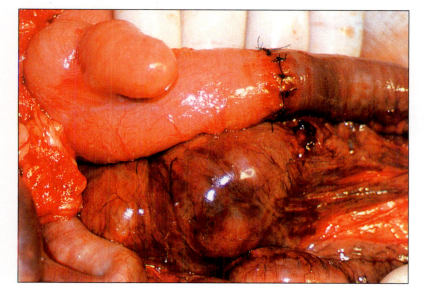

Figure 3-103. Intraoperative view of acute rejection. A marked, obvious difference in color can be easily seen between the host jejunum on the left compared with the blackened graft jejunum to the right and below the anastomosis in this dog model of transplantation 6 days following the transplantation. The darkened color results from the ischemic changes that accompany acute rejection and secondary sepsis. (*Courtesy of* Javier Tabasco-Minguillan, MD, William Hutson, MD, Atsushi Sugitani, MD, and James C. Reynolds, MD.)

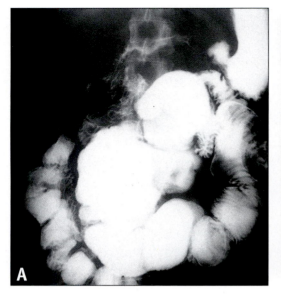

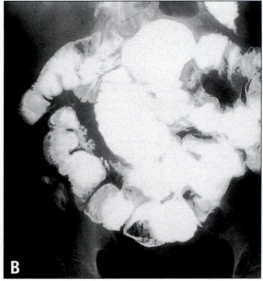

Figure 3-104. Post-transplantation bowel edema and dilatation. A barium study in a recipient of combined isolated small-bowel and liver transplantation showing normal gastric emptying (**panel A**) from the host stomach and dilated loops of the small-bowel graft (**panel A** and **panel B**). The transit of contrast material through the small intestine was markedly delayed. After a transit time of several hours, the leading edge of contrast reached the ostomy, and is shown in **panel B**. The study was requested to evaluate the cause of dilated loops of small-bowel graft. Adhesions were excluded, and histologic analysis of biopsies later confirmed the presence of acute cellular rejection. (*Courtesy of* Javier Tabasco-Minguillan, MD, William Hutson, MD, Atsushi Sugitani, MD, and James C. Reynolds, MD.)

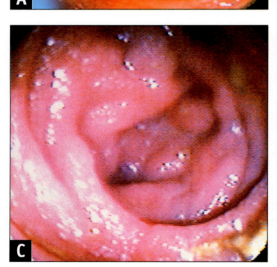

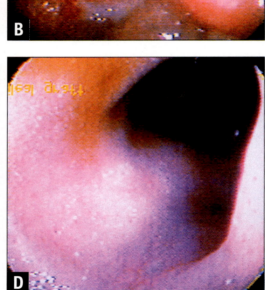

Figure 3-105. Sequence of endoscopic findings in a patient with acute cellular rejection in the graft ileum. In clinical practice, the observation of patients with small-bowel transplantation is achieved by periodic endoscopic surveillance of the allografts that provide histologic sampling and allows the visual inspection of the intestine. This surveillance is illustrated in the series of endoscopic photographs (**A–E**) with their histologic correlates

(Continued on next page)

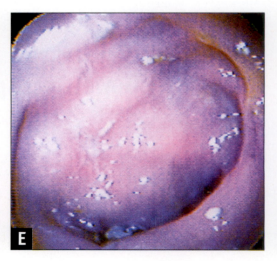

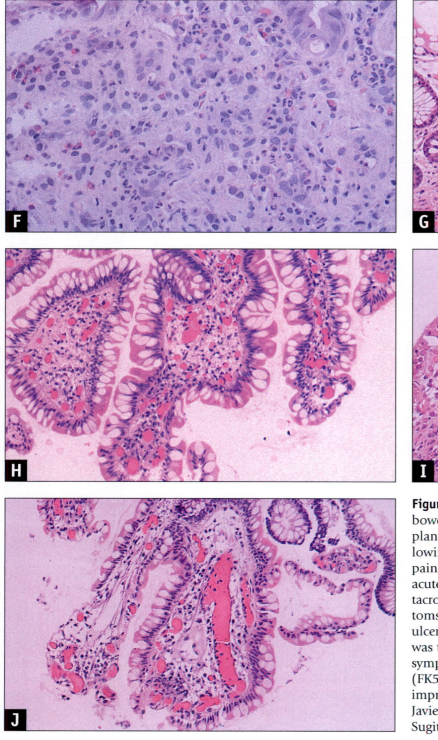

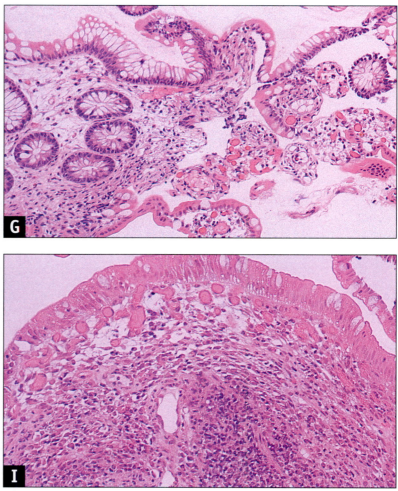

Figure 3-105. (F–J) from a patient who had undergone small-bowel transplantation. The patient was a 41-year-old woman transplanted for Gardner's syndrome who presented several months following an uneventful transplantation with diarrhea, abdominal pain, and abdominal distention. **A–B**, The initial studies showed acute cellular rejection, and she was treated with an increase in the tacrolimus (FK506) dose. She had some improvement in her symptoms. **C–D**, Follow-up endoscopy, however, showed persistent ulcerations. **E–F**, A week later she developed abdominal pain and was treated with bolus steroids. **G–H**, Despite her therapy, her symptoms persisted, thus necessitating increased tacrolimus (FK506) doses. **I–J**, Finally, her clinical and laboratory parameters improved and she was discharged from the hospital. (*Courtesy of* Javier Tabasco-Minguillan, MD, William Hutson, MD, Atsushi Sugitani, MD, and James C. Reynolds, MD.)

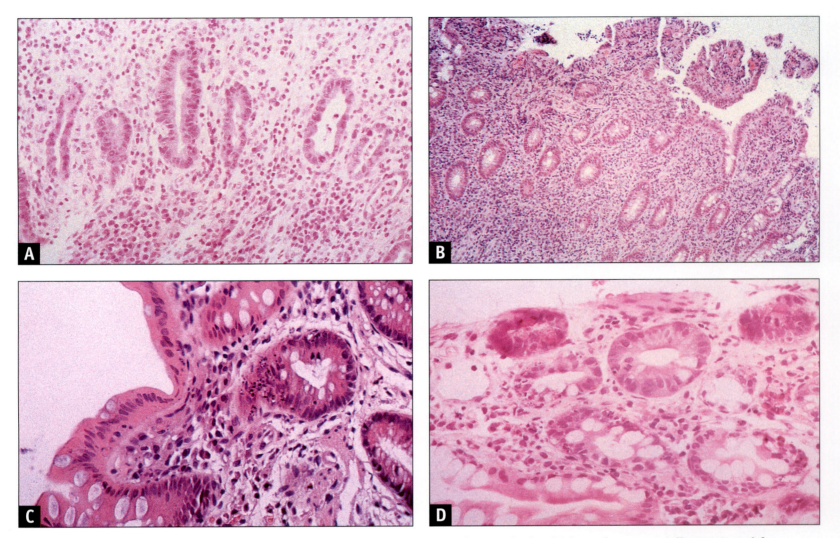

Figure 3-106. Characteristic histologic features of acute cellular rejection. During acute cellular rejection there are a variety of histologic abnormalities. There is damage to the mucosa with crypt loss and regeneration (**panel A**) and loss of mucosal integrity (**panel B**). There is also crypt cell damage and drop-out (apoptosis) (**panels C and D**), which can be sequentially monitored for diagnosis and response to therapy. (*Courtesy of* Javier Tabasco-Minguillan, MD, William Hutson, MD, Atsushi Sugitani, MD, and James C. Reynolds, MD.)

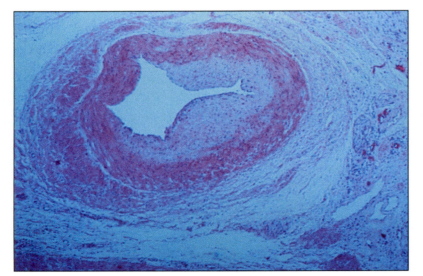

Figure 3-107. Obliterative arteriopathy in chronic rejection. A photomicrograph of a medium-sized mesenteric artery. As with other organs, the hallmark of chronic rejection is obliterative arteriopathy. The specimen was obtained at autopsy of an allograft with obliterative arteriopathy that was lost to chronic rejection. (*Courtesy of* Javier Tabasco-Minguillan, MD, William Hutson, MD, Atsushi Sugitani, MD, and James C. Reynolds, MD.)

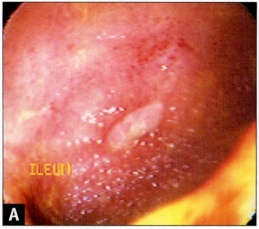
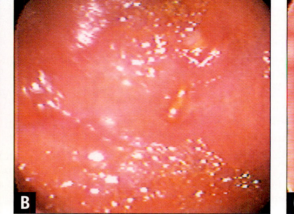
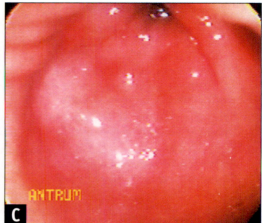

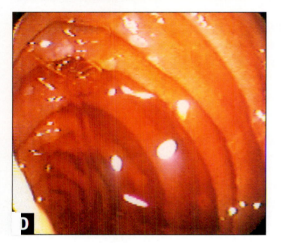

Figure 3-108. Characteristic endoscopic appearance of cytomegalovirus (CMV) infection of the graft. **A–B,** CMV infection of the graft ileum with erythema and ulcerations. **C,** The infection did not affect the native stomach. **D,** No effect in the graft jejunum. (*Courtesy of* Javier Tabasco-Minguillan, MD, William Hutson, MD, Atsushi Sugitani, MD, and James C. Reynolds, MD.)

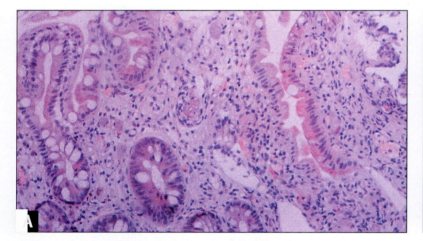
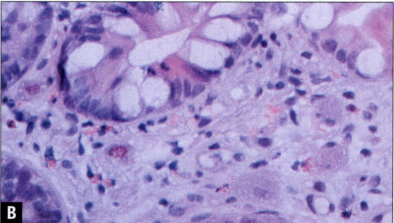

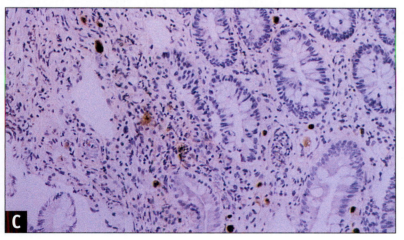

Figure 3-109. Histologic characteristics of cytomegalovirus (CMV) enteritis. **A,** CMV infection of the small-bowel graft. **B,** A magnified view of the biopsy specimen shows intracytoplasmic inclusion bodies. **C,** Specimen that tested positive (brown) with a specific immunoperoxidase staining. (*Courtesy of* Javier Tabasco-Minguillan, MD, William Hutson, MD, Atsushi Sugitani, MD, and James C. Reynolds, MD.)

References

1. Musola R, Franzin G, Mora R, Manfrini C: Prevalence of gastroduodenal lesions in uremic patients undergoing dialysis and after renal transplantation. *Gastrointest Endosc* 1984, 30:343–346.

2. Silverstein F, Gilbert D, Tedesco F, *et al*.: The national ASGE survey on upper gastrointestinal bleeding. *Gastrointest Endosc* 1981, 27:80–93.

3. Summers RW, Anuras S, Green J: Jejunal manometry patterns in health, partial intestinal obstruction and pseudoobstruction. *Gastroenterology* 1983, 85:1290–1300.

4. Quigley EMM: Intestinal pseudoobstruction. In *Evolving Concepts in Gastrointestinal Motility*. Edited by Orr W, Champion MC. Oxford: Blackwell Science; 1996:171–199.

5. Holt PR, Hashim SA, Van Itallie TB: Treatment of malabsorption syndrome and exudative enteropathy with synthetic medium chain triglycerides. *Am J Gastroenterol* 1965, 43:549–559.

6. Rogers AI, David S: Intestinal blood flow and diseases of vascular impairment. In *Bockus Gastroenterology*, vol 2, edn 5. Edited by Haubrich WS, Fenton S. Philadelphia: WB Saunders; 1995:1212–1234.

7. American Gastroenterological Association: *Undergraduate Teaching Project in Gastroenterology and Liver Disease*. Timonium, Maryland: Milner-Fenwick; 1983.

8. Dodds WJ, Stewart ET, Goldberg HI: Pneumatosis intestinalis associated with hepatic portal venous gas. *Dig Dis* 1976, 21:992–995.

9. Pounder RE, Allison MC, Dhillon AP: *A Color Atlas of Digestive System* London: Wolfe Publishing Co., 1989:126–127.

10. Kim JY, Ha HK, Byun JY, *et al*.: Intestinal infarction secondary to mesenteric venous thrombosis: CT-pathologic correlation. *J Comput Assist Tomogr* 1993, 17:382–385.

11. Harris MT, Lewis BS: Systemic diseases affecting the mesenteric circulation. *Surg Clin North Am* 1992, 72:245–259.

12. Kurland B, Brandt LJ, Delany HM: Diagnostic tests for intestinal ischemia. *Surg Clin North Am* 1992, 72:97.

13. Sachar D, Peppercorn M, Sweeting J, Burrell M: American Gastroenterological Association Clinical Teaching Project: Inflammatory Bowel Disease. Timonium: Milner-Fenwick 1991.

14. Wexner S: General principles of surgery in ulcerative colitis and Crohn's disease. *Semin Gastrointest Dis* 1991, 2:90–106.

15. Greenstein A, Sachar D, Pasternack B, *et al*.: Reoperation and recurrence in Crohn's colitis and ileocolitis: Crude and cumulative rates. *N Engl J Med* 1975, 293:685–690.

16. Rutgeerts P, Geboes K, Vantrappen G, *et al*.: Predictability of postoperative course of Crohn's disease. *Gastroenterology* 1990, 99:956–963.

17. Caprilli R, Andreoli A, Capurso L, *et al*.: Oral mesalamine (Asacol) for the prevention of recurrence of postoperative Crohn's disease. *Aliment Pharmacol Ther* 1994, 8:35–43.

18. Brignola C, Cottone M, Pera A, *et al*.: An Italian Cooperative Study Group: Mesalamine in the prevention of endoscopic recurrence after intestinal resection for Crohn's Disease. *Gastroenterology* 1995, 108:345–349.

19. Galandiuk S, Hermann RES, Jagelman DG, *et al*.: Villous tumors of the duodenum. *Ann Surg* 1988, 207:234.

20. Kurtz RC, Sternberg SJ, Miller HH, DeCosse JJ: Upper gastrointestinal neoplasia in familial polyposis. *Dig Dis Sci* 1987, 32:459.

21. Offerhaus GJA, Giardiello FM, Krush AJ, *et al*.: The risk of upper gastrointestinal cancer in familial adenomatous polyposis. *Gastroenterology* 1992, 102:1980.

22. Sinar DR: Small bowel neoplasms (other than carcinoid and lymphoma). In *Gastrointestinal Disease*, edn 5. Edited by Sleisenger MH, Fordtran JH. Philadelphia: WB Saunders; 1993:1393.

23. Zollinger RM, Sternfeld WC, Schreiber H: Primary neoplasms of the small intestine. *Am J Surg* 1986, 151:654.

24. Tio TL: *Gastrointestinal TNM cancer staging by endosonography*. New York: Igaku-Shoin; 1995.

25. Lashner BA: Risk factors for small bowel cancers in Crohn's disease. *Dig Dis Sci* 1992, 37:1179.

26. Lance P: Tumors and other neoplastic diseases of the small bowel. In *Textbook of Gastroenterology*. Edited by Yamada T. Philadelphia: JB Lippincott; 1995:1696.

27. Tarazi RY, Hermann RE, Vogt DP, *et al*.: Results of surgical treatment of periampullary tumors: A thirty-five year experience. *Surgery* 1986, 100:716.

28. Maglinte DDT, Hall R, Miller RE, *et al*.: Detection of surgical lesions of the small bowel by enteroclysis. *Am J Surg* 1984, 147:225.

29. Nolan DJ: Radiology of the small intestine. In *Surgery of the Small Intestine*. Edited by Nelson RL, Nyhus LM. Norwalk: Appleton & Lange; 1987:59.

30. Godwin DJ: Carcinoid tumors: An analysis of 2,837 cases. *Cancer* 1975, 36:560.

31. MacGillivray DC, Snyder DA, Drucker W, ReMine SG: Carcinoid tumors: The relationship between clinical presentation and the extent of disease. *Surgery* 1991, 110:68.

32. Merrell DE, Mansbach C, Garbutt JT: Carcinoid tumors of the duodenum: Endoscopic diagnosis of two cases. *Gastrointest Endosc* 31:269–271.

33. Weingrad DN, DeCosse JJ, Sherlock P, *et al*.: Primary gastrointestinal lymphoma: A 30-year review. *Cancer* 1982, 49:1258.

34. List AF, Greer JP, Cousar C, *et al*.: Non-Hodgkin's lymphoma of the gastrointestinal tract: An analysis of clinical and pathologic features affecting outcome. *J Clin Oncol* 1988, 7:1125.

35. Lewis BS, Kornbluth A, Waye JD: Small bowel tumours: Yield of enteroscopy. *Gut* 1991, 32:763.

36. Akwari OE, Dozois RR, Weiland LH, Beahrs OH: Leiomyosarcoma of the small and large bowel. *Cancer* 1978, 41:1375.

37. Walker MJ: Sarcomas of the small intestine. In *Surgery of the Small Intestine*. Edited by Nelson RL, Nyhus LM. Norwalk: Appleton & Lange; 1987:243.

38. Allison DJ, Hemingway AP, Cunningham DA: Angiography in gastrointestinal bleeding. *Lancet* 1982, ii:30.

39. Weber HC, Orbuch M, Jensen RT: Diagnosis and management of Zollinger-Ellison syndrome. *Semin Gastrointest Dis* 1995, 6:79–89.

40. Termanini B, Gibril F, Reynolds JC, *et al*.: Value of somatostatin receptor scintigraphy: a prospective study in gastrinoma of its effect on clinical management. *Gstroenterology* 1997; 112:335–347.

41. Maton PN, O'Dorisio TM, Howe BA, *et al*.: Effect of a long acting somatostatin analogue (SMS 201-995) in a patient with pancreatic cholera. *N Engl J Med* 1985, 312:17–21.

42. Danzig JB, Brandt LJ, Reinus JF, Klein RS: Gastrointestinal malignancy in patients with AIDS. *Am J Gastroenterol* 1991, 86:715.

43. Patel K, Didolkar MS, Pickren JW, Moore RH: Metastatic pattern of malignant melanoma: A study of 216 autopsy cases. *Am J Surg* 1978, 135:807.

44. Luk GD: Colonic polyps: Benign and premalignant neoplasms of the colon. In *Textbook of Gastroenterology*. Edited by Yamada T, Alpers DH, Owyang C, *et al*. Philadelphia: JB Lippincott; 1991:1645.

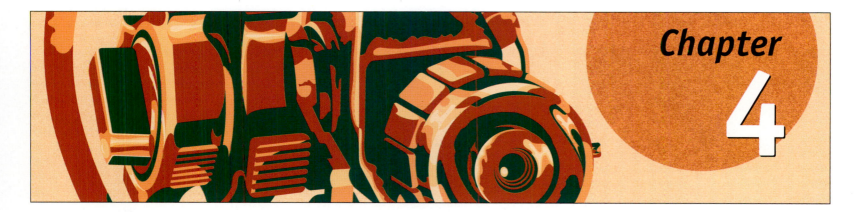

Colon and Rectum

● Normal Anatomy

Rectum, vascular detail . . . .

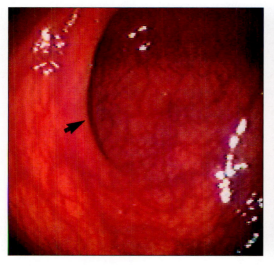

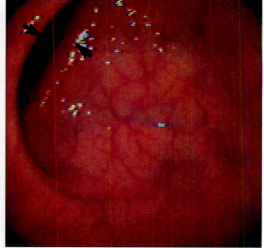

Figure 4-1. Colonoscopic evaluation of the rectum. Light reflection off the clear colonic mucosa should be glistening and not granular as shown. Venous channels as well as capillaries with many side branches are easily visible. This figure presents prominent subepithelial vascular detail with major subbranching. The first valve of Houston's valves (rectal valves) is shown on the left (*arrow*). (*Courtesy of* Timothy T. Nostrant, MD.)

Figure 4-2. A mucosa with less prominent vascular detail and longer capillary channels. Venous vessels are easily seen and clearly demarcated. The first two rectal valves are visible on the left (*arrows*). The lumen of the rectum is much wider than the sigmoid, descending, and transverse colon. Examination behind each of the rectal valves is mandatory to exclude lesions. (*Courtesy of* Timothy T. Nostrant, MD.)

Rectum, with retroflexion of the endoscope ....

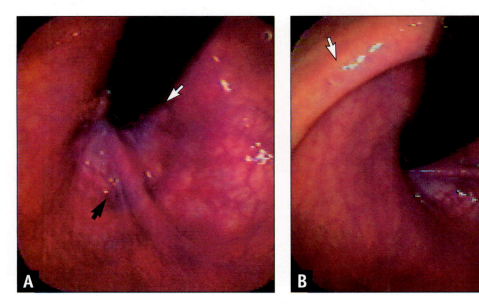

Figure 4-3. Retroflexion of the colonoscope in the rectum. This maneuver can be accomplished easily by raising the tip of the colonoscope upward and backward. As the maneuver is accomplished, the colonoscope can be advanced and torqued such that the distal rectal and anal mucosa are directly visualized. **A,** Pushing the colonoscope further in will bring the anal canal closer. The anal canal and scope (*open arrow*) are easily visible. The anal venous plexus and anal folds (*closed arrows*) are seen with puckering of the anal mucosa. No internal hemorrhoids are observed. The heavy density of vessels as the colonoscope approaches the anus is again appreciated. **B,** Pulling out the colonoscope gives a more panoramic view, with the first rectal valve easily seen at the top (*arrow*). (*Courtesy of* Timothy T. Nostrant, MD.)

Anus, with hemorrhoidal plexus ....

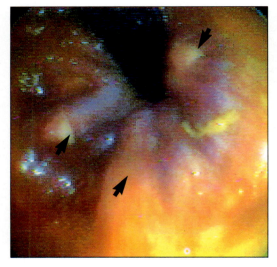

Figure 4-4. Skin tags can be seen at the beginning of the hemorrhoidal plexus. Skin tags (*arrows*) are particularly common in patients with internal hemorrhoids that prolapse. These skin tags usually represent squamous hyperplasia secondary to continuous movement irritation. If they enlarge, they can become polypoid and be mistaken for colon polyps. If biopsied or cauterized, skin tags can be painful because they maintain normal anal or skin innervation. (*Courtesy of* Timothy T. Nostrant, MD.)

Rectosigmoid ....

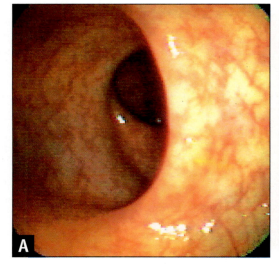 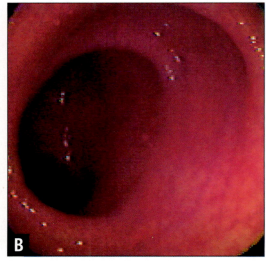

Figure 4-5. Approaching the rectosigmoid junction. As the colonoscope proceeds up the rectum, mucosal vessels become less prominent, and all three rectal valves can be seen (**A**). Just beyond these three rectal valves is the rectosigmoid junction (**B**). (*Courtesy of* Timothy T. Nostrant, MD.)

Sigmoid colon. . . . .

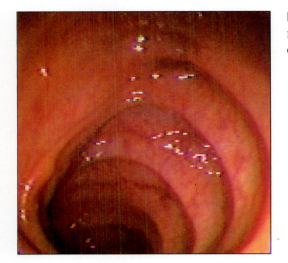

Figure 4-6. The sigmoid colon. Passing into the sigmoid colon, the caliber of the lumen narrows and becomes more tubular. Folds are usually thin and easily seen continuing deeper in the colon. (*Courtesy of* Timothy T. Nostrant, MD.)

Splenic flexure . . . .

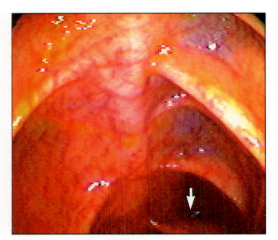

Figure 4-7. Approaching the splenic flexure, a focal discrete area of bluish hue is seen through the colonic mucosa. The hue is produced by the impression of the spleen on the colon. A large turn is visible at the bottom right of the mucosa (*arrow*). (*Courtesy of* Timothy T. Nostrant, MD.)

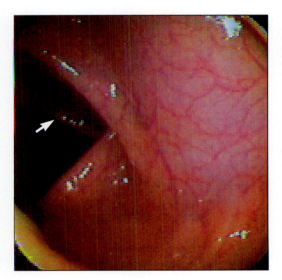

Figure 4-8. The splenic flexure may be redundant and offer both true and false passages. Endoscopists should pay close attention to detail and appreciate the fact that the true passage is almost always found by following the direction of the folds. The transverse colon is seen in the left upper quadrant (*arrow*). (*Courtesy of* Timothy T. Nostrant, MD.)

Transverse colon . . . .

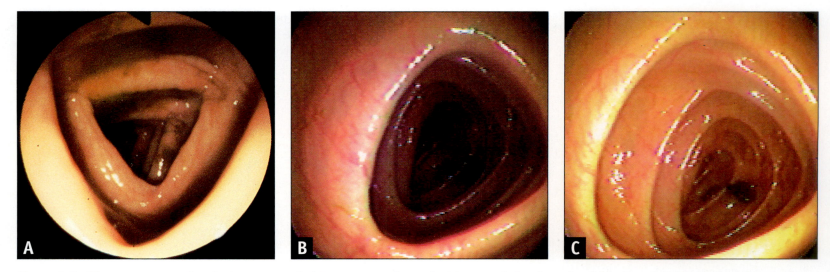

Figure 4-9. The transverse colon is the most varied in contour of all of the colon sections. **A,** Bound by the splenic flexure on the left and the hepatic flexure on the right, the transverse colon can have the characteristic triangular folds. **B** and **C,** Variants of this configuration include a more tubular transverse colon presented here. (*Courtesy of* Timothy T. Nostrant, MD.)

Hepatic flexure. . . . .

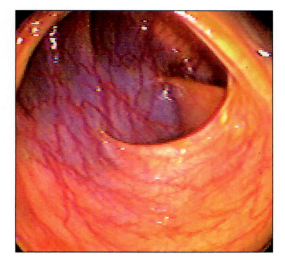

Figure 4-10. Hepatic flexure is similar in configuration to the splenic flexure but is usually less redundant. Once again a bluish hue is seen secondary to hepatic impression. (*Courtesy of* Timothy T. Nostrant, MD.)

Ascending colon . . . .

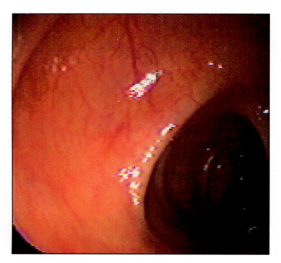

Figure 4-11. The ascending colon is more capacious than the transverse and left colon. Mucosal vessels are harder to see. Compared with the left and transverse colons, folds in the right colon are usually semilunar or incomplete. Similar to the transverse colon, triangular folds can be visible in the right colon. (*Courtesy of* Timothy T. Nostrant, MD.)

Cecum . . . .

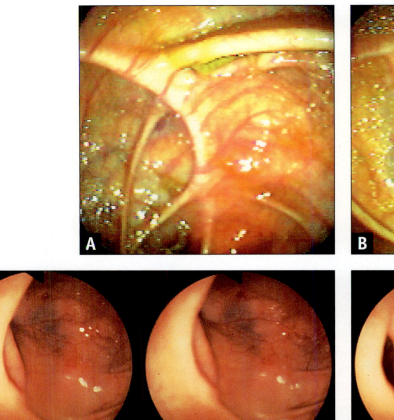

Figure 4-12. The cecum is identified by three different characteristics: fusing of the taeniae coli, the ileocecal valve, and the appendiceal orifice. **A**, The fusing of the taeniae coli is depicted. The taeniae coli represent the three longitudinal muscular strands that begin in the base of the appendix, run to the anus, and fuse into the longitudinal muscle of the external anal sphincter. **B**, The ileocecal valve (distal lip) and the fusion of the taeniae coli. The appearance of the proximal cecum may appear cuplike or dome-shaped if the taeniae coli fuse with the lips of the ileocecal valve.

A small notch (*arrow*) signifies the superior aspect of the ileocecal valve. **C** and **D**, The distal and proximal lips of the ileocecal valve. The valve is usually approached in this position, and the scope tip is turned into the valve and will usually pop into the terminal ileum. With modern instrumentation, the terminal ileum can be intubated if necessary in 80% or more of cases. Biopsy forceps placed into the terminal ileum may allow the endoscopist to pull the scope into the small bowel in difficult cases. (*Courtesy of* Timothy T. Nostrant, MD.)

Cecum with appendix and ileocecal valve . . . .

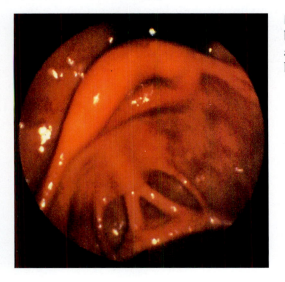

Figure 4-13. The appendix, taeniae coli fusion, and ileocecal valve. This view is produced by retroflexing the colonoscope tip in the cecum. Although this position allows good visualization, colonoscopic biopsy and entrance into the terminal ileum may not be possible because of instrument angulation. (*Courtesy of* Timothy T. Nostrant, MD.)

Terminal ileum . . . .

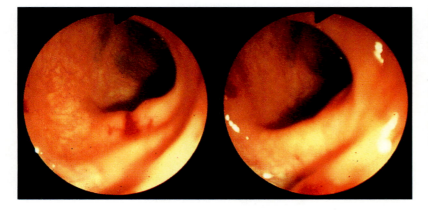

Figure 4-14. The terminal ileum is usually easily differentiated from the colon. Kerching rings are usually seen but are not as prominent as in the duodenum. The mucosa is less glistening and more villous and dull than the colon, similar to the duodenum. Active peristalsis and contractions moving toward the colonoscope tip point to the small bowel over colon. Kerching rings and a dull mucosa are depicted in this figure of the terminal ileum. The red spots are secondary to biopsy artifact. (*Courtesy of* Timothy T. Nostrant, MD.)

Diverticula

Diverticula, sigmoid colon . . . .

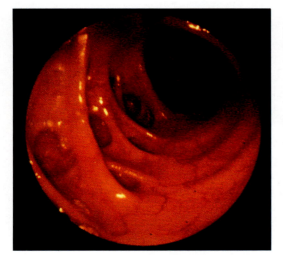

Figure 4-15. Diverticula with fold thickening should be closely evaluated in the sigmoid colon. Knowledge of the existence of diverticula is important in evaluating patients with left lower quadrant pain. (*Courtesy of* Timothy T. Nostrant, MD.)

Diverticula, barium enema . . . .

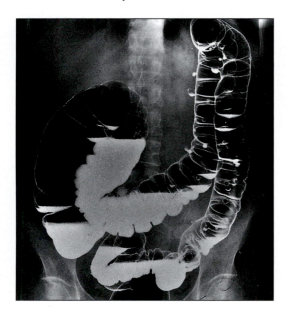

Figure 4-16. An air-contrast barium enema demonstrates scattered diverticulosis of the left colon. Most of the 30 million Americans with diverticulosis have no symptoms [1,2]. The prevalence of diverticulosis increases from 5% in patients over 40 years of age to 50% in patients over 80 years of age [3]. Only 1% to 2% of the population under 30 years of age has diverticulosis [4]. (*Courtesy of* David A. Rothenberger, MD, Carlos Belmonte-Montes, MD, and J. Javier Perez-Ramirez, MD.)

Sigmoid diverticulitis, barium enemas . . . .

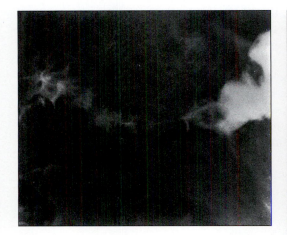

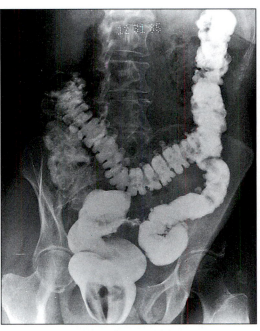

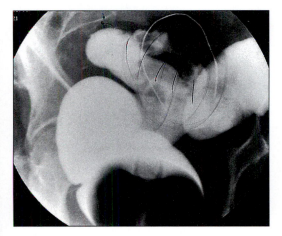

Figure 4-17. This barium enema demonstrates a classic case of acute sigmoid diverticulitis. Note the long segment of colon involved in the inflammatory process and the lumenal narrowing secondary to the inflammation. Endoscopic examination would reveal intense spasm and edema at the rectosigmoid junction. (*Courtesy of* David A. Rothenberger, MD, Carlos Belmonte-Montes, MD, and J. Javier Perez-Ramirez, MD.)

Figure 4-18. Sigmoid diverticulitis can mimic a carcinoma. Careful endoscopic examination of the sigmoid after resection of the acute phase of the illness may be possible and is necessary to exclude carcinoma. If the stricture and obstructive symptoms resolve as the inflammation subsides and if other pathology can be excluded, nonoperative management is usually indicated, especially after the initial episode of diverticulitis. A high-residue diet supplemented with bulk agents may decrease the lumenal pressure and may decrease the risk of perforation of diverticula. There is some evidence that a high-fiber diet can decrease recurrences of acute diverticulitis and prevent its complications [5]. (*Courtesy of* David A. Rothenberger, MD, Carlos Belmonte-Montes, MD, and J. Javier Perez-Ramirez, MD.)

Figure 4-19. This case of sigmoid diverticulitis has produced a stricture that causes obstructive symptoms and dilation of the proximal colon. After antibiotic treatment of the acute diverticulitis, the obstructive symptoms and dilation may resolve. If partial obstructive symptoms persist, if a recurrent pattern of diverticulitis develops, or if the patient develops another major complication of perforating diverticular disease, an elective resection is indicated. Today, this elective resection is almost always accomplished as a one-stage procedure with resection and primary anastomosis. (*Courtesy of* David A. Rothenberger, MD, Carlos Belmonte-Montes, MD, and J. Javier Perez-Ramirez, MD.)

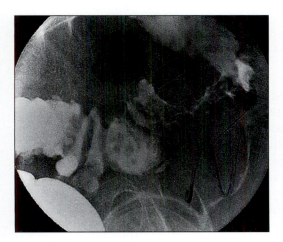

Figure 4-20. This case of sigmoid diverticulitis produced a chronic stricture and persistent obstructive symptoms. A modified mechanical bowel preparation is usually possible in these circumstances, thus increasing the likelihood of a single-stage resection and colorectal anastomosis. If bowel preparation is impossible or inadequate, the surgeon can consider an on-table lavage preparation to enhance the safety of a primary anastomosis. Alternatively, a resection and primary anastomosis followed by lavage through the terminal ileum or appendical stump can be used. Occasionally, the obstruction is so severe that a primary anastomosis is contraindicated. In such cases, resection and diversion are necessary. (*Courtesy of* David A. Rothenberger, MD, Carlos Belmonte-Montes, MD, and J. Javier Perez-Ramirez, MD.)

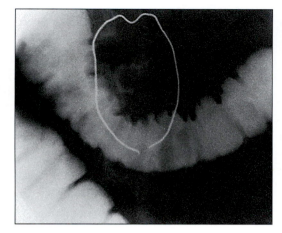

Figure 4-21. Pericolic extravasation is noted in this contrast study. Diverticular disease rarely results in free perforation and diffuse peritonitis. Most often, as in this case, the perforation is contained and the infection is localized to the pericolic tissues. The degree of peritonitis has a major influence on the decision to perform a staged procedure. If diffuse fecal or purulent peritonitis is present, the operation of choice is almost always resection of the perforated segment of colon, including the distal sigmoid and construction of an end-descending colostomy with closure of the rectum as a Hartmann's pouch. With lesser degrees of peritonitis, other operative options including resection and anastomosis with or without proximal diversion are viable. The traditional three-staged delayed resection approach is almost never used today. (*Courtesy of* David A. Rothenberger, MD, Carlos Belmonte-Montes, MD, and J. Javier Perez-Ramirez, MD.)

Diverticulitis, complicated ·······························

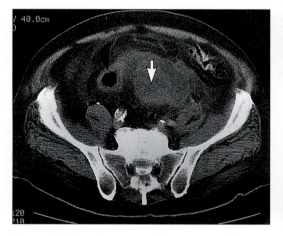

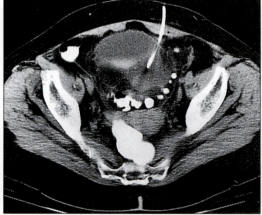

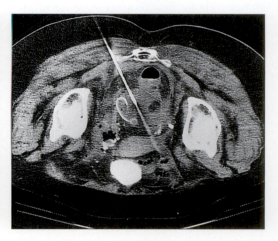

Figure 4-22. A computed tomographic scan of a patient with acute diverticulitis and signs of sepsis demonstrates a large pelvic abscess. The abscess is indicated by the *open arrow* and the distended loop of bowel is indicated by the *closed arrow*. The computed tomographic scan is the most sensitive and specific test to diagnose the inflammatory complications of diverticular disease. (*Courtesy of* David A. Rothenberger, MD, Carlos Belmonte-Montes, MD, and J. Javier Perez-Ramirez, MD.)

Figure 4-23. Drainage of diverticular abscesses. Percutaneous drainage of diverticular abscesses under computed tomographic guidance has become a highly successful method of controlling sepsis in such situations. Drainage catheters are left in place until the drainage ceases and the patient's sepsis is controlled. Sinograms obtained by injection via the catheter can be used to demonstrate complete drainage and collapse of the abscess cavity. The drain can then be removed. (*Courtesy of* David A. Rothenberger, MD, Carlos Belmonte-Montes, MD, and J. Javier Perez-Ramirez, MD.)

Figure 4-24. Abscesses located deep within the pelvis can also be drained by computed tomographic guidance. Here, a posterior approach is used to achieve abscess drainage. The patient is in a prone position. The needle enters the abscess from the left posterolateral approach. (*Courtesy of* David A. Rothenberger, MD, Carlos Belmonte-Montes, MD, and J. Javier Perez-Ramirez, MD.)

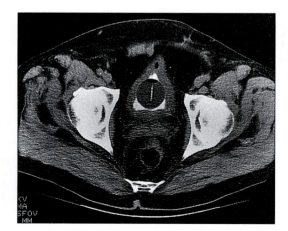

Figure 4-25. Colovesical fistula diagnosis. Fistulas to other viscera are present in 8% to 42% of patients undergoing surgery for diverticular disease. Colovesical fistulas are the most common type of diverticular disease, accounting for approximately half of all such fistulas. Computed tomographic scanning is the best imaging procedure to establish the diagnosis of colovesical fistula. This computed tomographic scan demonstrates an air-fluid level within the bladder in a patient who presented with sepsis and pneumaturia. Systemic sepsis is usually controlled in such patients as the diverticular abscess drains itself into the bladder. Urosepsis is controlled with antibiotics until an elective colon resection is possible [6]. (*Courtesy of* David A. Rothenberger, MD, Carlos Belmonte-Montes, MD, and J. Javier Perez-Ramirez, MD.)

Diverticulitis, with colovaginal fistula . . . .

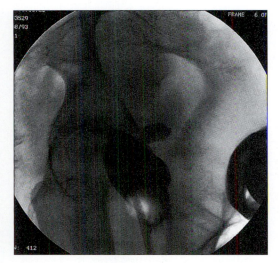

Figure 4-26. Colovaginal fistula. This anterior-posterior reversed contrast study demonstrates filling of the vagina via a diverticular fistula from the sigmoid colon. Colovaginal fistulas are the second most common type of diverticular fistula. (*Courtesy of* David A. Rothenberger, MD, Carlos Belmonte-Montes, MD, and J. Javier Perez-Ramirez, MD.)

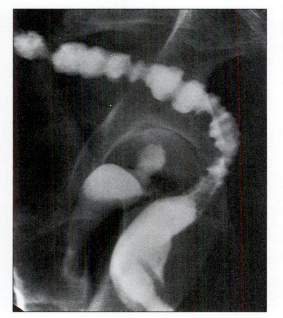

Figure 4-27. This lateral contrast enema demonstrates a colovaginal fistula. Approximately half of colovaginal fistulas can be identified by barium enema. Vaginography can often confirm the presence of a colovaginal fistula, even if the barium enema shows no fistula. (*Courtesy of* David A. Rothenberger, MD, Carlos Belmonte-Montes, MD, and J. Javier Perez-Ramirez, MD.)

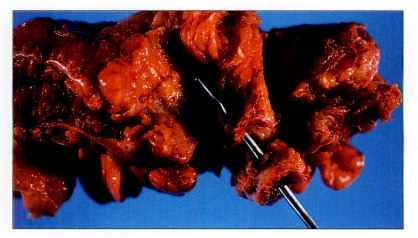

Figure 4-28. The operative specimen from the case shown in Figure 4-27. The probe demonstrates the diverticular fistula that perforated into the vagina. Fifty percent of women with colovesical fistulas and 83% of women with colovaginal fistulas have had a prior hysterectomy. (*Courtesy of* David A. Rothenberger, MD, Carlos Belmonte-Montes, MD, and J. Javier Perez-Ramirez, MD.)

Ulcerative Colitis

Ulcerative colitis, variable severity ....

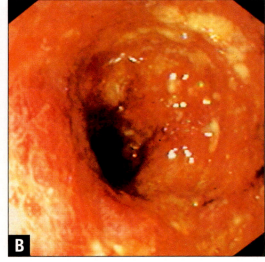

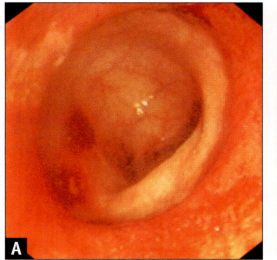

and, when severe, frank mucopurulent exudate. Inflammation invariably begins in the rectum and extends proximally for varying extents. The chronicity of the process is suggested by the loss of colonic haustrations; otherwise, the endoscopic picture is nonspecific and could be consistent with acute infectious colitis, chronic ulcerative or Crohn's colitis, or any number of other specific causes of colitis. **A,** Mild distal ulcerative colitis with diffuse erythema and friability well demarcated from the normal mucosa more proximally is depicted. **B,** This example shows moderately severe ulcerative colitis with irregular, inflamed, ulcerated mucosa and a patchy exudate. (*Courtesy of* Lawrence S. Friedman, MD, Fiona Graeme-Cook, MD, and Robert H. Shapiro, MD.)

Figure 4-29. Endoscopic features of active ulcerative colitis. Findings include diffusely erythematous, edematous, and granular mucosa with areas of submucosal hemorrhage

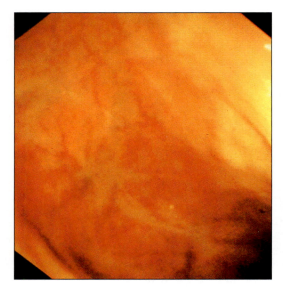

Figure 4-30. Endoscopic view of ulcerative colitis in remission. The normal vascular pattern is absent and a white scar indicates the site of a previous ulcer. (*Courtesy of* Lawrence S. Friedman, MD, Fiona Graeme-Cook, MD, and Robert H. Shapiro, MD.)

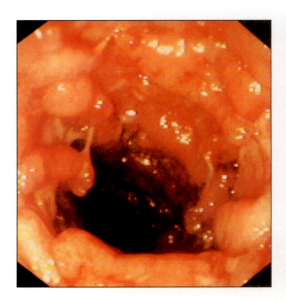

Figure 4-31. Severe ulcerative colitis seen endoscopically. The mucosa shows extensive ulceration and diffuse thickening with an inflammatory infiltrate. In contrast to Crohn's colitis, the ulceration lacks depth. (*Courtesy of* Lawrence S. Friedman, MD, Fiona Graeme-Cook, MD, and Robert H. Shapiro, MD.)

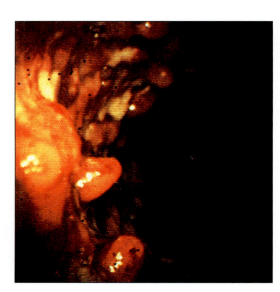

Figure 4-32. Severe ulcerative colitis with pseudopolyps viewed endoscopically. In addition to severe mucosal ulceration and inflammation, chronic ulcerative colitis is often associated with the formation of pseudopolyps, which represent islands of regenerating mucosa and exuberant inflammation amidst diffuse mucosal destruction. Pseudopolyps have no malignant potential. (*Courtesy of* Lawrence S. Friedman, MD, Fiona Graeme-Cook, MD, and Robert H. Shapiro, MD.)

Ulcerative colitis, barium enemas . . . .

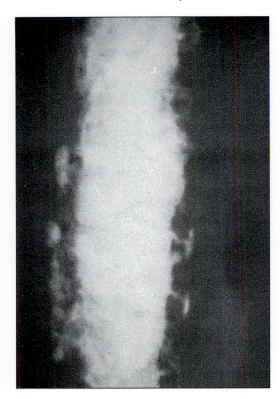

Figure 4-33. Radiographic appearance of severe ulcerative colitis. This single contrast barium enema demonstrates the typical ragged and ulcerative appearance of the mucosa in active ulcerative colitis. Characteristic collarbutton or undermining ulcers are seen. In general, barium enema and colonoscopy should be avoided in fulminant ulcerative colitis because of the possibility of precipitating toxic megacolon. (*Courtesy of* Lawrence S. Friedman, MD, Fiona Graeme-Cook, MD, and Robert H. Shapiro, MD.)

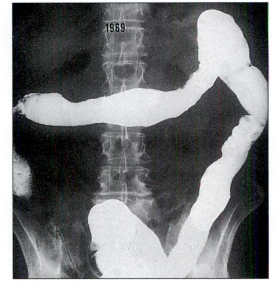

Figure 4-34. Radiographic appearance of chronic ulcerative colitis. Long-standing chronic ulcerative colitis, as shown in this single contrast barium enema, is characterized by shortening and straightening of the colon with loss of haustrations, resulting in the appearance of a featureless tube. No ulcerations are seen. (*Courtesy of* Lawrence S. Friedman, MD, Fiona Graeme-Cook, MD, and Robert H. Shapiro, MD.)

Ulcerative colitis, severe, gross specimen . . . .

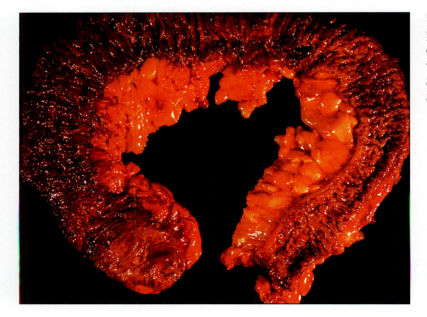

Figure 4-35. Gross pathologic specimen of resected colon from a patient with severe ulcerative colitis. Inflammation is diffuse and continuous, involving the mucosa and extending from the rectum without interruption to the ascending colon. (*Courtesy of* Lawrence S. Friedman, MD, Fiona Graeme-Cook, MD, and Robert H. Shapiro, MD.)

Ulcerative colitis, microscopic pathology . . . .

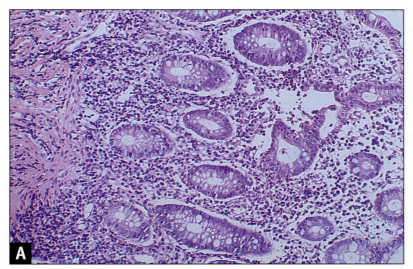

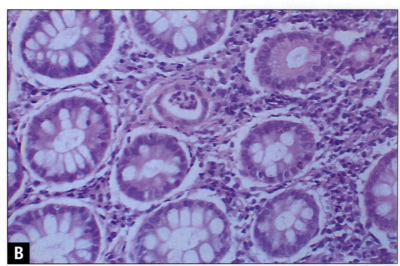

Figure 4-36. Microscopic features of the specimen shown in Figure 4-35. **A,** There is diffuse acute and chronic inflammation with architectural distortion and destruction of some glands, depletion of mucin from goblet cells, and crypt abscesses. Inflammation is limited to the mucosa. **B,** A higher power microscopic feature showing diffuse inflammation and a crypt abscess. (*Courtesy of Lawrence S. Friedman, MD, Fiona Graeme-Cook, MD, and Robert H. Shapiro, MD.*)

Ulcerative colitis, pathology . . . .

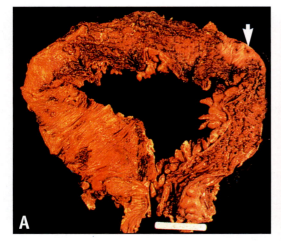

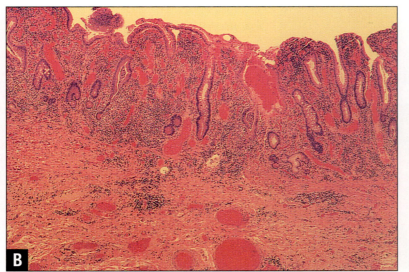

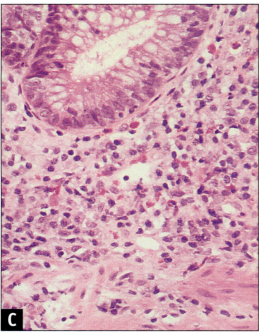

Figure 4-37. Ulcerative colitis. **A,** This total colectomy specimen shows a normal mucosal pattern in the terminal ileum and cecum (*arrow*) with diffuse involvement from the transverse colon to the rectum. The distal mucosa is erythematous and friable with many ulcers and erosions. **B,** This low-power photomicrograph shows diffuse chronic inflammation of the lamina propria with crypt distortion. These two features are important in differentiating ulcerative colitis from acute "self-limited" colitis. **C,** This high-power view depicts the base of a single distorted colonic crypt. There are large number of "basal" plasma cells between the crypt and the muscularis mucosae. This finding is another important feature that helps differentiate acute from chronic colitis.

(*Continued on next page*)

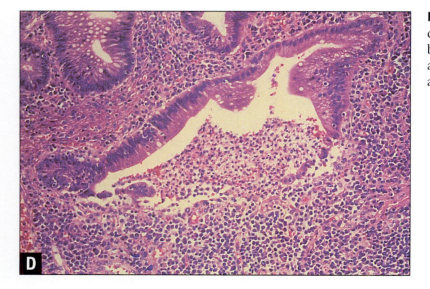

Figure 4-37. *(Continued)* **D,** This photograph shows a single crypt abscess. The bottom of this distorted crypt has been destroyed by an aggregate of neutrophils. This finding is not specific for ulcerative colitis; Crohn's disease and other active forms of colitis may also have crypt abscesses. (*Courtesy of* Joel K. Greenson, MD.)

Dysplasia-associated mass lesion with dysplasia . . . .

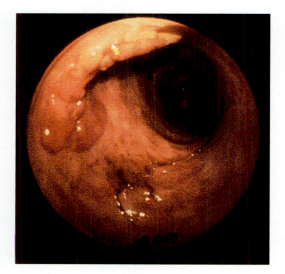

Figure 4-38. Dysplasia-associated mass lesions seen at colonoscopy in a patient with ulcerative colitis. Such lesions may be plaquelike or polypoid and contain dysplastic epithelium. These lesions are highly associated with synchronous carcinoma of the colon. (*Courtesy of* Robert S. Bresalier, MD.)

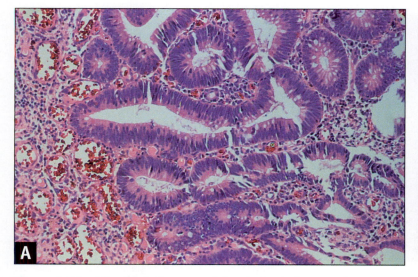

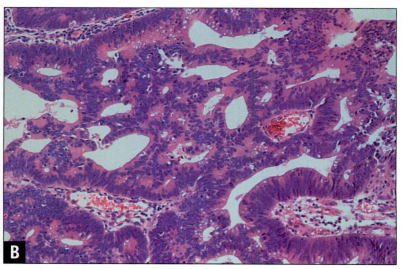

Figure 4-39. Histologic features of dysplasia. **A,** Low-grade dysplasia characterized by nuclear enlargement, crowding, and hyperchromasia in the colonic epithelial cells. Nuclei are stratified but remain in the basal half of the cells. There is some depletion of mucin. **B,** In high-grade dysplasia, the changes are more pronounced. Nuclei are stratified to the surface, and there is a marked increase in nuclear pleomorphism. A branching of cribriform pattern to the glands and scattered cell necrosis is shown. No mucin goblets are evident. (*Courtesy of* Lawrence S. Friedman, MD, Fiona Graeme-Cook, MD, and Robert H. Shapiro, MD.)

Ulcerative colitis and adenocarcinoma . . . .

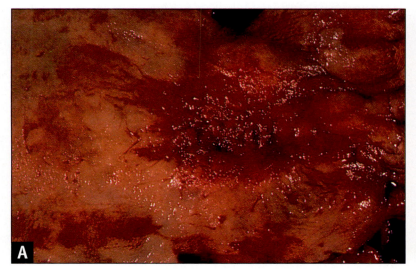 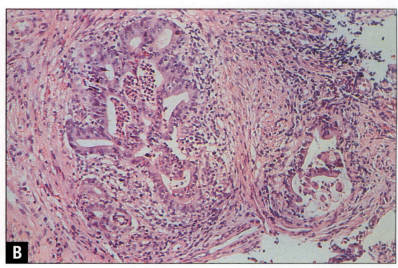

Figure 4-40. Colonic carcinoma in ulcerative colitis. **A**, Gross resected specimen of the rectum showing frank rectal carcinoma in the setting of diffuse ulcerative colitis. The rectum has a loss of mucosal folds and a granular hemorrhagic surface surrounding a deeply invasive carcinoma. **B**, Microscopic section showing an infiltrating adenocarcinoma arising in a background of chronic ulcerative colitis with a surrounding desmoplastic stroma. (*Courtesy of* Lawrence S. Friedman, MD, Fiona Graeme-Cook, MD, and Robert H. Shapiro, MD.)

Crohn's Disease

Crohn's disease, mild. . . . .

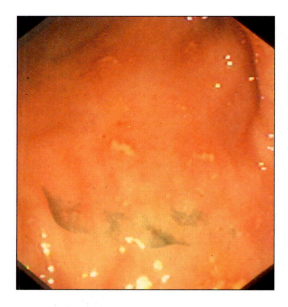

Figure 4-41. Endoscopic features of early Crohn's disease. The earliest lesion of Crohn's disease, shown on colonoscopy, is aphthous ulceration, a focal mucosal defect with surrounding erythema. This finding is nonspecific and may also be seen in herpesvirus infection, cytomegalovirus infection, Yersinia infection, tuberculosis, schistosomiasis, and Behcet's disease. (*Courtesy of* Lawrence S. Friedman, MD, Fiona Graeme-Cook, MD, and Robert H. Shapiro, MD.)

Crohn's disease, severe ·

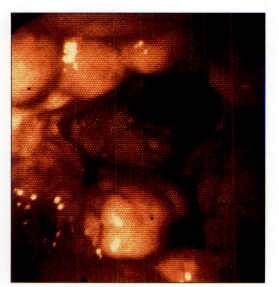

Figure 4-42. Endoscopic view of severe Crohn's colitis. A characteristic "cobblestone" appearance is the result of multiple longitudinal ulcers and exuberant inflammation with pseudopolyp formation as well as thickening of the intestinal wall because of transmural inflammation. (*Courtesy of* Lawrence S. Friedman, MD, Fiona Graeme-Cook, MD, and Robert H. Shapiro, MD.)

Crohn's disease, terminal ileum. ·

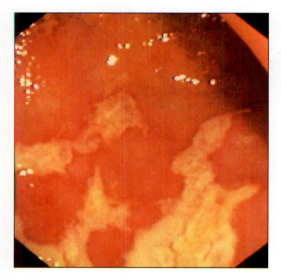

Figure 4-43. Endoscopic features of Crohn's disease of the terminal ileum. A diffuse inflammation is depicted with characteristic large irregular ulcers that are often stellate or longitudinal. (*Courtesy of* Lawrence S. Friedman, MD, Fiona Graeme-Cook, MD, and Robert H. Shapiro, MD.)

Crohn's disease, ileocolonic anastomosis ·

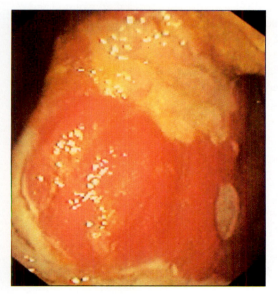

Figure 4-44. Crohn's disease at an ileocolonic anastomosis. Endoscopic recurrence of disease following surgical resection is invariable and first occurs on the ileal side of an ileocolonic anastomosis, although clinical recurrence may not necessarily follow. Typical Crohn's ulcers in the neoterminal ileum at an ileorectal anastomosis are shown. (*Courtesy of* Lawrence S. Friedman, MD, Fiona Graeme-Cook, MD, and Robert H. Shapiro, MD.)

Crohn's disease, in remission ....

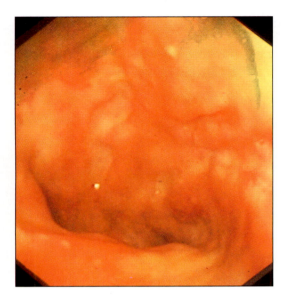

Figure 4-45. Crohn's colitis in remission seen endoscopically. Patchy erythema surrounds areas in which epithelialization of previous sites of ulceration has taken place. There is no active ulceration. (*Courtesy of* Lawrence S. Friedman, MD, Fiona Graeme-Cook, MD, and Robert H. Shapiro, MD.)

Crohn's disease of small bowel, radiographs ....

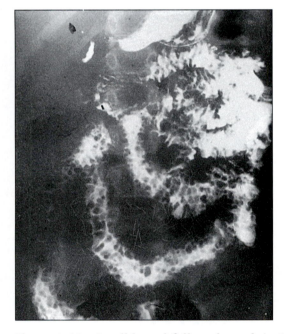

Figure 4-46. Small bowel follow through in Crohn's disease. In addition to diffuse nodularity of the small intestine, lumens of involved loops of bowel appear to be widely separated as a result of a marked increase in the thickness of the bowel wall, resulting from transmural inflammation and mesenteric edema and hyperemia. (*Courtesy of* Lawrence S. Friedman, MD, Fiona Graeme-Cook, MD, and Robert H. Shapiro, MD.)

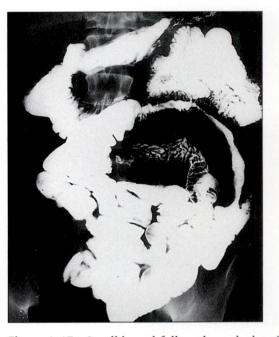

Figure 4-47. Small bowel follow through showing an isolated segment of Crohn's disease of the jejunum, the so-called "string sign." Lumen of the involved segment is narrowed as a result of either diffuse inflammation of the bowel wall with spasm or a fibrotic stricture from previous inflammation. (*Courtesy of* Lawrence S. Friedman, MD, Fiona Graeme-Cook, MD, and Robert H. Shapiro, MD.)

Crohn's colitis, microscopic pathology ·····························

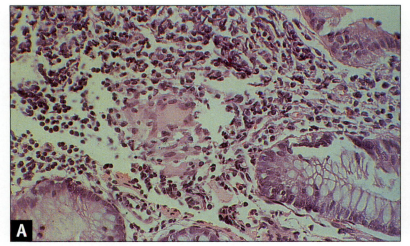

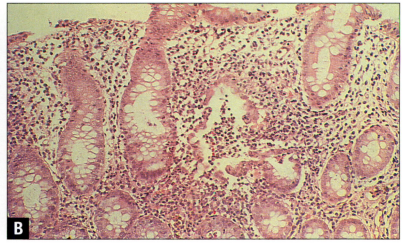

Figure 4-48. Microscopic specimen from a patient with Crohn's colitis. **A**, The specimen has diffuse inflammation of the mucosa and submucosa with a small granuloma in the center. **B**, Patchy inflammation with marked enlargement of crypts and a focal abscess can be seen. In contrast to ulcerative colitis, the mucin is relatively preserved. (*Courtesy of* Lawrence S. Friedman, MD, Fiona Graeme-Cook, MD, and Robert H. Shapiro, MD.)

Crohn's disease, pathology ·······························

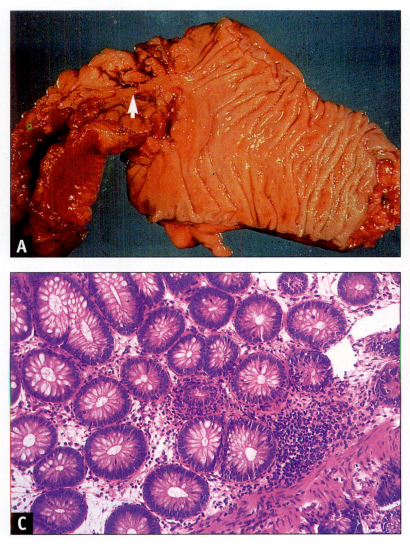

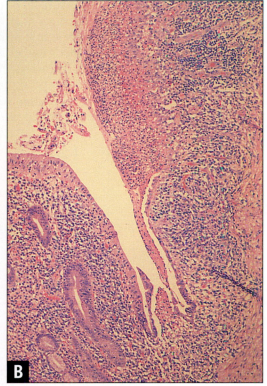

Figure 4-49. Crohn's disease. **A**, This segment of colon shows a stricture in the right colon (*arrow*) with normal appearing mucosa in the distal portion of the specimen. Strictures in the right colon may be seen in both Crohn's disease and ischemic colitis [7]. **B**, Photomicrograph of a fissuring ulcer is shown overlying a lymphoid aggregate (aphthous ulcer). Aphthous lesions can be seen in Crohn's disease as well as infectious colitis. **C**, This low-power view shows a single inflamed distorted crypt that appears much smaller than the more normal adjacent crypts. Focal lesions such as this lesion are often seen in smoldering Crohn's disease.

(Continued on next page)

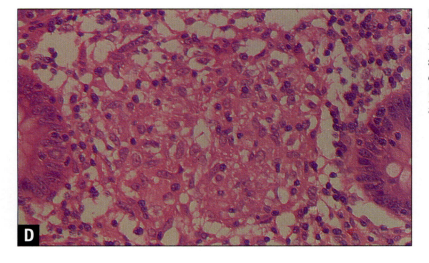

Figure 4-49. *(Continued)* **D,** An epithelioid granuloma between two colonic crypts is depicted. Although the presence of a granuloma may help establish the diagnosis of Crohn's disease in endoscopic biopsy specimens, serial sections must be examined to be certain that a granuloma is not caused by a ruptured crypt abscess (so-called mucin granuloma). The latter finding may be seen in any active colitis. (*Courtesy of* Joel K. Greenson, MD.)

Ischemic colitis

Ischemic colitis, endoscopic appearance.

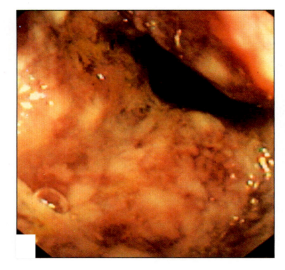

Figure 4-50. Endoscopic appearance of ischemic colitis. In elderly persons, in particular, ischemic colitis enters into the differential diagnosis of inflammatory bowel disease. The etiology is usually nonocclusive ischemic damage to the colon as a result of hypotension or hypoperfusion. Iatrogenic injury to or ligation of the inferior mesenteric artery may also result in ischemic colitis. In contrast with ulcerative colitis, the rectum is typically spared, colonic involvement is segmental, and the symptoms are acute and self-limited. Typical endoscopic features include ulceration, which is patchy and in severe cases, as shown here, associated with necrosis and exudation. In some cases, resolution may be followed by stricture formation. (*Courtesy of* Lawrence S. Friedman, MD, Fiona Graeme-Cook, MD, and Robert H. Shapiro, MD.)

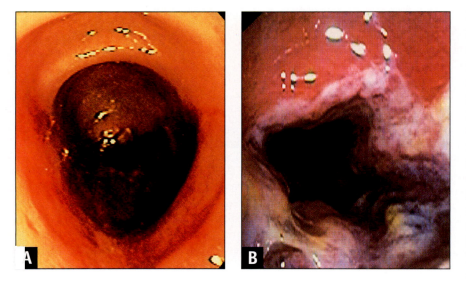

Figure 4-51. Ischemic colitis seen endoscopically. Most patients with ischemic colitis present with abdominal pain, however, 15% to 25% of patients may present with overt rectal bleeding. Complete absence of bleeding, including occult bleeding, is uncommon. Bleeding is occasionally massive. Endoscopy is the diagnostic procedure of choice. Endoscopically, rectal sparing is typical because of the middle rectal artery collateral circulation. Ischemic proctitis has primarily been reported in patients with extensive pelvic surgery and presumed disruption of rectal blood flow. **A,** The mucosa may be pale, edematous, and friable in early disease. **B,** The mucosa may also show a blue-black discoloration signifying mucosal necrosis and submucosal hemorrhage if the disease is extensive. The areas most commonly affected are the watershed areas of the splenic flexure and sigmoid colon, which are at the periphery of the inferior mesenteric artery circulation. Most patients with ischemic colitis have a self-limited course with spontaneous recovery. However, transmural necrosis and peritonitis may develop, and this possibility necessitates careful clinical observation. In some cases, healing may occur with subsequent stricture formation. (**A,** *Courtesy of* D. Johnson, MD; **B,** *courtesy of* R. Goulet, MD.)

Ischemic colitis, pathology..

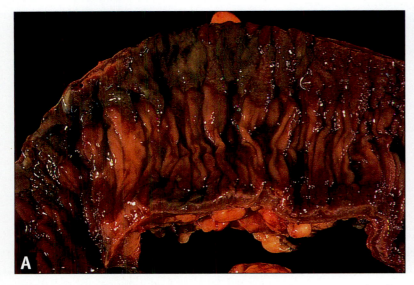

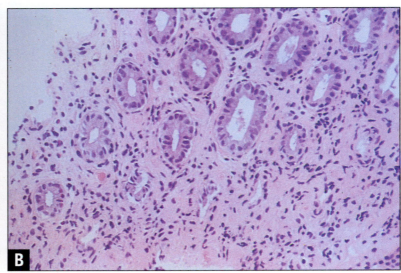

Figure 4-52. Pathologic features of ischemic colitis. **A,** Grossly, the mucosa is inflamed and hemorrhagic with scattered deep ulcers and a greenish pseudomembrane representing sloughed mucosa. **B,** Microscopic examination shows little if any inflammation. There is scattered gland dropout, small fibrin thrombi in arterioles, and fibrin in the stroma. In some cases of ischemic colitis, inflammation with crypt abscesses may be present, simulating ulcerative colitis. (*Courtesy of* Lawrence S. Friedman, MD, Fiona Graeme-Cook, MD, and Robert H. Shapiro, MD.)

Radiation Colitis

Radiation colitis, endoscopic and microscopic images ....

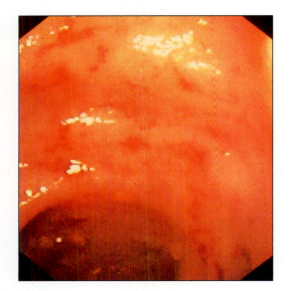

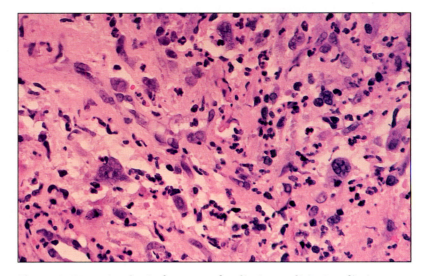

Figure 4-53. Endoscopic features of radiation colitis. Radiation colitis is seen most commonly as a complication of pelvic irradiation for gynecologic malignancy. The endoscopic appearance may be indistinguishable from that of ulcerative colitis, but common characteristic mucosal telangiectatic lesions are seen. Luminal narrowing is frequent and solitary ulcers may occur. (*Courtesy of* Lawrence S. Friedman, MD, Fiona Graeme-Cook, MD, and Robert H. Shapiro, MD.)

Figure 4-54. Histologic features of radiation colitis. Irradiation leads to mural fibrosis that often contains large, atypical mesenchymal cells with a typical pleomorphic and hyperchromatic nuclei. In addition, obliterative vascular changes are seen in the muscular arteries which can, in turn, lead to ischemia and mucosal ulceration. (*Courtesy of* Randall G. Lee, MD.)

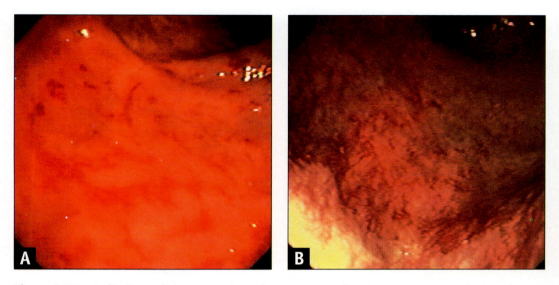

Figure 4-55. Radiation colitis. Approximately 2% to 5% of patients receiving radiation therapy for gynecologic, prostate, bladder, or rectal cancer will develop chronic radiation injury to the rectum and sigmoid colon. The extent and severity of the injury depends on the total dose of radiation and the volume of the bowel exposed. The pathogenesis of the injury is believed to involve radiation-induced vascular changes of the bowel wall with resultant tissue ischemia. Because of its fixed position in the pelvis, the rectum is damaged in 70% to 90% of all patients with intestinal radiation injuries. Patients usually present with intermittent rectal bleeding, tenesmus, and altered bowel habits. The bleeding may be slow, resulting in iron deficiency anemia, or occasionally, massive. **A** and **B**, Endoscopically there is mucosal erythema, edema, friability, and diffuse telangiectasias. An effective therapy for hemorrhage from radiation proctitis is endoscopic laser ablation or electrocautery of telangiectasias. Decreased transfusion requirements can be achieved using the Nd:YAG (neodymium:yttrium=aluminum=garnet) laser or argon laser. Medical therapy of radiation proctitis has met with limited success. Oral or rectal steroids and sulfasalazine, sucralfate enemas, intrarectal formalin, and hyperbaric oxygen have all been used, but no controlled trials of these modalities have been performed. Surgery is seldom used for radiation injury because of a substantial risk of complications. (*Courtesy of* Chistopher S. Cutler, MD, and Douglas K. Rex, MD.)

Radiation proctitis, bleeding ....

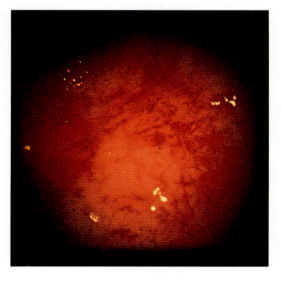

Figure 4-56. Sigmoidoscopic view of bleeding radiation proctitis. After an upper gastrointestinal source of bleeding has been excluded, anoscopy and sigmoidoscopy should be the next diagnostic steps in the evaluation of lower gastrointestinal bleeding. Anoscopy is the most sensitive test to diagnose anal fissures and hemorrhoids. Sigmoidoscopy is used to evaluate the distal colonic mucosa for inflammatory bowel disease, polyps, or malignancies. Pictured is an endoscopic view of bleeding radiation proctitis of a patient undergoing flexible sigmoidoscopy for hematochezia. (*Courtesy of* Christopher S. Cutler, MD, and Douglas K. Rex, MD.)

Pseudomembranous Colitis

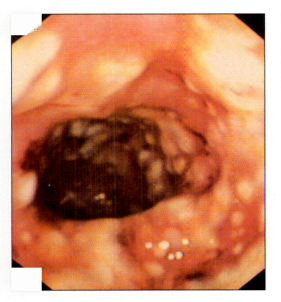

Figure 4-57. Endoscopic appearance of pseudomembranous colitis. Pseudomembranous colitis characteristically results from the use of antibiotics and is caused by the toxin produced by *Clostridium difficile*. The characteristic appearance is yellow-white pseudomembranes on a background of diffuse colonic inflammation. (*Courtesy of* Lawrence S. Friedman, MD, Fiona Graeme-Cook, MD, and Robert H. Schapiro, MD.)

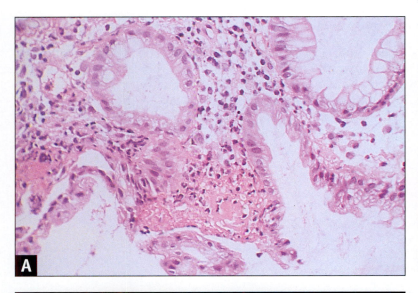

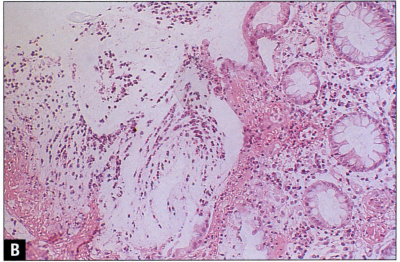

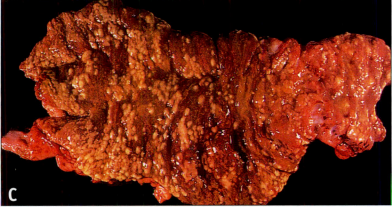

Figure 4-58. Pathologic features of pseudomembranous colitis. **A**, Histologically, the early lesion is characterized by fibrin deposition and an infiltration of neutrophils under the surface epithelium. **B**, Subsequently, a characteristic volcano lesion may be seen in which crypts erupt as mucus and neutrophils stream from the destroyed gland. Surrounding crypts may appear normal. **C**, The gross appearance demonstrates the characteristic yellow-white plaquelike pseudomembranes. (*Courtesy of* Lawrence S. Friedman, MD, Fiona Graeme-Cook, MD, and Robert H. Shapiro, MD.)

● Polyps

Large pedunculated polyp, tubular adenoma . . . .

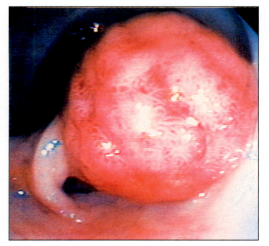

Figure 4-59. Large pedunculated polyp seen at colonoscopy. The polyp extends from the colonic mucosa by way of a fibrovascular stalk (*See* Figure 4-60.) (*Courtesy of* Robert S. Bresalier, MD.)

Pathology of tubular adenoma . . . .

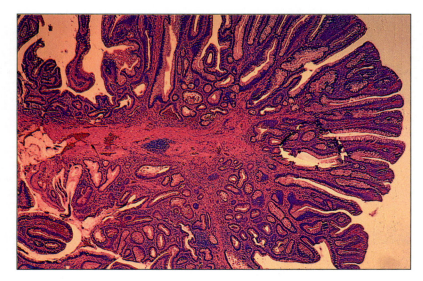

Figure 4-60. Photomicrograph of tubular adenoma of the colon cut in cross section to demonstrate stalk. Tubular adenomas are characterized by a complex network of branching adenomatous glands. (*Courtesy of* Robert S. Bresalier, MD.)

Pathology of tubular adenoma with foci adenocarcinoma . . . .

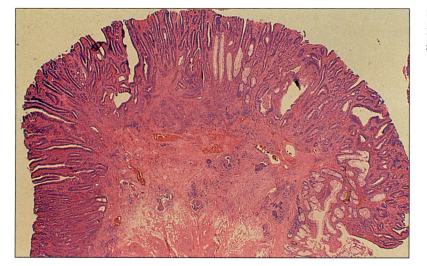

Figure 4-61. Low-power photomicrograph of pedunculated adenoma containing focus of adenocarcinoma. Malignant glands can be seen invading stalk. (*Courtesy of* Robert S. Bresalier, MD.)

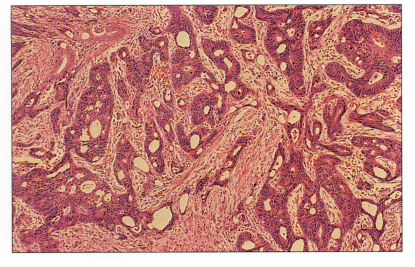

Figure 4-62. High-power view of the stalk of polyp seen in Figure 4-61. Well-differentiated carcinomatous glands are seen invading the polyp stalk. (*Courtesy of* Robert S. Bresalier, MD.)

Adenocarcinoma invading neck of tubular adenoma. . . . .

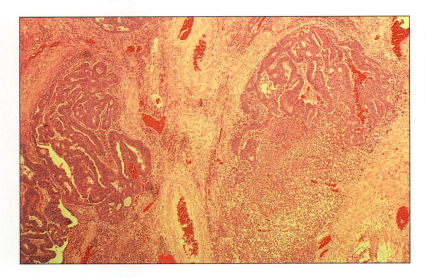

Figure 4-63. Well-differentiated adenocarcinoma invading the neck of an adenomatous polyp (*ie*, submucosal invasion). Malignant glands are seen in close proximity to vascular structures and are at the resection margin, indicating high likelihood of extension beyond the confines of the polyp. (*Courtesy of* Robert S. Bresalier, MD.)

Large sessile polyp, villous adenoma. . . . .

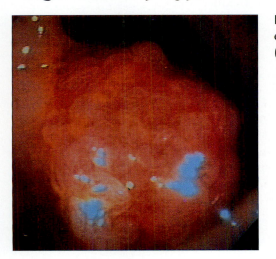

Figure 4-64. Large sessile polyp seen at colonoscopy (villous adenoma). The polyp extends directly from the colonic wall. This large polyp was found to be a villous adenoma (*See* 4-66B). (*Courtesy of* Robert S. Bresalier, MD.)

Sessile polyp, barium enema

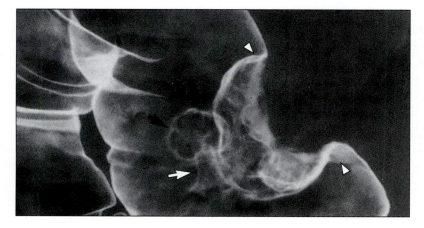

Figure 4-65. Sessile adenocarcinoma and adjacent pedunculated adenomatous polyp. This single film from an air-contrast examination with malignant lesions as well as benign lesions. The larger ses-sile polyp originates from the mucosa; it is slightly nodular, and its dimensions are large enough to suspect malignant disease. Although the surface characteristics cannot predict malignancy in the absence of obvious ulceration, the size alone makes this lesion highly likely to be invasive carcinoma, which was present on removal. Notice the undercut margins (*arrowheads*) that support the mucosal origin of this tumor. The second smaller lesion is a very nicely displayed pedunculated polyp on a short stalk (*white arrow*). The head of the polyp is slightly irregular along the surface (*black arrows*). This lesion represents a benign adenomatous polyp and demonstrates the exquisite detail that can be seen on this double-contrast examination in these types of lesions. The coexistence of adenocarcinoma with other neoplastic polyps is common. At least 50% of patients will have additional lesions once the index polyp is identified. It is extremely important to exclude other synchronous lesions whenever a polypoid lesion is found in the colon either endoscopically or radiographically. (*From* Stewart and Dodds [8]; with permission.)

Pathology of tubulovillous adenoma

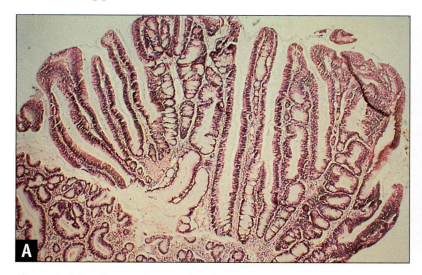

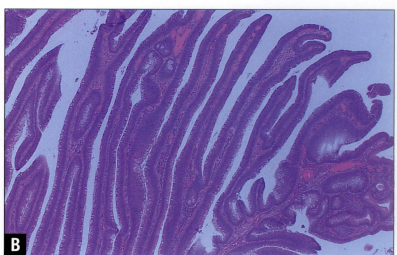

Figure 4-66. Photomicrograph of a tubulovillous adenoma (**A**). This polyp has the characteristics of a tubular adenoma as well as adenomatous glands that extend straight down from the surface to the center of the polyp and are characteristic of villous adenomas (**B**). (*Courtesy of* Robert S. Bresalier, MD.)

Endoscopic polypectomy

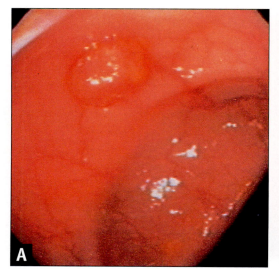

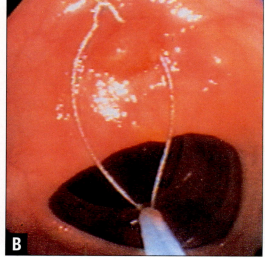

Figure 4-67. Endoscopic polypectomy. A, Colonic polyp. B, A polypectomy snare placed around the polyp. The snare is closed around the base of the polyp and gently pulled away from the wall into the lumen.

(*Continued on next page*)

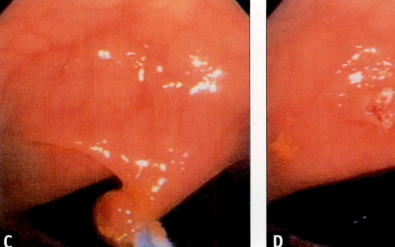

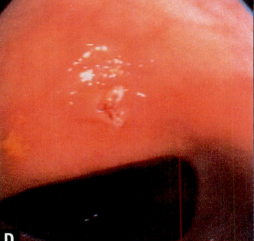

Figure 4-67. *(Continued)* **C,** Current is applied to cut the stalk and cauterize the site. **D,** The polypectomy site after removal of polyp. (*Courtesy of* Robert S. Bresalier, MD.)

 ## Carcinomas

Adenocarcinomas of colon

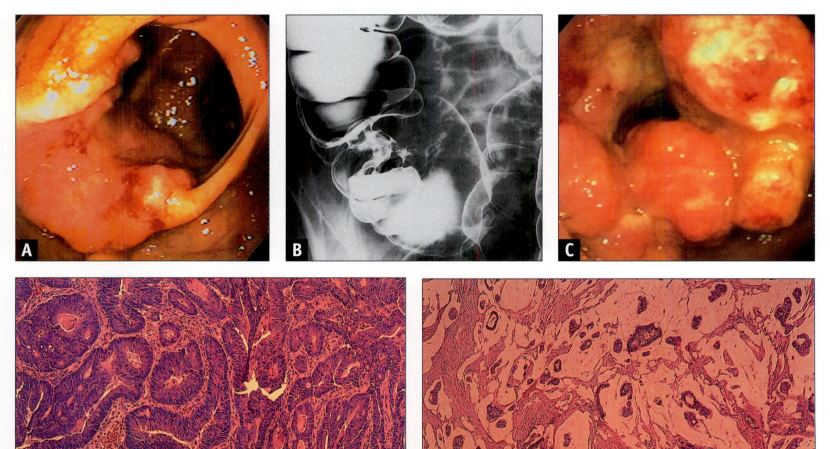

Figure 4-68. Miscellaneous adenocarcinomas and carcinomas affecting the colon. **A,** Adenocarcinoma of the colon infiltrating a gross colonic fold seen at colonoscopy. **B,** Air-contrast barium enema demonstrating mucosal involvement by cecal carcinoma. **C,** An obstructing polypoid carcinoma of the colon seen at colonoscopy. **D,** Well-differentiated adenocarcinoma of the colon. This histologic section demonstrates crowded neoplastic glands. **E,** Colloid carcinoma of the colon with scattered nests of tumor cells floating in "lakes of mucin." (*Courtesy of* Robert S. Bresalier, MD.)

Napkin-ring adenocarcinoma of colon . . . .

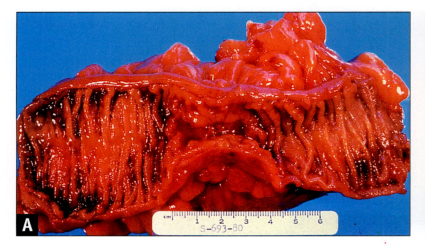

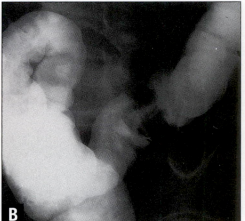

Figure 4-69. **A**, A gross surgical specimen of annular constricting or napkin ring carcinoma of the colon. **B**, Full-column barium enema demonstrating the annular constricting lesions. (*Courtesy of* Robert S. Bresalier, MD.)

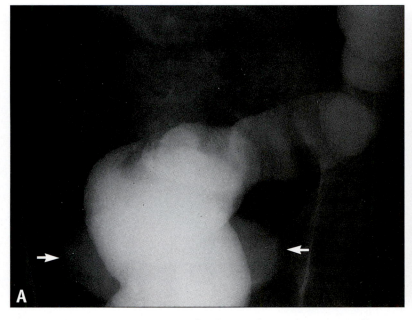

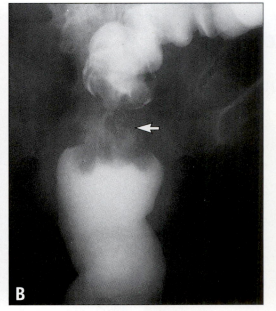

Figure 4-70. The importance of radiographic techniques is illustrated in this patient who has a circumferential adenocarcinoma of the rectosigmoid junction. **A**, In the anterior-posterior view, the tumor is largely hidden by the redundancy of the bowel on the single-contrast examination. There is also some retained contrast in the bladder from a coexistent excretory urogram (*arrows*). During the performance of positive-contrast examinations, it is important to display redundant portions of the colon so that lesions are identified or excluded. **B**, An angled view of the rectum with the overhead tube angled toward the feet very nicely uncovers the redundant areas and allows much better discrimination of this infiltrating annular carcinoma, which shows the tumor almost obliterating the lumen of the colon (*arrow*). Despite the size and obvious

nature of the lesion on this film, it is not nearly as well defined in the projection shown in *A*.

Redundancy of the colon is a problem for the radiologists as well as the endoscopists. Because at least half of the neoplastic lesions encountered will be located somewhere between the rectum and the descending colon, it is important to adequately define this area; this area is the location where redundancy, smooth muscle hypertrophy, and diverticulosis is most common. In order to minimize perceptive or technical misses, it is the radiologist's responsibility to make sure that redundancy is reduced and filming and fluoroscopic examination is adequate to see all areas of the colon. (*Courtesy of* Edward T. Stewart, MD.)

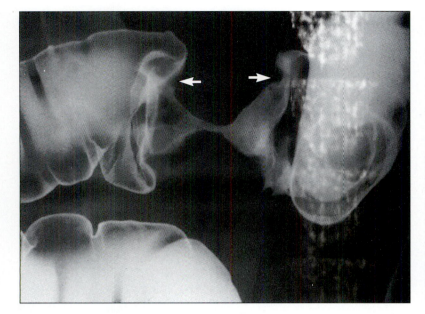

Figure 4-71. As malignancies advance and encompass the lumen of the colon, the annular appearance, often referred to as the *apple core lesion*, may be seen on positive-contrast studies. In this figure, the features of a malignant-circumferential carcinoma are well displayed. Notice the circumferential luminal narrowing of the colon. Sharp margins with overhanging edges are seen on both ends of the lesion (*arrows*). This lesion is probably superficially ulcerated, but this superficial ulceration is not well demonstrated.

Not only does this case graphically demonstrate the morphologic appearance of an infiltrating annular carcinoma, it also demonstrates that it is not likely that an endoscope will pass through the luminal narrowing of this tumor. The remainder of the colon is therefore the domain of the radiologist to exclude synchronous lesions. To remove this lesion without confirming the absence of any other pathology of the colon would be a major error in management. Patients with high-grade colonic obstruction with diverting colostomies must have the proximal colon examined some time during the initial management. (*From* Stewart and Dodds [8]; with permission.)

Adenocarcinoma, bleeding . . . .

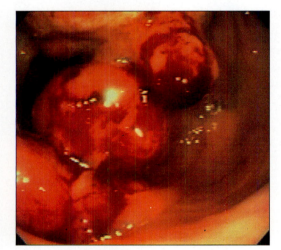

Figure 4-72. Colonoscopic view of bleeding colon cancer. Colorectal cancers may present with gross bleeding (hematochezia) or result in the presence of occult blood in the stool. (*Courtesy of* Robert S. Bresalier, MD.)

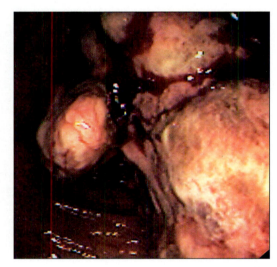

Figure 4-73. An exophytic rectal mass with oozing red blood. An endoscopic view from a patient undergoing flexible sigmoidoscopy for hematochezia. (*Courtesy of* Christopher S. Cutler, MD, and Douglas K. Rex, MD.)

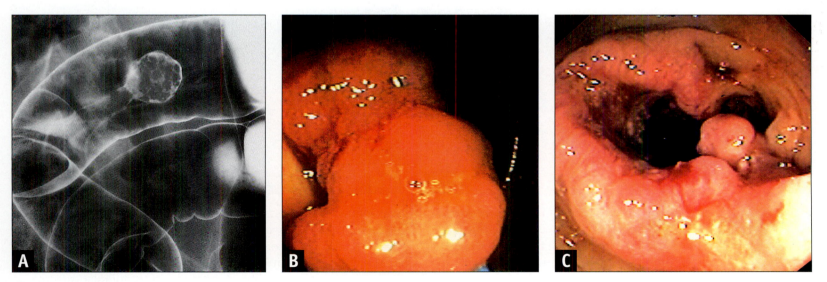

Figure 4-74. Bleeding adenocarcinomas. Most bleeding from colorectal polyps and cancer is occult or mild and intermittent. Rarely polyps and cancer may cause significant lower gastrointestinal hemorrhage. Left-sided and rectal neoplasms are more likely to cause gross bleeding than right-sided lesions. Diagnosis is made by endoscopy or barium enema. Treatment for bleeding polyps or cancer is usually by colonoscopic removal or surgery. This figure depicts a pedunculated sigmoid polyp (**A**). A descending colon adenocarcinoma (**B**) and an annular rectal adenocarcinoma (**C**) are also shown. (**A**, *Courtesy of* J. Lappas, MD; **B** and **C**, *courtesy of* Christopher S. Cutler, MD, and Douglas K. Rex, MD.)

● Familial Polyposis Coli

Familial polyposis coli, pathology specimen and barium enema ● ● ● ● ● ● ● ● ● ● ● ● ● ● ● ● ●

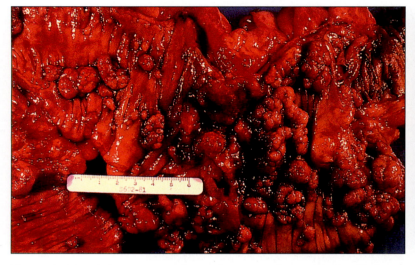

Figure 4-75. Colectomy specimen from a patient with familial adenomatous polyposis coli. In this syndrome, hundreds to thousands of adenomatous polyps arise in the colon. This disease is inherited as an autosomal dominant gene located on chromosome 5q (*APC*). If the colon is not removed in these individuals, the development of colon cancer is inevitable. (*Courtesy of* Robert S. Bresalier, MD.)

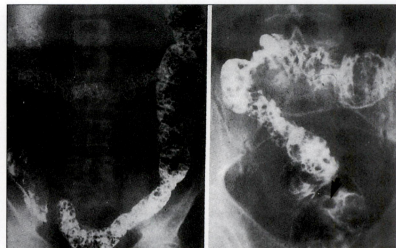

Figure 4-76. Radiograph of a barium enema from a patient with familial adenomatous polyposis. Thousands of polyps are seen as filling defects in the barium column. The *arrow* points to a carcinoma arising in this setting. (*Courtesy of* Robert S. Bresalier, MD.)

Gardner's syndrome ●

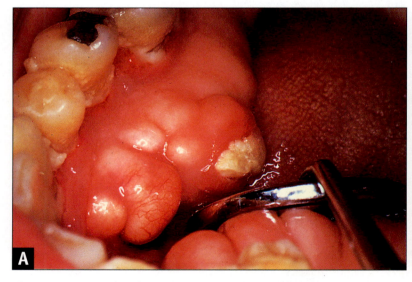

A

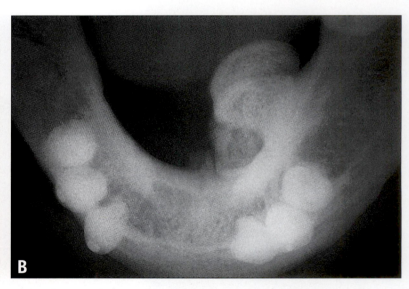

B

Figure 4-77. Gardner's syndrome is a subset of familial adenomatous polyposis. Familial adenomatous polyposis and Gardner's syndrome are variable manifestations of a disease that may be traced to a single gene locus. The primary features of this syndrome are colonic polyposis, osteomas (particularly in the skull and mandible),

and soft-tissue tumors. Periampullary tumors of the duodenum including carcinomas are also common. Soft-tissue tumors include epidermoid cysts, fibromas, lipomas, and desmoid tumors. **A,** Mandibular osteoma in a patient with Gardner's syndrome. **B,** Radiograph of a mandible demonstrating mandibular osteoma.

(*Continued on next page*)

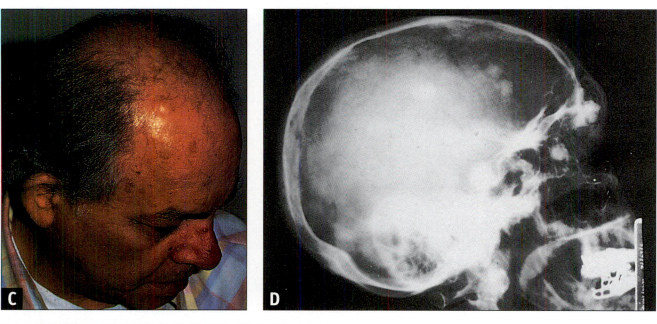

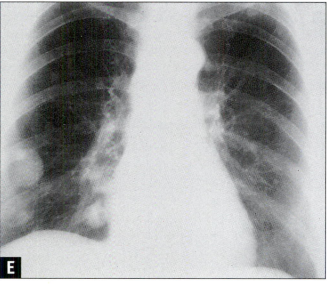

Figure 4-77. *(Continued)* **C**, Osteoma of the skull in a patient with gross Gardner's syndrome. **D**, Skull radiograph showing multiple osteomas. **E**, Fibroma seen as soft-tissue density on chest radiograph in a patient with Gardner's syndrome. (*Courtesy of* Robert S. Bresalier, MD.)

Peutz-Jeghers syndrome

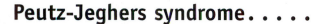

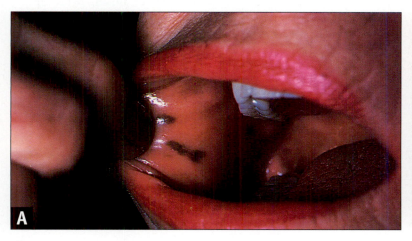

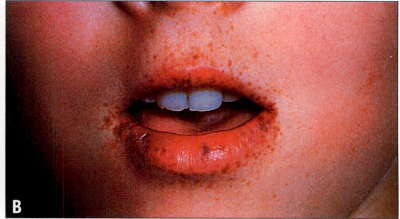

Figure 4-78. Peutz-Jeghers syndrome. Hamartomatous polyposis syndromes are characterized by multiple hamartomatous polyps of the gastrointestinal tract, including the colon. Although the hamartomas themselves carry no malignant potential, carcinomas of the colon do arise in adenomatous tissue associated with juvenile polyposis, the Peutz-Jeghers syndrome, and the Cronkhite-Canada syndrome. **A** and **B**, Mucocutaneous pigmentation is depicted in a patient with Peutz-Jeghers syndrome. Hamartomas of gastrointestinal tract and mucocutaneous pigmentation define this familial syndrome (autosomal dominant with variable penetrance). Carcinomas of the colon and small intestine may arise in associated adenomatous epithelium. (*Courtesy of* Robert S. Bresalier, MD.)

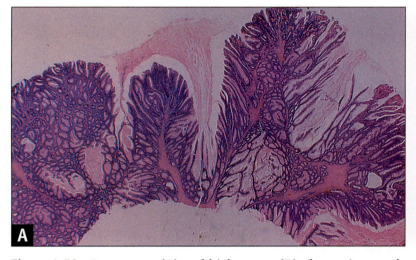 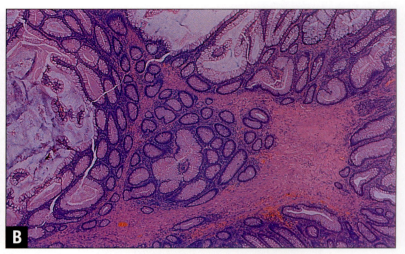

Figure 4-79. Low-power (**A**) and high-power (**B**) photomicrograph of a Peutz-Jeghers polyp. In this type of polyp the glandular epithelium is supported by an arborizing framework of well-developed smooth muscle that is contiguous with the muscularis mucosae. (*Courtesy of* Robert S. Bresalier, MD.)

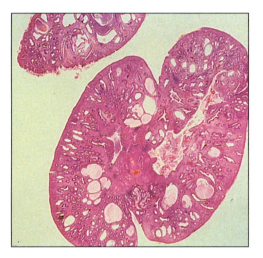

Figure 4-80. Juvenile polyp. This low-power photomicrograph demonstrates a hamartomatous polyp with dilated mucus-filled glands and extensive edema and inflammation in the lamina propria. Hamartomas of the colon, small intestine, and stomach characterize familial juvenile polyposis. The risk of colon cancer is increased in this syndrome caused by the presence of synchronous adenomatous polyps. (*Courtesy of* Robert S. Bresalier, MD.)

Peutz-Jeghers, pathology . . . .

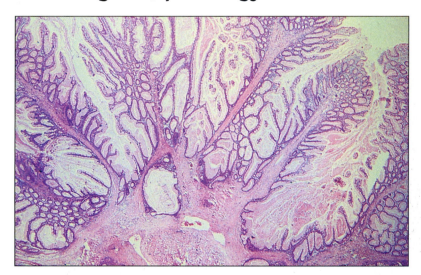

Figure 4-81. Peutz-Jeghers polyp. A hamartomatous polyp that exhibits arborizing branches of smooth muscle arising from the muscularis mucosae, which are covered by nonneoplastic colonic epithelium. These lesions may be isolated polyps but are usually found scattered throughout the gastrointestinal tract in patients with mucocutaneous pigmentation (Peutz-Jeghers syndrome) [9]. (*Courtesy of* Joel K. Greenson, MD.)

Miscellaneous Colonic Lesions

Pneumotosis cystoides. . . . .

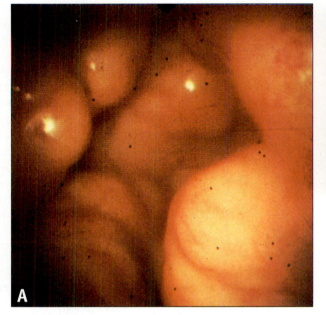

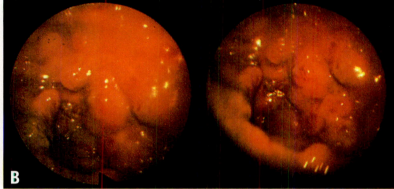

Figure 4-82. Endoscopic views of pneumatosis cystoides. Pneumotosis cystoides intestinalis is an uncommon condition characterized by multiple gas-filled endothelial-lined cysts occurring either in the subserosa or submucosa of the intestinal tract. Proposed mechanisms include forced passage of air from the colon lumen or pulmonary alveoli into the colon walls. The second mechanism is anaerobic fermentation and trapping of diffused gas. **A,** Submucosal gas is presented. Biopsy will usually cause the bleb to disappear. **B,** Submucosal or subserosal gas accumulation is shown. Biopsy specimens may show overlying inflammation. Biopsy specimens demonstrate firm tissue; their appearance may mimic neoplastic disease. Radiographs or computed tomography may confirm the diagnosis. (*Courtesy of* Timothy T. Nostrant, MD.)

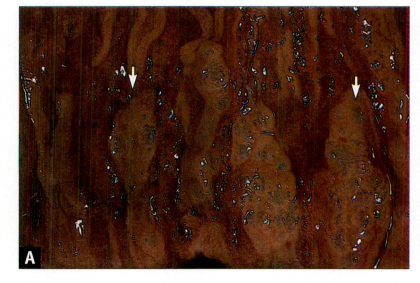

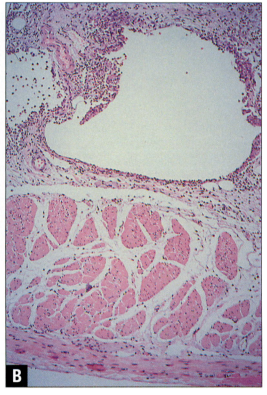

Figure 4-83. Pneumatosis coli. **A,** Numerous gas-filled cysts can be seen in this surface view of the mucosa (*arrows*). These lesions may be seen throughout the small and large intestine owing to several different conditions. Pulmonary emphysema and gastric outlet obstruction may both cause this condition secondary to the escape of air via the retroperitoneum. In the colon, gas-producing bacteria have also been implicated as a possible etiologic agent. **B,** A large gas-filled cyst is seen in the submucosa. These cysts are usually lined by multinucleated giant cells. Cysts may also be present in the subserosa [10–13]. (*Courtesy of* Joel K. Greenson, MD.)

Melanosis coli. . . . .

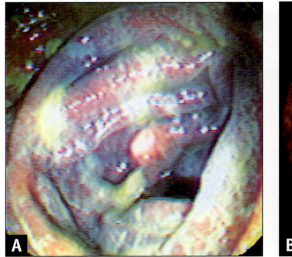

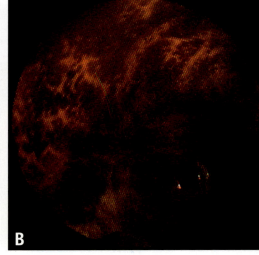

colonic crypt epithelium. Pigment can also be seen in the deeper bowel layers and lymph nodes. Degenerated lipid membranes damaged by the anthraquinone laxatives (senna, cascara, danthron, aloe) are the source for the pigmentation. Distribution is variable, but most often predominates in the cecum and rectum. Polyps and cancers do not pigment and therefore are easily seen against the dark background. The condition is benign and usually takes a year to both accumulate or disappear with taking or abstaining from laxatives. **Panel A** demonstrates mild "tigroid" pigmentation predominantly on the folds, whereas **Panel B** demonstrates heavy accumulation of pigment and "black bowel". (*Courtesy of* Timothy T. Nostrant, MD.)

Figure 4-84. Endoscopic views of melanosis coli. Melanosis coli is an accumulation of pigmented lipofuscin-like pigment in macrophages in the lamina propria below the

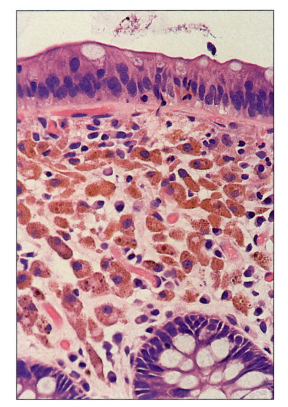

Figure 4-85. Melanosis coli. The superficial lamina propria is filled with macrophages that contain brown granular pigment. These macrophages impart a brown color to the mucosa when present in sufficient quantity. Most cases of melanosis coli are thought to be caused by the use of anthracene-containing laxatives. It should be noted that normal colon biopsy specimens may contain an occasional pigmented macrophage, but not to the degree seen in melanosis coli. (*Courtesy of* Joel K. Greenson, MD.)

Solitary rectal ulcer. . . . .

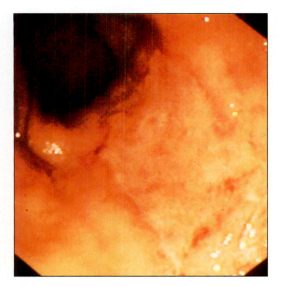

Figure 4-86. Solitary rectal ulcer syndrome. A solitary ulcer in the rectum may represent the solitary rectal ulcer syndrome when no other causes can be identified. The pathogenesis is related to the combination of prolonged straining at stool, resulting in mucosal prolapse, and inappropriate external anal sphincter and puborectalis muscle contraction during defecation. Anorectal pain and bleeding may result. Ulcers, which may be multiple, are usually on the anterior rectal wall. Occasionally a nodular elevation rather than an ulcer is observed. Characteristic histologic findings include fibrous obliteration of the lamina propria, thickening of the muscularis mucosa, regenerative changes in the crypt epithelium, and mucosal ulceration. (*Courtesy of* Lawrence S. Friedman, MD, Fiona Graeme-Cook, MD, and Robert H. Shapiro, MD.)

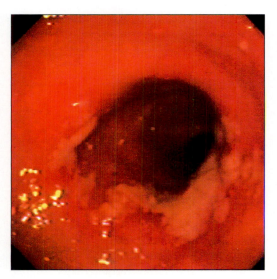

Figure 4-87. Solitary rectal ulcer. Eighty-five percent to 95% of patients with solitary rectal ulcer syndrome present with hematochezia, usually of low volume and associated with mucus. Symptoms may also include anorectal pain, altered bowel movements, and straining with defecation. It is believed that solitary rectal ulcer syndrome is related to prolonged straining during bowel movements and difficulty initiating defecation. Classically, at sigmoidoscopy, there is a shallow, discrete 1-cm ulcer with hyperemic margins 7 to 10 cm from the anal verge on the anterior wall. Lesions, however, may be multiple or vary in size and location. These ulcers follow a benign course, and two thirds of patients improve with conservative measures, including a high-fiber diet, laxatives, and avoidance of straining. Diagnosis is histologic, and the characteristic histologic findings may be seen in patients whose endoscopic findings are only rectal polyps. Pictured is a solitary rectal ulcer seen during flexible sigmoidoscopy. (*Courtesy of* Christopher S. Cutler, MD, and Douglas K. Rex, MD.)

Diversion colitis . . . .

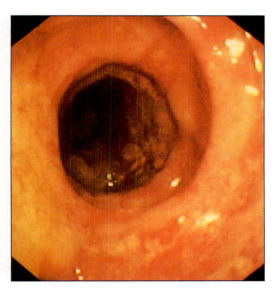

Figure 4-88. Endoscopic appearance of diversion colitis. Diversion colitis occurs in 50% to 100% of cases in which the distal colon is excluded and the fecal stream diverted, depriving the distal colon of short-chain fatty acids, the preferred metabolic substrate of colonic epithelium. Endoscopic findings are nonspecific and include edema, erythema, friability, granularity, erosions, and exudates. Histologically, the inflammation is limited largely to the mucosa but may be associated with fibrosis of the lamina propria and thickening of the muscularis mucosa. The findings may be indistinguishable from those of ulcerative colitis but reverse promptly when bowel continuity is reestablished or with topical short-chain fatty acid therapy. (*Courtesy of* Lawrence S. Friedman, MD, Fiona Graeme-Cook, MD, and Robert H. Shapiro, MD.)

Diversion colitis, pathology

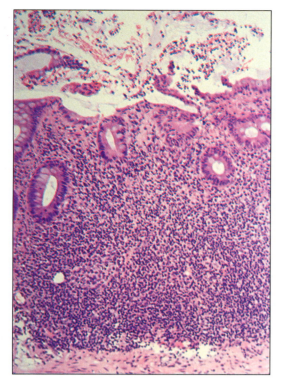

Figure 4-89. Diversion colitis. An expanded lymphoid follicle with patchy cryptitis and an overlying erosion is depicted. A modest increase in lamina propria mononuclear cells is often seen as well. These findings may show overlap with those of smoldering inflammatory bowel disease, but the inflammation resolves once fecal flow is reestablished to the diverted segment [14]. (*Courtesy of* Joel K. Greenson, MD.)

Lower Gastrointestinal Bleeding

99m technetium-labeled red blood cell scan

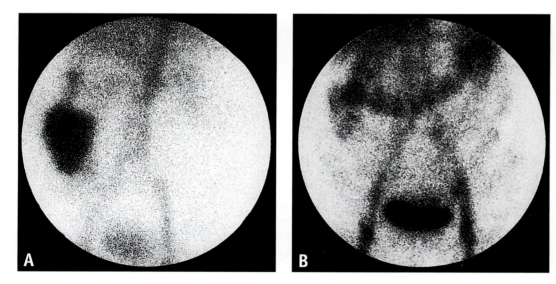

Figure 4-90. Two radionuclide techniques are used for localization of gastrointestinal bleeding [15]. One technique is the technetium sulfur colloid scan. This radionuclide is injected intravenously and is rapidly cleared from the intravascular compartment by the reticuloendothelial system. Because of a very short half-life, positive scans are seen only with active bleeding at the time of injection. This method can detect bleeding at rates as low as 0.1 mL/min. Unfortunately, because of the prerequisite for active bleeding, the sensitivity ranges from 8% to 12%. A preferred radionuclide scan is the 99m technetium-labeled red blood cell scan. In this test, autologous red blood cells are labeled in vitro with technetium and injected into the patient. Images are obtained every 5 minutes for 30 minutes and then every few hours for 24 hours. The cells remain in the vascular pool for the life of the circulating red blood cells. Thus, this method is a sensitive test for diagnosis of intermittent gastrointestinal bleeding. Some studies have shown a sensitivity of 93% and a specificity of 95% for tagged red blood cell studies. As in the case of the sulfur colloid scan, tagged red blood cell scans can detect bleeding rates as low as 0.1 mL/min. A major deficit of this method is that delayed scans are often performed at wide intervals. Extravasation of radionuclide into the gut can be followed by considerable transit down the gut prior to the next scan, resulting in misleading information about the location of the bleed. Bleeding cecal diverticula (**A**) and ascending colon angiodysplasia (**B**) are shown. (*Courtesy of* Christopher S. Cutler, MD, and Douglas K. Rex, MD.)

Mesenteric angiography, bleeding ascending colon diverticulum ....

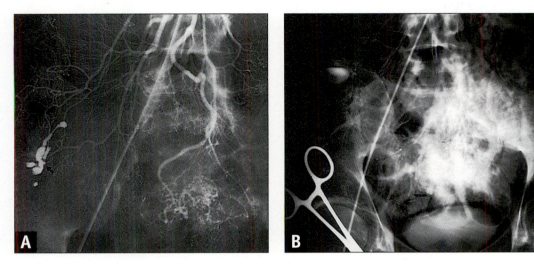

Figure 4-91. Mesenteric angiography is sometimes useful for the diagnosis of lower gastrointestinal bleeding. It can provide precise anatomic localization of the bleeding site and requires no bowel preparation. Extravasation of contrast may be seen with arterial bleeding rates as low as 0.5 mL/min [15]. Sensitivities for diagnosing lower gastrointestinal bleeding range from 14% to 86% in various series. In most clinical practices, the actual sensitivity is near the lower end of this range. Because a considerable amount of diverticular bleeding and almost all angiodysplasia bleeding occurs in the superior mesenteric artery distribution, selective cannulation should begin with this vessel, followed by the inferior mesenteric artery, and then the celiac artery. The complication rate ranges from 2% to 4%. Complications include arterial thrombosis, embolization, acute renal failure, and complications related to the catheter itself [16]. These figures represent an actively bleeding ileocolonic anastomosis in a patient with Crohn's disease (**A**), and a bleeding ascending colon diverticula (**B**). (**A**, *Courtesy of* J. Lappas, MD; **B**, *courtesy of* Christopoher S. Cutler, MD, and Douglas K. Rex, MD.)

Mesenteric angiography, bleeding descending colon diverticulum ....

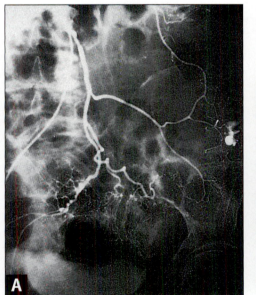
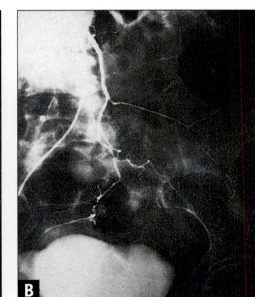

Figure 4-92. Selective mesenteric angiography is effective in the diagnosis of active diverticular bleeding. Extravasation of contrast into a diverticula is the diagnostic radiographic finding. Angiographic infusion of vasopressors may halt diverticular bleeding in 80% to 90% of patients [17]. Typical infusion doses in the superior mesenteric artery range from 0.2 to 0.3 units per minute and in the inferior mesenteric artery from 0.1 to 0.2 units per minute. Fifteen percent to 25% of these patients rebleed and eventually require surgery. Angiographic embolization may also be used, but below the ligament of Treitz, there is a 30% incidence of bowel ischemia or infarction. Figures of a patient with an actively bleeding diverticula of the descending colon (**A**) and following intra-arterial vasopressin infusion (**B**) are shown. (*From* Dietzen and Pemberton [18]; with permission.)

Angiodysplasias, endoscopic images ·····················

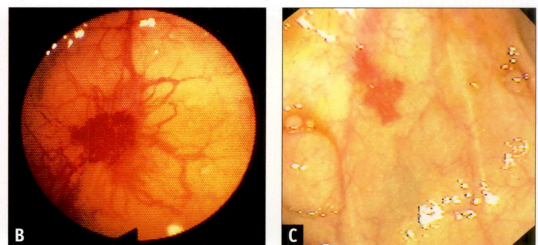

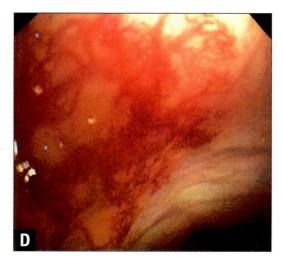

Figure 4-93. Colonoscopy detects approximately 80% of colonic angiodysplasia. Lesions appear flat or slightly raised, red, and 2 to 10 mm in diameter. They may be round, stellate, or fernlike [19]. There may be a prominent feeding vessel or a pale mucosal halo (**A–D**). Many lesions may mimic angiodysplasia, including lesions of hereditary hemorrhagic telangiectasia, ischemia, radiation colitis, and suction artifacts. Lesions may be missed if the patient is anemic or volume depleted. The effect of narcotics on the endoscopic appearance of angiodysplasia is controversial. Narcotics may lead to vasoconstriction and decreased mucosal blood flow, thus obscuring angiodysplasia, whereas naloxone hydrochloride may act to reverse these vasoconstrictive effects [20]. (*Courtesy of* Christopher S. Cutler, MD, and Douglas K. Rex, MD.)

Angiodysplasias, angiographic images ·····················

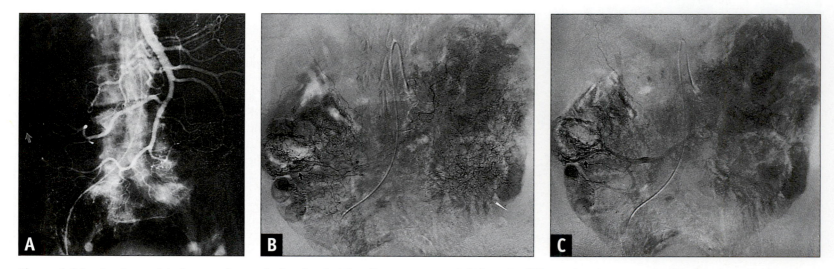

Figure 4-94. Angiographic images for angiodysphasia. The diagnostic yield of angiography for angiodysplasia is 17% to 20%. Classic findings include late draining veins (85% to 90%) representing obstructed submucosal veins (**A**), vascular tufts (70% to 75%) (**B**), early filling veins (60% to 80%) indicative of arteriovenous communication (**C**), and extravasation of contrast (6% to 20%)(not pictured) [19]. (*Courtesy of* N. Harris, MD.)

Anal Disorders

External hemorrhoids

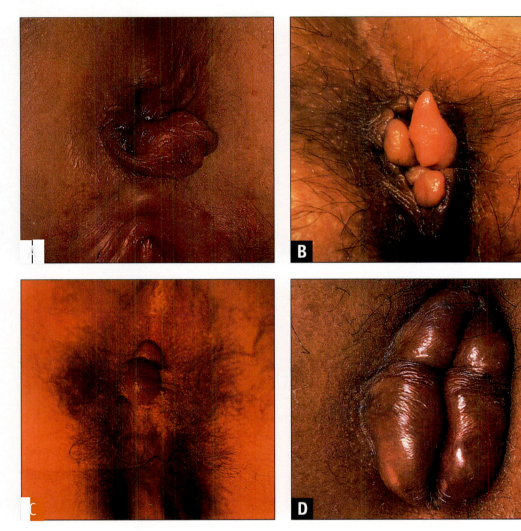

Figure 4-95. External or perianal skin tags are soft, fleshy folds of fibrous connective tissue. They are often the sequelae after the clot from a thrombosed external hemorrhoid has resolved. External hemorrhoids arise from the inferior hemorrhoidal plexus and are located below the dentate line; they are covered by squamous epithelium. External hemorrhoids are usually asymptomatic unless thrombosis occurs. Internal hemorrhoids are submucosal vascular cushions arising from above the dentate line and are covered by rectal mucosa. Internal and external hemorrhoids may coexist as a mixed hemorrhoid. **A,** An external or perianal skin tag. Skin tags may interfere with adequate anal hygiene and may worsen anal irritation or pruritus. Surgical excision is rarely necessary. **B,** Prominent fibroepithelial anal canal tags. **C,** An acutely thrombosed external hemorrhoid. A thrombosed external hemorrhoid may be quite painful, and bleeding may occur if the overlying skin ulcerates and the hematoma is expressed. Most respond to conservative management, but if acute and painful, local incision and clot evacuation afford immediate relief. **D,** Acutely prolapsed large, bilateral external and internal (mixed) hemorrhoids. (*Courtesy of* R. Burney, MD.)

Internal hemorrhoids

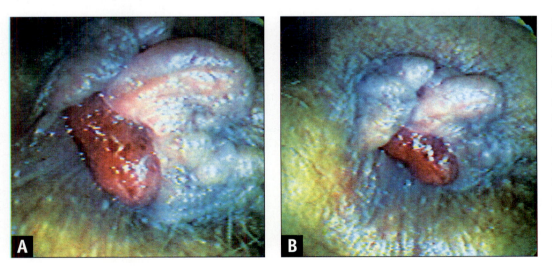

Figure 4-96. Internal hemorrhoids may be associated with pruritus, fecal soiling, discomfort, or no symptoms at all. However, bleeding and prolapse are the most typical complaints and bring the patient to the physician. Internal hemorrhoids may be graded by bleeding and degree of prolapse. With first degree hemorrhoids, the patient experiences painless, defecatory bleeding without significant prolapse of tissue. The hemorrhoids may be barely visible in the anal canal with straining, and they are best seen through the anoscope. Bleeding and prolapse occur at the time of defecation with second degree hemorrhoids, but the hemorrhoid reduces spontaneously back into the rectum after straining. Bleeding and prominent prolapse after defecation or straining that requires digital reduction characterize third degree hemorrhoids. Large, usually acute, hemorrhoids that cannot be persistently reduced and are at risk for strangulation are considered fourth degree hemorrhoids.

A and **B,** Prolapsed internal hemorrhoid. This friable internal hemorrhoid was the cause of hematochezia during defecation. External hemorrhoidal skin tags are also shown.

(*Continued on next page*)

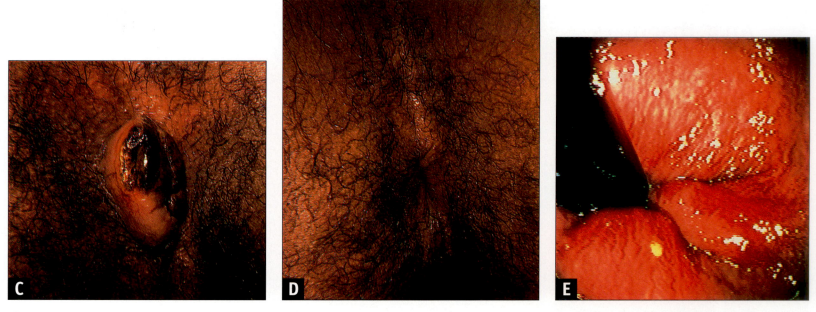

Figure 4-96. *(Continued)* Ulcerated, prolapsing internal hemorrhoids before (**C**) and after (**D**) reduction are depicted. **E,** This figure shows the view of internal hemorrhoids looking through the retroflexed sigmoidoscope. (**A, B** and **E,** *Courtesy of* Jeffrey L. Barnett, MD; **C** and **D,** *courtesy of* R. Burney, MD.)

Anorectal varices.

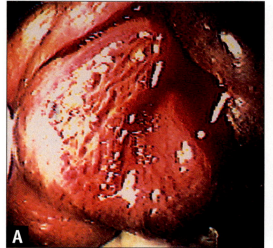

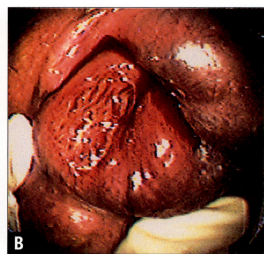

Figure 4-97. **A** and **B,** Anorectal varices. These large vascular lesions may be mistaken for large external or mixed hemorrhoids. However, in contrast to external hemorrhoids, varices are compressible and refill rapidly. Hemorrhoids and anorectal varices are unrelated. The incidence of hemorrhoids is similar in those with and without portal hypertension, and hemorrhoids have no direct connection to the portal system. Bleeding may be massive. Nonsurgical means (banding, sclerotherapy, etc.) have been used to treat anorectal varices, but surgical ligation is probably safer and more effective. (*Courtesy of* Jeffrey L. Barnett, MD.)

Excoriated anus secondary to pruritus ani

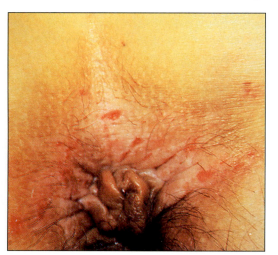

Figure 4-98. Intense perianal itching and burning discomfort is called *pruritus ani.* Causes include local irritants or sensitivities, benign and malignant dermatoses, infections, and anorectal diseases that lead to fecal contamination or leakage. This excoriated perianal skin was a result of idiopathic pruritus ani. (*Courtesy of* R. Burney, MD.)

Anal fissure . . . .

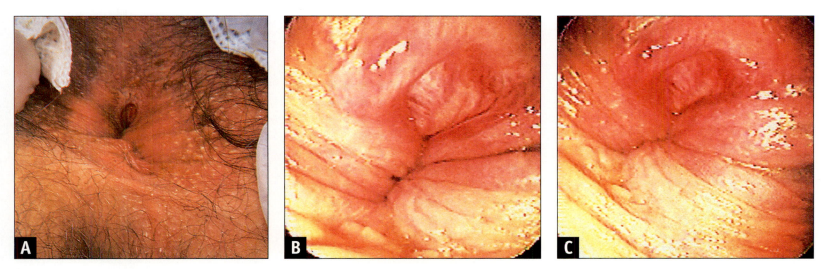

Figure 4-99. Anal fissures. An anal fissure is a painful, linear defect in the anal canal oriented perpendicularly to the dentate line. It is usually caused by a tearing that occurred during passage of a stool. The vast majority are located in the posterior midline; the remainder are anteriorly placed. A fissure located laterally should arouse suspicion of an underlying condition such as inflammatory bowel disease. An anal fissure is best identified by gentle but forceful lateral traction of the buttocks (after topical application of an anesthetic if necessary). Most acute anal fissures will heal with conservative medical management and time. Persistent acute fissures and most chronic fissures require definitive surgery, usually a lateral internal sphincterotomy to reduce resting sphincter tone. **A**, Typical fissure in ano located in the posterior midline. **B** and **C**, Large, painful anal fissure that failed to heal on medical therapy. (*Courtesy of* Jeffrey L. Barnett, MD.)

Anal condyloma . . . .

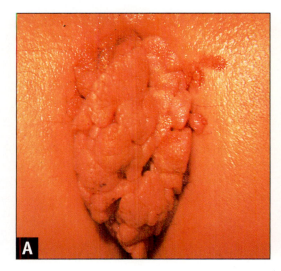
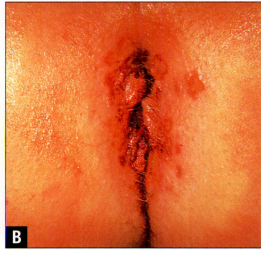

Figure 4-100. Anal condylomata acuminata. Anal warts are caused by the human papilloma virus (HPV type 6). Spread is usually through anal intercourse, but autoinoculation from the genitals may also occur. Despite treatment with caustic agents or fulguration, recurrence and reinfection rates are high. Extensive, verrucous perianal condyloma before (**A**) and after (**B**) surgical excision. Bulky disease such as this disease may be confused with squamous cell carcinoma. Biopsy is required to make the distinction. (*Courtesy of* R. Burney, MD.)

Anal neoplasm ·

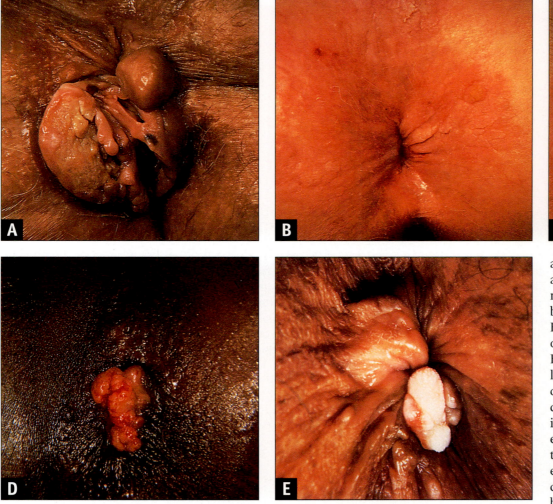

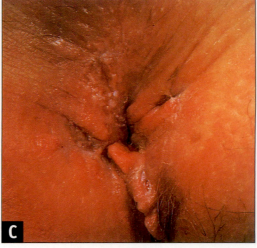

Figure 4-101. Anal neoplasms. The most common malignancies of the anal margin and anal canal are of the squamous cell type. Presenting symptoms include bleeding and discomfort, but nearly 25% of malignancies are found incidentally during routine examination. Occasionally, a surgical specimen for benign anorectal disease is found to contain previously unsuspected carcinoma. Risk factors for anal cancer include cigarette smoking, anal intercourse, genital warts and other venereal diseases, and chronic anal inflammation and scarring. Small lesions of the anal margin may be surgically excised, but extensive anal canal tumors are now usually treated with radiation and chemotherapy. Nonepidermoid anal malignancies are rare. They include adenocarcinoma of the anal canal, extra-mammary Paget's disease, Bowen's disease, basal cell cancer, and anal melanoma. **A,** Extensive, bulky squamous cell carcinoma of the anus. **B,** This figure is an example of Bowen's disease. This subtle, slow-growing lesion represents intradermal squamous cell carcinoma and may be mistaken for dermatitis or pruritus ani. Local excision is usually curative. **C,** This figure is an example of Paget's disease. This glandular tumor seen in the elderly appears as an eczematoid plaque. Similar to Bowen's disease, it is also easily mistaken for a benign anal condition. **D,** Protruding, cloacogenic polyp on a stalk is shown. This nonmalignant lesion was removed under local anesthesia. **E,** This firm, white, nodular growth was excised for fear of a small squamous cell carcinoma. However, the lesion was benign, revealing only thick hyperkeratosis and acanthosis. (*Courtesy of* R. Burney, MD.)

References

1. Almy TP, Howel DA: Diverticula of the colon. *N Engl J Med* 1980, 302:324–331.

2. Connell AM: Pathogenesis of diverticular disease of the colon. *Adv Intern Med* 1977, 22:377–395.

3. Parks TG: Natural history of diverticular disease of the colon. *Clin Gastroenterol* 1975, 4:53–69.

4. Rege RV, Nahrwold DL: Diverticular disease. *Curr Probl Surg* 1989, 26:133–189.

5. Hyland JMP, Taylor I: Does a high fibre diet prevent the complications of diverticular disease? *Br J Surg* 1980, 67:771–779.

6. Woods RJ, Lavery IL, Fazio VW, *et al.*: Internal fistulas in diverticular disease. *Dis Colon Rectum* 1988, 31:591–596.

7. Shepherd NA: Pathological mimics of chronic inflammatory bowel disease [Review]. *J Clin Pathol* 1991, 44:726–733.

8. Stewart ET, Dodds WJ: Neoplastic colonic lesions. In *Margulis and Burhenne's Alimentary Tract Radiology*, vol 1, edn 5. Edited by Freeny PC, Stevenson GW. St. Louis–Year Book; 1994:762–800.

9. Matuchansky C, Babin P, Coutrot S, *et al.*: Peutz-Jeghers syndrome with metastasizing carcinoma arising from a jejunal hamartoma. *Gastroenterology* 1979, 77:1311–1315.

10. Chippindale AJ, Desai S: Two unusual cases of pneumatosis coli. *Clin Radiol* 1991, 43:180–182.

11. Johansson K, Lindstrom E: Treatment of obstructive pneumatosis coli with endoscopic sclerotherapy: Report of a case. *Dis Colon Rectum* 1991, 34:94–96.

12. McCollister DL, Hammerman HJ: Air, air, everywhere: Pneumatosis cystoides coli after colonoscopy [Letter]. *Gastrointest Endosc* 1990, 36:75–76.

13. Spigelman AD, Williams CB, Ansell JK, *et al.*: Pneumatosis coli: A source of diagnostic confusion. *Br J Surg* 1990, 77:155.

14. Geraghty JM, Charles AK: Aphthoid ulceration in diversion colitis. *Histopathology* 1994, 24:395–397.

15. Shapiro MJ: The role of the radiologist in the management of gastrointestinal bleeding. *Gastroenterol Clin North Am* 1994, 23:123–179.

16. Gelfand DW, Routh WD, Cowan RJ: Diagnostic imaging in gastrointestinal hemorrhage. In *Gastrointestinal Bleeding*. Edited by Sugawa C, Schuman BM, Lucas CE. New York: Igaku-Shoin; 1992:205–221.

17. Reinus JF, Brandt LJ: Vascular ectasias and diverticulosis. Common causes of lower intestinal bleeding. *Gastroenterol Clin North Am* 1994, 23:1–20.

18. Dietzen CD, Pemberton JH: Diverticulitis. In *Atlas of Gastroenterology*. Edited by Yamada T. Philadelphia: JB Lippincott; 1992:279–285.

19. Fouch PG: Angiodysplasia of the gastrointestinal tract. *Am J Gastroenterol* 1993, 88:807–818.

20. Deal SE, Zfass AM, Duckworth PF, *et al.*: Arteriovenous malformation (AVMs). Are they concealed by meperidine [Abstract]? *Am J Gastroenterol* 1991, 86:1351.

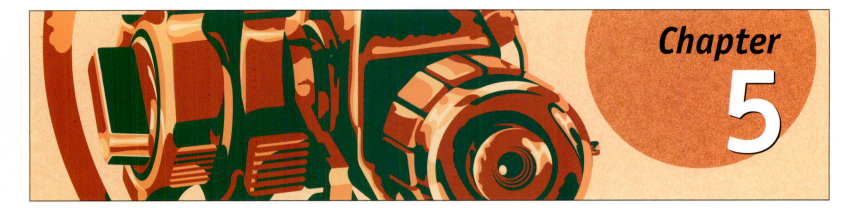

Gallbladder and Bile Ducts

 Normal Anatomy

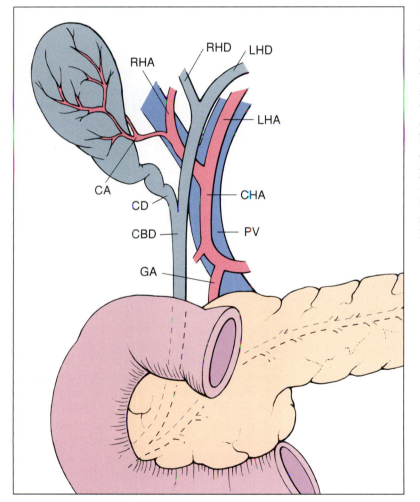

Figure 5-1. Extrahepatic bile ducts. The right hepatic duct (RHD) and left hepatic duct (LHD) emerge from the porta hepatis and in most instances join together after about 0.5 to 1 cm to form the common hepatic duct, which further descends in the free edge of the lesser omentum anterior to the foramen of Winslow. At a variable distance (from 1 to 5 cm) the cystic duct (CD) enters to form the common bile duct (CBD) (*see* Fig. 5-2). The latter continues downward in the hepatoduodenal fold of the peritoneum, passes behind the first part of the duodenum and the pancreas, then curves or bends to the right to enter in an oblique way the second part of the duodenum on its posteromedial side [1] (*see* Figs. 5-2, 5-7, and 5-8). CA—cystic artery; CHA—common hepatic artery; GA—gastroduodenal artery; GB—gallbladder; LHA—left hepatic artery; PV—portal vein; RHA—right hepatic artery. (*Adapted from* Frierson [1].)

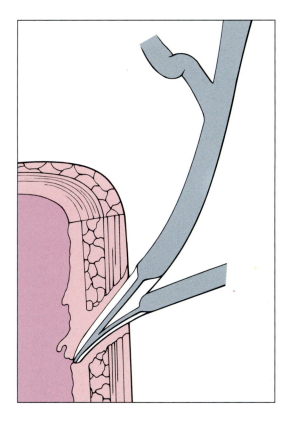

Figure 5-2. Common bile duct. The common bile duct is the extrahepatic bile duct segment between the junction of the cystic duct and the papilla of Vater (*see* Fig. 5-1). Although of variable length, the common bile duct usually measures 5 to 8 cm, with a mean diameter of 0.66 cm [1]. It is anatomically divided into supraduodenal, retro-duodenal, pancreatic, and intraduodenal segments.

The pancreatic segment is embedded to a variable extent in the posterior side of the pancreas and is partly or wholly covered by pancreatic tissue in 85% of cases. During its passage downward there may be a slight narrowing of its diameter until a point just outside the duodenal wall where the lumen is suddenly reduced. This narrowing is not obvious on external examination because it is the result of a marked increase in the thickness of the wall by the addition of muscle fibers. The junction between the upper broader and the lower narrower portion is marked by a characteristic notch, which corresponds with the upper margin of the choledochal sphincter of Boyden (*see* Fig. 5-8). This notch lies 2 mm outside the duodenal wall, so that the greater part of this terminal tapered portion of the common bile duct is related to the muscular and submucous layers of the duodenal wall [2]. The length of this terminal segment varies between 11 mm and 27 mm, with an average of 16 mm. Based on these findings it has been suggested that the previously mentioned anatomic segments of the common bile duct be replaced by a division into only two segments: an upper thin-walled portion and a lower narrow-lumened, thick-walled portion (the so-called Vaterian segment) [2]. Just above the notch the pancreatic duct approaches the common bile duct; both ducts become surrounded by a common sheath of connective tissue and smooth muscle but are separated by a fibromuscular septum. Both ducts pass obliquely through the choledochal window of the duodenal wall on its posteromedial side. (*Adapted from* Hand [2].)

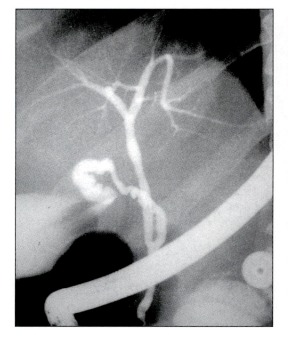

Figure 5-3. This endoscopic retrograde cholangiogram shows normal biliary anatomy. The endoscope is the radiopaque tube in the left lower portion of the figure. Valves of Heister are visible in the neck of the gallbladder. (*Courtesy of* David Reid, MD.)

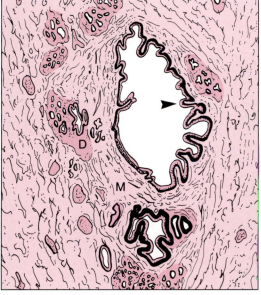

Figure 5-4. The extrahepatic bile ducts have tubuloalveolar glands that are located in the connective tissue of the lamina propria, some of them inside, but most of them outside the thin and incomplete muscle layer. The glands are mostly serous, although some are mucous. They are surrounded by a denser layer of connective tissue and communicate with the extra-hepatic bile duct lumen through an epithelium-lined duct. Along the intra-hepatic parts of the right and left hepatic ducts, the periductal glands are arranged in two rows on opposite sides of the duct, similar to the barbs of a feather [3]. Along the common bile duct, the glandular ducts run obliquely towards the bile duct and open into the periphery of shallow depressions of the bile duct mucosa. These openings are called the sacculi of Beale.

In children, the glandular acini are evenly distributed throughout the thickness of the common bile duct wall, whereas in adults they occur in clusters in the outer layers of the wall. The number of acini increases throughout the fetal period to reach its maximum within the first year after birth. Because of the progressive increase in diameter and surface area of the wall of the common bile duct, the concentration of acini per mm^2 decreases progressively from the fetal stage to adulthood. The glands are involved in protective mucin secretion and apparently also serve as regeneration centers after desquamation of the mucosal surface epithelium [4]. Arrowhead indicates mucosal fold; D—duct of small gland; M—muscle bundles. (*Adapted from* Elias and Sherrick [3].)

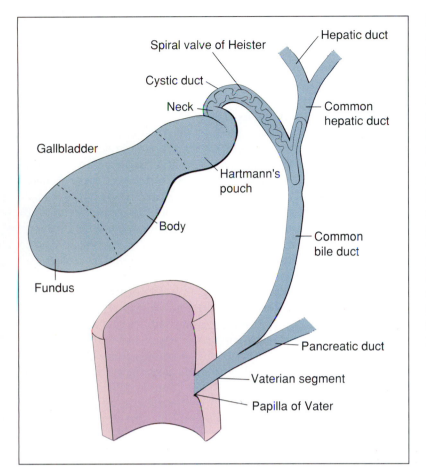

Spiral valve of Heister

Hepatic duct

Cystic duct

Neck

Gallbladder

Common
hepatic duct

Hartmann's
pouch

Body

Fundus

Common
bile duct

Pancreatic duct

Vaterian segment

Papilla of Vater

Figure 5-9. Gallbladder. The gallbladder is a pear-shaped sac located under the right lobe of the liver lateral to the quadrate lobe; it lies in a depression of the liver surface in contact with the interlobular connective tissue of the liver (facies visceralis). It is covered to a variable extent by peritoneum reflected off the liver. In more than 50% of patients the gallbladder may reach 0.5 to 1 cm beyond the anterior hepatic edge, contacting the anterior abdominal wall. The gallbladder measures up to 10 cm long and 3 to 4 cm wide in adults and has a volume of about 50 mL. It consists of a fundus with a blind end, a central body, and a narrow neck that connects to the cystic duct. The body is the largest segment; it narrows to an infundibulum as it joins the neck. The cholecystoduodenal ligament is a peritoneal fold that attaches the infundibulum to the first portion of the duodenum. In its normal location, the body passes upward and backwards into the neck. Hartmann's pouch is a dilatation in the neck region that may become adherent to the common hepatic duct. It is thought to be a consequence of disease processes and not a normal anatomic configuration [11]. The gallbladder neck is S-shaped, measures 5 to 7 mm in length, and narrows towards its connection with the cystic duct. (*Courtesy of* Valeer J. Desmet, MD, Tania Roskams, MD, and Rita De Vos, PhD.)

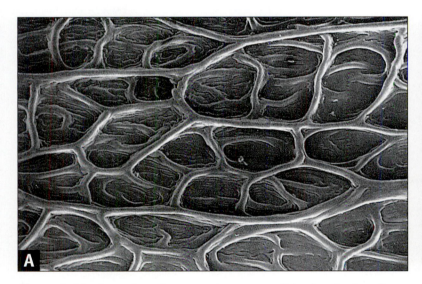

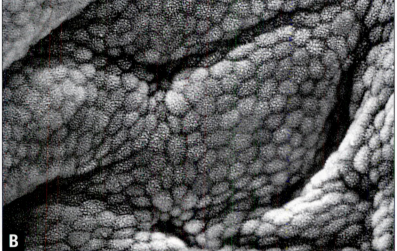

A **B**

Figure 5-10. Scanning electron microscopy of the luminal surface of rabbit gallbladder mucosa. **A,** The mucosal surface of the gallbladder is characterized by ridge-like projections of various heights. These ridges interconnect with each other, creating a polygonal pattern. The highest folds delineate larger polygonal compartments, whereas lower ridges divide the latter into smaller compartments. (× 55.) **B,** Scanning electron microscopy at higher magnification (× 1450) reveals the dome-shaped tops of individual epithelial cells that are studded with numerous regular microvilli. (*From* Castellucci and Caggiati [12]; with permission.)

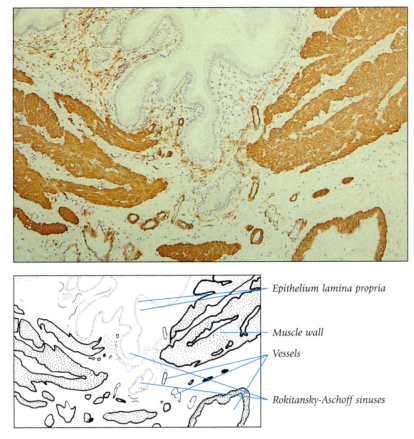

Figure 5-11. *Epithelium lamina propria*

Muscle wall

Vessels

Rokitansky-Aschoff sinuses

Figure 5-11. The mucosal folds consist of a lining columnar epithelium over a core of lamina propria. The single layer of tall cylindrical cells rests on a basement membrane. The cells have a pale or slightly eosinophilic cytoplasm and uniform oval nuclei located at the base of, or more centrally in, the cells. Occasional cylindrical cells with narrow diameter and dark eosinophilic

cytoplasm are designated "pencil-like cells." Rare basal cells have elongated nuclei lying just above, and parallel to, the basement membrane. The normal epithelium shows positive immunostaining for α_1-antitrypsin and α_1-antichymotrypsin, focal weak positivity on the apical lining of some cells for carcinoembryonic antigen, and strong immunoreactivity for epithelial membrane antigen, low molecular weight cytokeratins [1] and carbonic anhydrase II [13].

The epithelium may herniate quite deeply into the lamina propria and even into the muscle layer and subserosa. These herniations are known as *Rokitansky-Aschoff sinuses*. Approximately 40% of normal gallbladders have a small number of these sinuses, which are confined to the lamina propria [14]. Their number appears to increase with aging, and they are thought to result from increased intraluminal pressure and extreme contractions of the gallbladder. The *ducts of Luschka* are bile ducts of microscopic size in the perimuscular connective tissue of the gallbladder on its hepatic side. They are observed in about 10% of routine examinations of cholecystectomy specimens, in both normal and diseased gallbladders. The ducts of Luschka are thought to represent embryonic remnants, single or anastomosing channels that are surrounded by a dense layer of connective tissue and that communicate with intrahepatic bile ducts but apparently not with the gallbladder lumen. In the gallbladder neck, near the cystic duct, the lining epithelium invaginates into the lamina propria to form tubuloalveolar glands. The latter are characterized by a wide lumen, are lined by mucous cells secreting sulfated mucin, and contain no neuroendocrine cells [15]. These glands are different from those observed in the fundus region of chronically irritated gallbladders ("pseudopyloric glands") but similar to those found in the cystic duct. (Immunostain for α–smooth muscle actin; counterstained with hematoxylin. Smooth muscle and vessel walls brown. $\times$ 62.5.) (*Courtesy of* Valeer J. Desmet, MD, Tania Roskams, MD, and Rita De Vos, PhD.)

Gallstones and Cholecystitis

Types of Gallstones			
	Cholesterol	**Black pigment**	**Brown pigment**
Location	Gallbladder	Gallbladder	Bile ducts
Pathogenesis	Physical-Chemical	Physical-Chemical	Infectious
Composition: Cholesterol	+++	+	++
Calcium and Bilirubin Content	+	+++	++

Figure 5-12. The three major classes of gallstones—cholesterol stones, black pigment stones, and brown pigment stones—differ in their pathogenesis as well as in their composition [16,17]. Cholesterol and black pigment stones form only in the gallbladder, but brown pigment stones are formed in the bile ducts after bacterial infection of the biliary tree. They are essentially an infectious disease of the biliary tree, and as such, their only major risk factor is mechanical bile stasis because of obstruction or, in some cases, a duodenal diverticula. In contrast, the formation of cholesterol and black pigment stones depends on a physical chemical problem,

that is, the presence of an excess of insoluble constituents of bile. Hence, the composition of these three types of gallstones differs. Cholesterol is the major constituent of cholesterol gallstones, which also contain small amounts of inorganic calcium salts and the calcium salt of bilirubin. Black pigment stones contain large amounts of calcium and bilirubin, whereas brown pigment stones are composed of calcium salts of lipids degraded by bacteria, such as fatty acid soaps, as well as smaller amounts of bilirubin and cholesterol. (*Courtesy of* Joanne M. Donovan, MD.)

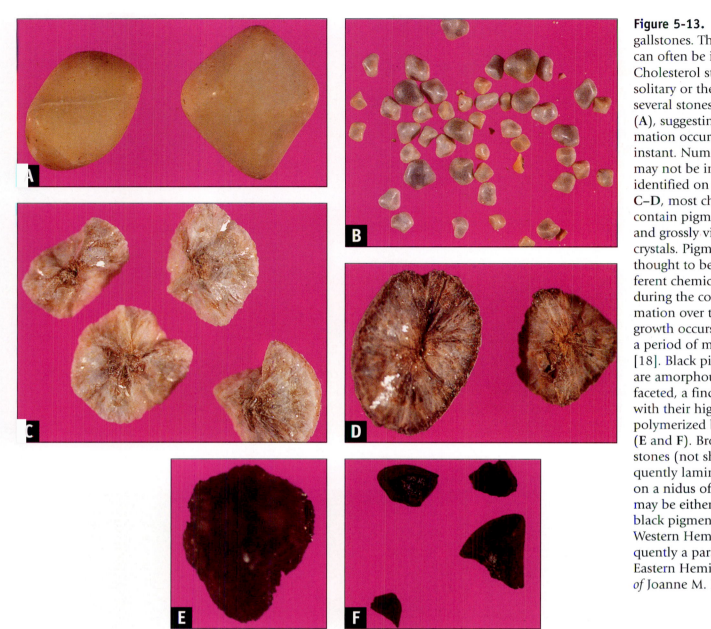

Figure 5-13. Appearance of gallstones. The type of stone can often be identified visually. Cholesterol stones may be solitary or they may occur as several stones of similar size (**A**), suggesting that stone formation occurred at a single instant. Numerous tiny stones may not be individually identified on ultrasound (**B**). **C–D**, most cholesterol stones contain pigment at the center and grossly visible cholesterol crystals. Pigmented rings are thought to be secondary to different chemical stimulations during the course of stone formation over time because growth occurs over a period of months to years [18]. Black pigment stones are amorphous, but may be faceted, a finding consistent with their high content of polymerized bilirubin pigment (**E** and **F**). Brown pigment stones (not shown) are frequently laminated and occur on a nidus of infection, which may be either a cholesterol or black pigment stone in the Western Hemisphere or frequently a parasite in the Eastern Hemisphere. (*Courtesy of* Joanne M. Donovan, MD.)

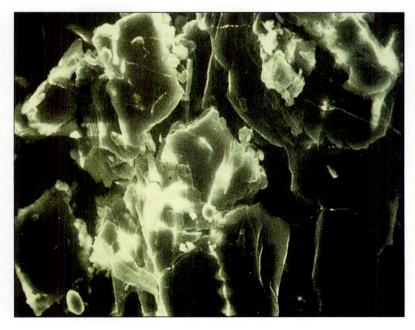

Figure 5-14. Structure of cholesterol gallstones. Scanning electron microscopy of a cholesterol stone demonstrates that the stone is largely composed of flat rhomboidal cholesterol monohydrate crystals, which are cemented together by amorphous material. The crystals can be identified macroscopically, and are typically arranged in a radial pattern (*see* Figs. 5-13C and 5-13D). Analysis of cholesterol stones has shown that a mucin matrix is almost universally present and is likely to be the scaffolding on which cholesterol crystals are cemented together [19]. (*From* Malet *et al.* [20]; with permission.)

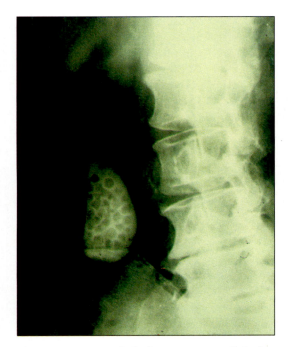

Figure 5-15. Oral cholecystogram of cholesterol gallstones. Gallstones can be visualized by an oral cholecystogram. Here, the gallbladder is filled with multifaceted lucencies, similar to those seen in Figure 5-13A. In contrast to black pigment stones, whose high calcium content renders them radiodense, most cholesterol stones are radiolucent. (*From* Donovan and Carr-Locke [21]; with permission.)

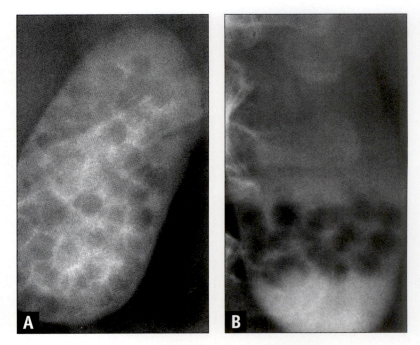

Figure 5-16. Stones that float (layer) above more dense oral radiopaque contrast medium are cholesterol stones (**A, B**). If the stones are radiolucent on CT scan, they usually can be completely dissolved. (*Courtesy of* Johnson L. Thistle, MD.)

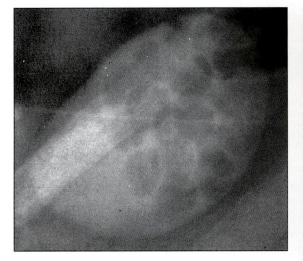

Figure 5-17. This patient with several smooth faceted stones of equal size almost certainly has cholesterol stones. (*Courtesy of* Johnson L. Thistle, MD.)

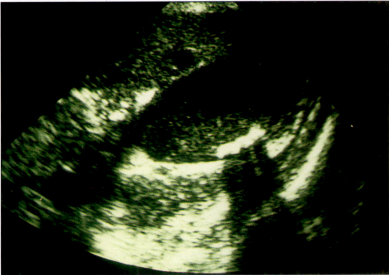

Figure 5-18. Gallstones and biliary sludge. Ultrasound is the preferred technique for identifying gallstones; it has a sensitivity and specificity of more than 95%. Three gallstones with acoustic shadowing are shown here. Biliary sludge can be identified as a discrete echogenic, mobile layer within the gallbladder, which lacks the acoustic shadowing that is characteristic of gallstones. This ultrasonographic appearance results from microscopic and larger crystals of cholesterol and granules of calcium bilirubinate that are trapped in a thick mucin gel [22]. (*From* Donovan and Carr-Locke [21]; with permission.)

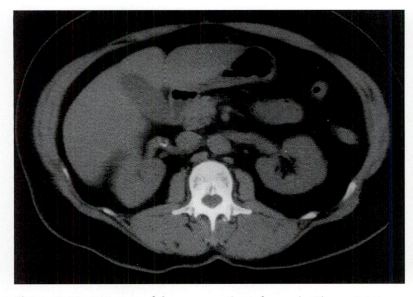

Figure 5-19. CT scan of the same patient shown in Figure 5-17 demonstrates that the stones are isodense with bile, which is diagnostic of noncalcified cholesterol stones. These stones dissolved completely without residual debris when direct contact dissolution with methyl *tert*-butyl ether was used. (*Courtesy of* Johnson L. Thistle, MD.)

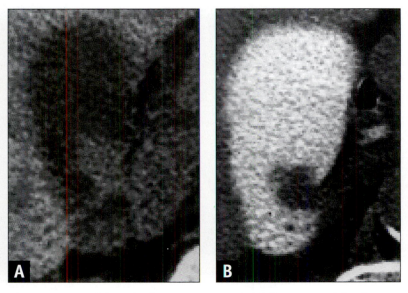

Figure 5-20. Although this patient was initially reported by the radiologist to have a radiolucent gallstone, it is apparent on close scrutiny that this radiodensity is unusually irregular and may be attached to the wall. This figure illustrates CT scans without (**A**) and with (**B**) gallbladder opacification. (*Courtesy of* Johnson L. Thistle, MD.)

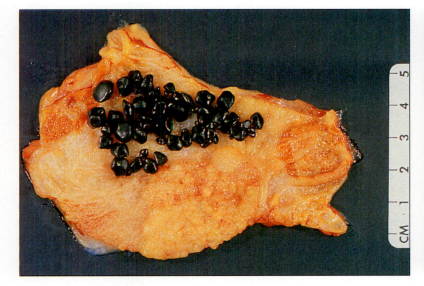

Figure 5-21. This patient did indeed have cholesterol stones with a thin surface layer of black pigment, but of most importance is the grade 2 adenocarcinoma in the neck of the gallbladder. Although it is unusual for a neoplasm to exist in addition to stones, this consideration must be kept in mind and the therapeutic plan reassessed if a neoplasm is suspected. (*Courtesy of* Johnson L. Thistle, MD.)

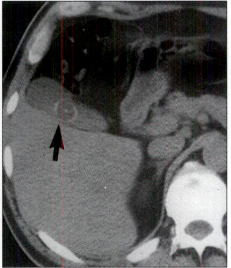

Figure 5-22. Gallstone characterization. The presence of any calcium visible by CT scan (*arrow*) excludes a stone from being dissolved by oral bile acid therapy, but direct contact dissolution may be used. (*Courtesy of* Johnson L. Thistle, MD.)

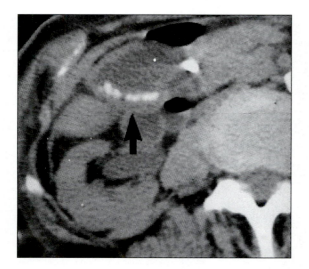

Figure 5-23. Gallstone characterization. Pigment stones are usually detectable on CT scan (*arrow*). If there are only a few small stones, it is important to make thin slices (*eg*, 3 mm) to avoid missing a small part of the gallbladder that may contain all of the stones. Rapid scanning CT allows complete coverage of the gallbladder without respiratory variation. Oral cholecystography radiopaque media may require 10 days to completely clear from the gallbladder and, if retained, may mask or be misinterpreted as stone calcification. Because oral contrast in the duodenum adjacent to the gallbladder also may be confused with stone calcification, avoidance of all contrast is optimal. (*Courtesy of* Johnson L. Thistle, MD.)

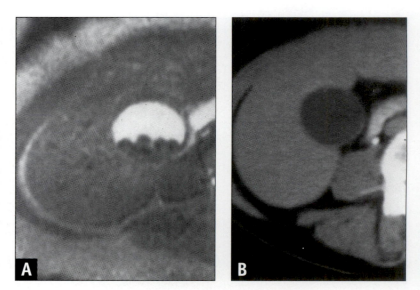

Figure 5-24. Cholesterol stones. **A**, MR imaging shows several smooth, round stones of similar size and shape that are strongly characteristic, if not diagnostic, of cholesterol stones. **B**, CT scan of the same patient shows no evidence of stones; thus, it is virtually certain that these are almost pure cholesterol stones. Note also the globular obstructed appearance of the gallbladder. (*Courtesy of* Johnson L. Thistle, MD.)

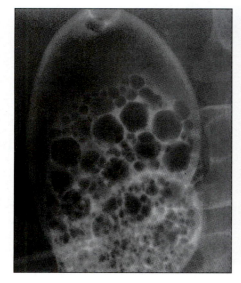

Figure 5-25. After a percutaneous transhepatic catheter was placed in the patient shown in Figure 5-24, several families of cholesterol stones were apparent. In addition, several stones were in the gallbladder neck and one stone obstructed the proximal cystic duct. (*Courtesy of* Johnson L. Thistle, MD.)

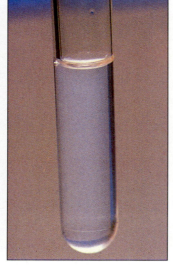

Figure 5-26. The white bile obtained on aspiration from the gallbladder shown in Figure 5-24 was diagnostic of complete obstruction. (*Courtesy of* Johnson L. Thistle, MD.)

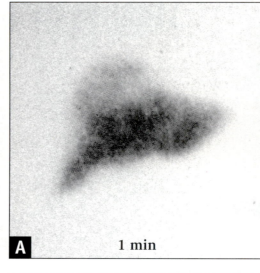

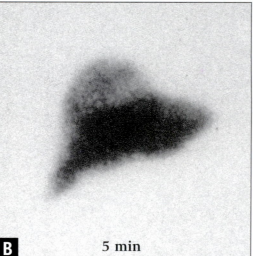

Figure 5-27. A–H, This representative cholescintigram [23] shows where bile goes during fasting. Sequential g-camera images show uptake by the liver 30 minutes (min) after injection of the radiolabel (^{99m}technetium [Tc] hepatoiminodiacetic acid), filling of the gallbladder, and entry into the duodenal sweep.

(Continued on next page)

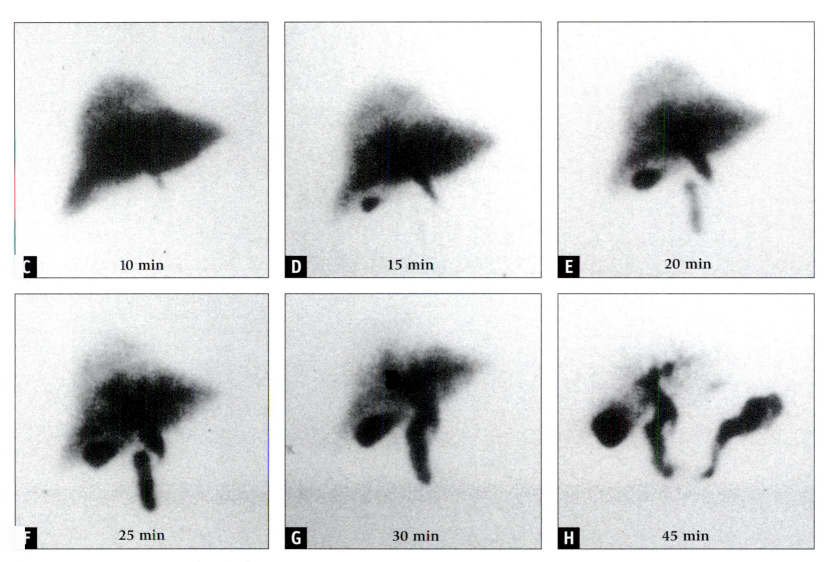

C 10 min

D 15 min

E 20 min

F 25 min

G 30 min

H 45 min

Figure 5-27. *(Continued)* An infusion of cholecystokinin (here at 0.02 GIH units/kg/minute for 30 minutes) causes diminution of activity over the gallbladder and the subsequent appearance of the radiopharmaceutical in the small intestine [23]. Thereafter, swallowing of ^{99m}Tc sulfur colloid locates the position of the stomach. (*Courtesy of* Eldon A. Shaffer, MD.)

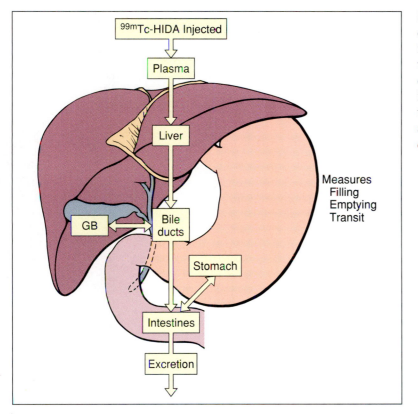

^{99m}Tc-HIDA Injected

Plasma

Liver

GB ← Bile ducts

Stomach

Measures
Filling
Emptying
Transit

Intestines

Excretion

Figure 5-28. Principle of quantitative cholescintigraphy. This diagram represents the excretion of ^{99m}technetium (Tc) hepato-iminodiacetic acid (HIDA). After being injected into the plasma, the radiopharmaceutical is principally taken up by the liver then excreted into the bile ducts and finally into the gallbladder or (GB) intestines. Bile may then reflux into the stomach. Extraneous activity in the blood pool, renal uptake, and excretion into the bladder are excluded from the determination of where bile goes. (*Courtesy of* Eldon A. Shaffer, MD.)

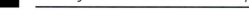

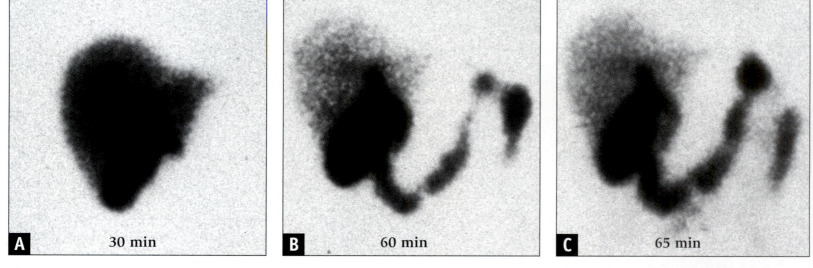

Figure 5-29. Changes in activity over time in the biliary tract of a healthy subject. These are the dynamic curves from a ⁹⁹ᵐtechnetium hepatoiminodiacetic acid cholescintigraphic study. Radioactivity is expressed as absolute counts per minute, corrected for background activity, natural decay of the isotope, and superimposed areas. Net activity is given for three areas of interest: the liver, the gallbladder, and the duodenum. The dynamic curves for the liver show a prompt uptake and a steady loss as the radioactivity is excreted into the biliary tree and then into the gallbladder and duodenum. The gallbladder shows little uptake for 15 minutes, the time necessary to traverse the ductal system from the hepatocyte to the entrance of the cystic duct. Thereafter, gallbladder filling is evident as a steady increase in radioactivity. Cholecystokinin (CCK) infused at 0.02 GIH units per kilogram per minute causes a prompt fall in activity from the gallbladder. The duodenum similarly has little activity until 15 to 20 minutes; thereafter it steadily rises. By 60 minutes, there are fewer counts per minute in the duodenum compared with the gallbladder, indicating a greater proportion of the hepatic bile has filled the gallbladder rather than the duodenum. The infusion of CCK continues the rise of activity in the duodenum and small intestine. Cholescintigraphy does not measure the concentrating function of the gallbladder or gallbladder volume changes. (*Courtesy of* Eldon A. Shaffer, MD.)

Figure 5-30. Hepatoiminodiacetic acid cholescintigraphic study-sequential g-camera images of a healthy subject (control) compared with those of a patient with cholelithiasis (see Figure 5-31). A–D, For the control person, the liver is visualized first. Within

30 minutes there is sufficient radioactivity in the gallbladder for it to be visualized. By 60 minutes the radiopharmaceutical agent has begun to clear significantly from the liver and to enter the small intestine. With the infusion of cholecystokinin (CCK) the

(*Continued on next page*)

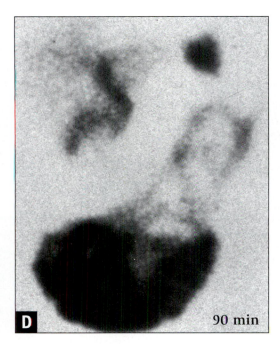

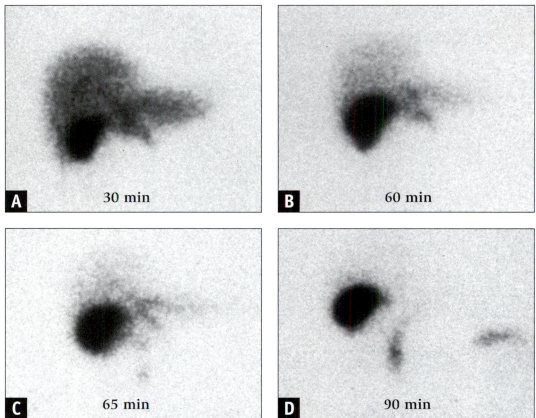

Figure 5-30. *(Continued)* gallbladder empties its radiolabeled contents and largely disappears. The remainder of the radioactive material moves on into the distal small bowel. (*Courtesy of* Eldon A. Shaffer, MD.)

Figure 5-31. A–D, In the patient with cholelithiasis, the radiolabel fills the gallbladder by 30 minutes (in this case very little entered the duodenum), then is retained despite an infusion of CCK (0.2 GIH units/kg/minute over 30 minutes). A subgroup of patients with cholesterol gallstones have impaired gallbladder emptying similar to this [24]. (*Courtesy of* Eldon A. Shaffer, MD.)

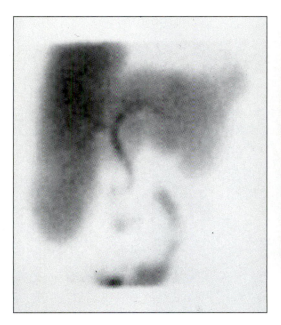

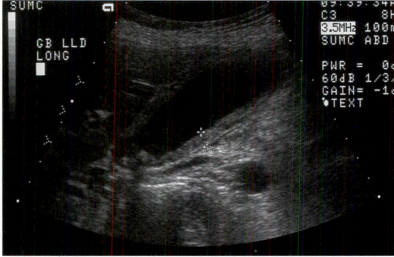

Figure 5-32. Cholescintigram compatible with acute cholecystitis. This patient had acute cholecystitis, and this HIDA study shows uptake by the liver and excretion of isotope into the biliary tree and duodenum, but no visualization of the gallbladder. (*Courtesy of* Brooke Jeffrey, MD.)

Figure 5-33. Ultrasound showing acute cholecystitis. This patient's ultrasound demonstrates findings compatible with acute cholecystitis, including thickening of the gallbladder wall and gallstones in the dependent portion of the gallbladder. The gallstones are seen as an echogenic focus within the gallbladder lumen, and posterior acoustical shadowing in present. (*Courtesy of* Brooke Jeffrey, MD.)

Choledocholithiasis

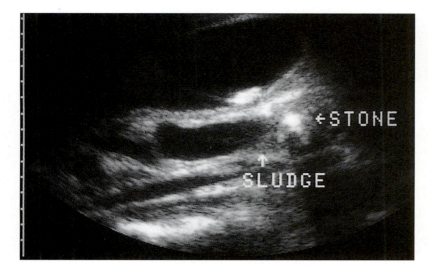

Figure 5-34. Choledocholithiasis diagnosis with ultrasonography. Several noninvasive imaging modalities are currently available. Selection of the most appropriate technique requires knowledge of the sensitivities and limitations of each study. Ultrasonography has a sensitivity for detection of common bile duct stones ranging from 10% to 81%, whereas computed tomography (CT) has a sensitivity of 50% to 90%. The data for magnetic resonance cholangiopancreatography are not yet available. Intravenous cholangiography and nuclear scintigraphy do not have well defined roles in the diagnosis and management of patients with known or suspected choledocholithiasis. This ultrasonogram shows common bile duct dilatation, echogenic sludge, and a common bile duct stone with acoustic shadowing present distally. Although ultrasonography is the preferred modality for diagnosing suspected cholelithiasis, it is relatively insensitive with respect to documentation of stones in the common bile duct. (*Courtesy of* Alfred D. Roston, MD, and David L. Carr-Locke, MD.)

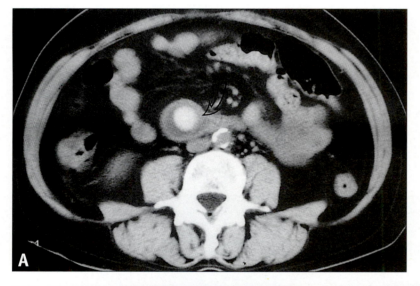

Figure 5-35. A, This CT scan shows a hyperdense focus (*arrow*) in the distal common bile duct, with surrounding hypodense bile within an enormously dilated common bile duct. **B**, The magnetic resonance cholangiopancreatogram reveals multiple filling defects of varying size throughout the entire extrahepatic biliary tree within a tortuous and dilated common bile duct and prominent intrahepatic ducts. **C**, The corresponding cholangiogram obtained at endoscopic retrograde cholangiopancreatography is shown. (**A**, **C**, *Courtesy of* Alfred D. Roston, MD, and David L. Carr-Locke, MD; **B**, *courtesy of* Robert Whitlock, MD.)

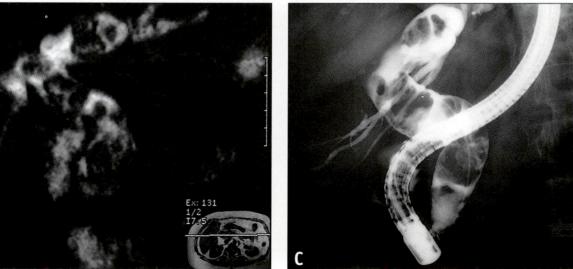

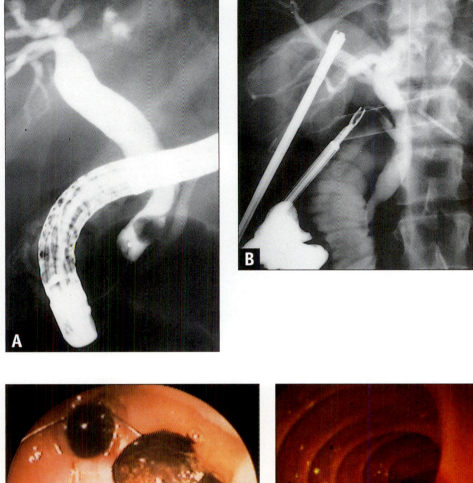

Figure 5-36. Diagnostic modalities. Endoscopic retrograde cholangiopancreatography is the most accurate invasive diagnostic modality and can clearly demonstrate intraluminal filling defects as well as ductal dilatation (**A**). Other diagnostic modalities, depending on availability and local expertise, include percutaneous cholangiography, intraoperative cholangiography (obtained laparoscopically in **panel B**), and common bile duct exploration, performed laparoscopically or by an open approach. Surgical and endoscopic ductal clearance rates are usually reported to be greater than 95%. Mortality rates for surgical series range from 0% to 28%, depending on the patient populations selected, and recurrence rates range from 5% to 21%. In contrast, endoscopic ductal clearance has a published mortality rate ranging from 0% to 3% and a recurrence rate of less than 5%. (*Courtesy of* Alfred D. Roston, MD, and David L. Carr-Locke, MD.)

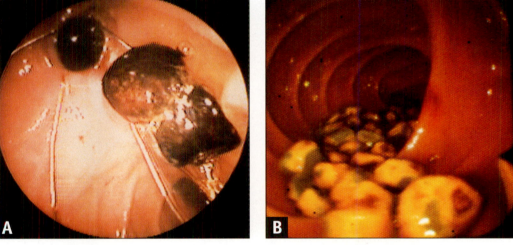

Figure 5-37. Common bile duct stones can be classified into primary (those arising de novo in the bile duct) and secondary (those forming in the gallbladder, and subsequently migrating into the common bile duct). **A**, Primary stones are rich in calcium bilirubinate and have less cholesterol content than do gallbladder stones. Contributors to their formation include bacterial or parasitic infection and stasis due to obstruction from stricture or papillary disease. **B**, In the Western world, secondary bile duct stones are more prevalent, and of these, cholesterol stones are the most common type. In Western choledocholithiasis, 80% to 90% of patients have concomitant gallbladder stones. In the era of open cholecystectomy, as many as 15% of all patients harbored bile duct stones. In patients undergoing open ductal exploration, up to 5% have retained bile duct stones. Although the majority of patients with gallbladder stones do not eventually develop symptoms, patients with bile duct stones characteristically develop complications that include pain, jaundice, pancreatitis, or cholangitis. This natural history thus argues for active intervention rather than observation after discovery of bile duct stones, whether they are symptomatic or asymptomatic. (*Courtesy of* Alfred D. Roston, MD, and David L. Carr-Locke, MD.)

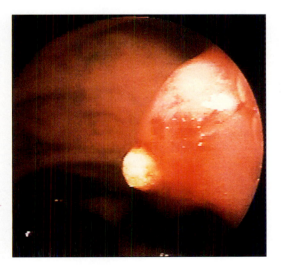

Figure 5-38. Endoscopic view of an impacted common bile duct stone in a 64-year-old patient who presented with severe acute biliary pancreatitis. At emergency endoscopic retrograde cholangiopancreatography the impacted stone, as well as a bulging and deformed papilla, were noted. Sphincterotomy and stone extraction were successfully performed. (*Courtesy of* Alfred D. Roston, MD, and David L. Carr-Locke, MD.)

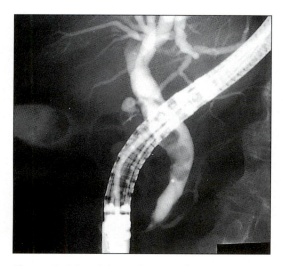

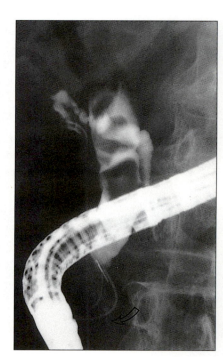

Figure 5-40. During endoscopic retrograde cholangiopancreatography a sphincterotome (*arrow*) is in position, and a sphincterotomy is in progress. Note the common bile duct dilatation, as well as the patent cystic duct, square common bile duct stones, and air in the proximal biliary tree. (*Courtesy of* Alfred D. Roston, MD, and David L. Carr-Locke, MD.)

Figure 5-39. This patient underwent endoscopic retrograde cholangiopancreatography after presenting with abnormal results in liver function tests, jaundice, and a long history of biliary pain. The cholangiogram revealed dilatation of the common bile duct to 12 mm and three rounded filling defects measuring 10 mm each. The cystic duct was patent and filled the gallbladder, which contained two large stones, each measuring approximately 2 cm. There is some residual contrast in the main pancreatic duct, which filled from the bile duct via a common channel. (*Courtesy of* Alfred D. Roston, MD, and David L. Carr-Locke, MD.)

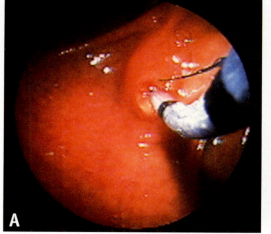

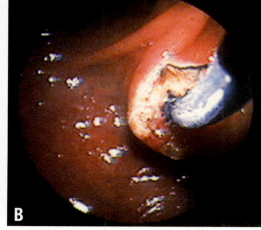

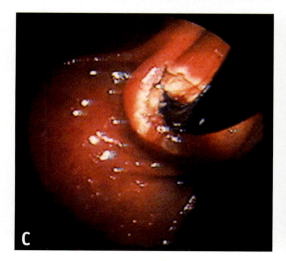

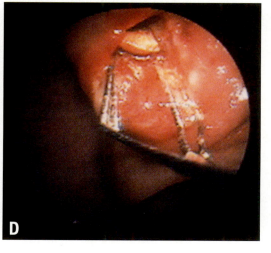

Figure 5-41. Endoscopic view of sphincterotomy and basket extraction of common bile duct stones. **A**, The sphincterotome is within the common bile duct. **B**, The sphincterotomy is performed using electrocautery and extended toward the 11 o'clock to 12 o'clock position. After completion of sphincterotomy, the basket catheter is deployed under fluoroscopic guidance (**C**) and withdrawn through the papilla along with several common bile duct stones (**D**). (*Courtesy of* Alfred D. Roston, MD, and David L. Carr-Locke, MD.)

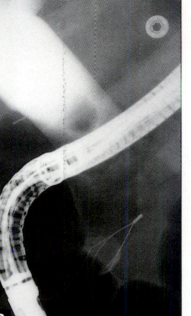

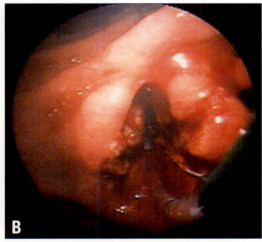

Figure 5-42. Radiographic view of the basket extraction of common bile duct stones shown in Figure 5-41. **A,** The biliary basket catheter has entrapped two common bile duct stones, each measuring approximately 18 mm. The proximal biliary tree is significantly dilated (27 mm). **B,** Delivery of one stone through the papilla is shown. (*Courtesy of* Alfred D. Roston, MD, and David L. Carr-Locke, MD.)

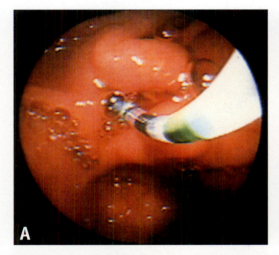

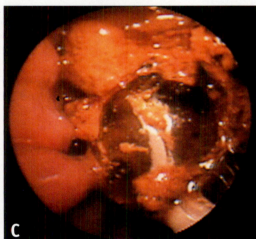

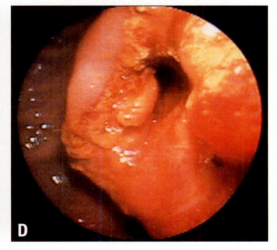

Figure 5-43. Balloon extraction of common bile duct stones after sphincterotomy. **A,** The bile duct is cannulated using a sphincterotome. **B,** Electrocautery is applied and sphincterotomy is performed in a 12 o'clock direction. The balloon catheter is inserted under fluoroscopic guidance, then inflated and withdrawn towards the endoscope. **C,** When the catheter is withdrawn, stone debris is seen emanating from the papilla. **D,** After sphincterotomy and stone extraction, the biliary orifice is patent. (*Courtesy of* Alfred D. Roston, MD, and David L. Carr-Locke, MD.)

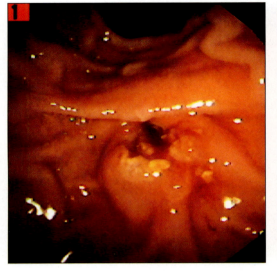

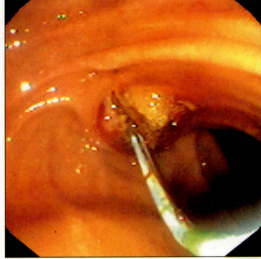

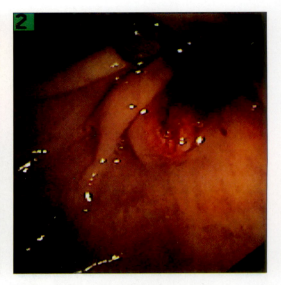

Figure 5-44. Status post sphincterotomy. This patient had a common bile duct stone that was treated with sphincterotomy and stone extraction. This image from the duodenum demonstrates a typical image of the papilla of Vater after sphincterotomy. (*Courtesy of* Harvey Young, MD.)

Figure 5-45. Sphincterotomy with sphincterotome in place. This duodenal image of the papilla of Vater demonstrates a sphincterotome with catheter and wire in place across the papilla of Vater. The initial cut has been made across the roof of the papilla of Vater. (*Courtesy of* Harvey Young, MD.)

Figure 5-46. Sphincterotomy with stone extraction. This patient has undergone a sphincterotomy of a papilla of Vater located next to a diverticulum in the duodenum. The sphincterotomy is seen in the foreground with a dark stone having been extracted and lying immediately above the sphincterotomy. (*Courtesy of* Harvey Young, MD.)

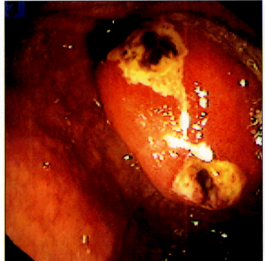

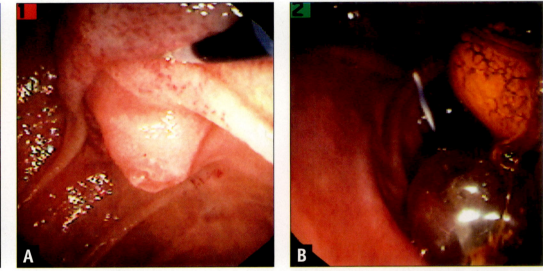

Figure 5-47. Stone eroding through papilla. An enlarged papilla of Vater with a stone in the superior portion eroding through the mucosa is demonstrated. The actual opening to the ampulla of Vater is inferior to the area of the eroding common bile duct stone. (*Courtesy of* Harvey Young, MD.)

Figure 5-48. Endoscopic sphincterotomy. **A,** An enlarged papilla of Vater is seen with the orifice in the center of the papilla, extending into the duodenum. **B,** A wire and balloon have been placed into the common bile duct with extraction of a stone seen off to the right in this image. (*Courtesy of* Harvey Young, MD.)

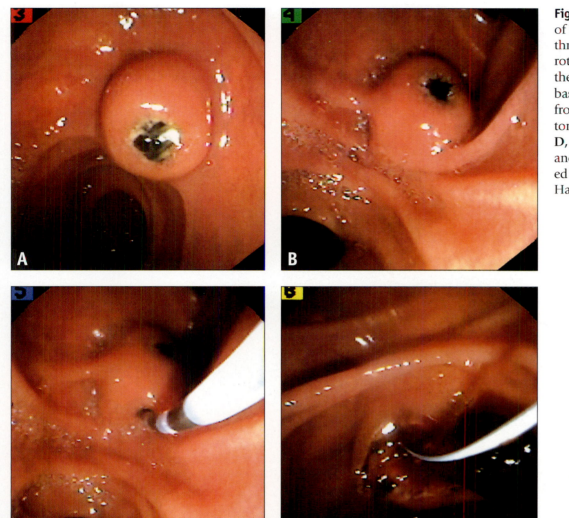

Figure 5-49. Stone eroding through papilla of Vater. **A,** A dark stone is seen eroding through an enlarged papilla of Vater. **B,** With rotation of the endoscope, the opening of the ampulla of Vater is vaguely seen at the base of the papilla of Vater, some distance from the eroding stone. **C,** The sphincterotome is inserted into the papilla of Vater. **D,** A sphincterotomy has been performed and a stone, off to the right, has been extracted from the common bile duct. (*Courtesy of* Harvey Young, MD.)

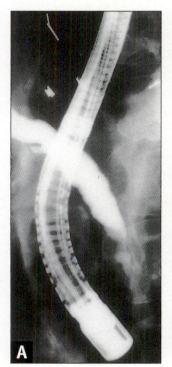
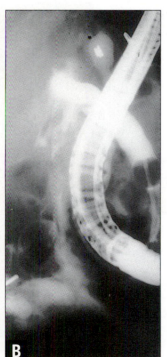

Figure 5-50. **A–B,** Endoscopic retrograde cholangiopancreatogram of the patient in Figure 5-43 shows inflated balloon catheter. Smaller stones can be removed after balloon dilation of the papilla without sphincterotomy. (*Courtesy of* Alfred D. Roston, MD, and David L. Carr-Locke, MD.)

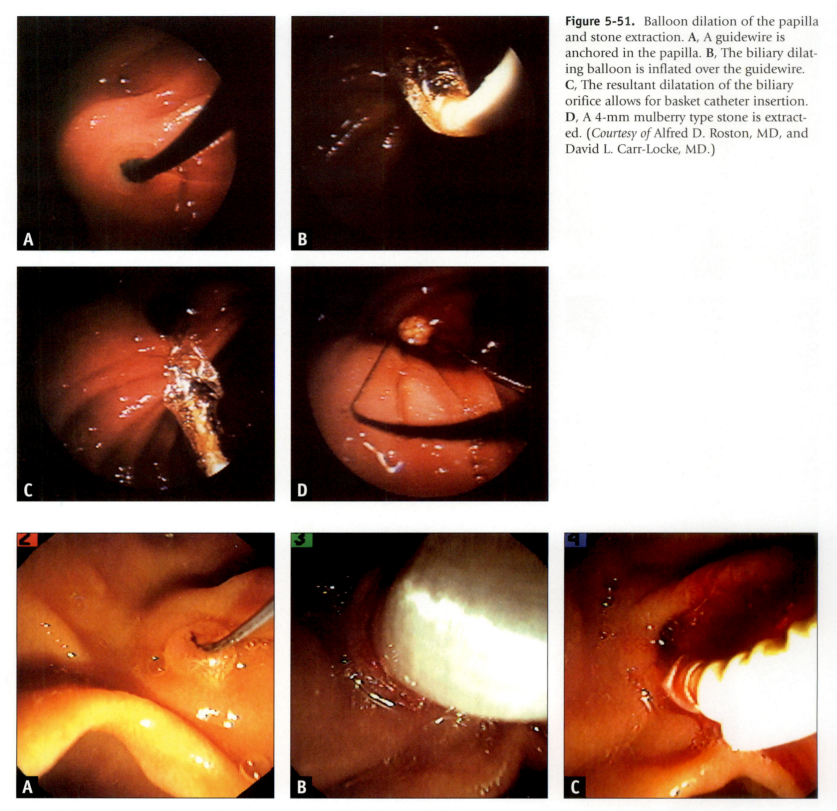

Figure 5-51. Balloon dilation of the papilla and stone extraction. **A,** A guidewire is anchored in the papilla. **B,** The biliary dilating balloon is inflated over the guidewire. **C,** The resultant dilatation of the biliary orifice allows for basket catheter insertion. **D,** A 4-mm mulberry type stone is extracted. (*Courtesy of* Alfred D. Roston, MD, and David L. Carr-Locke, MD.)

Figure 5-52. Balloon sphincteroplasty for treatment of choledocholithiasis. **A,** Catheter through papilla of Vater within the common bile duct. **B,** Sphincteroplasty is performed by inflating the balloon across the papilla of Vater. **C,** The balloon is now deflated while the catheter remains traversing the papilla of Vater.

(Continued on next page)

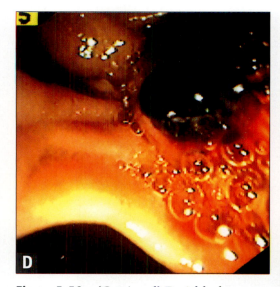

Figure 5-52. *(Continued)* **D,** A black stone has been extracted from the common bile duct and is seen laying on top of the papilla of Vater. (*Courtesy of* Harvey Young, MD.)

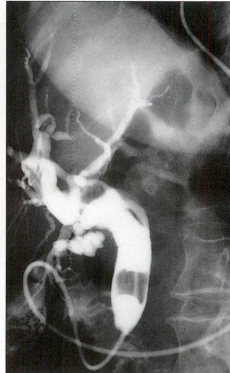

Figure 5-53. Cholangitis. In patients with calculous cholangitis, initial management consists of stabilization with intravenous fluids and antibiotics. After the patient responds appropriately, endoscopic retrograde cholangiopancreatography (ERCP) is indicated. If the patient cannot be stabilized within 24 hours (or presents with shock or mental status change), emergency ERCP should be undertaken. Options at ERCP include placement of a nasobiliary tube or endoprosthesis to establish bile duct drainage. This elderly patient presented with acute suppurative cholangitis. ERCP revealed a faceted stone that was not easily removable. A nasobiliary tube was placed and copious pus was drained until the patient was stabilized. The patient then underwent successful sphincterotomy with stone extraction. (*Courtesy of* Alfred D. Roston, MD, and David L. Carr-Locke, MD.)

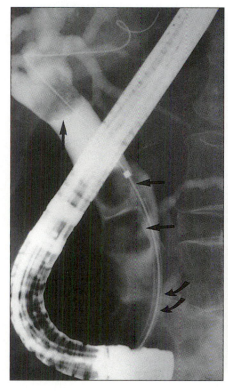

Figure 5-54. This patient presented with severe acute cholangitis and several large, square stones (*straight arrows*). A biliary endoprosthesis was placed (*curved arrows*). (*Courtesy of* Alfred D. Roston, MD, and David L. Carr-Locke, MD.)

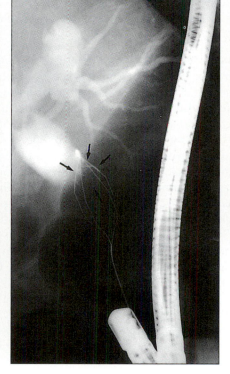

Figure 5-55. Extraction of common bile duct stones may be hindered by surgically altered anatomy. One example of altered anatomy is Billroth II partial gastrectomy, shown here with basket extraction of a common bile duct stone (*arrows*). (*Courtesy of* Alfred D. Roston, MD, and David L. Carr-Locke, MD.)

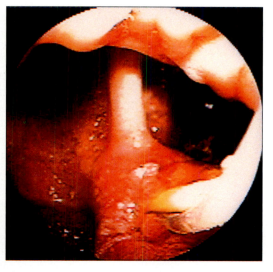

Figure 5-56. Another example is a periampullary diverticulum. Modified accessories and techniques, including needle-knife and reverse papillotomes, greatly facilitate access and ductal clearance rates in these circumstances. (*Courtesy of* Alfred D. Roston, MD, and David L. Carr-Locke, MD.)

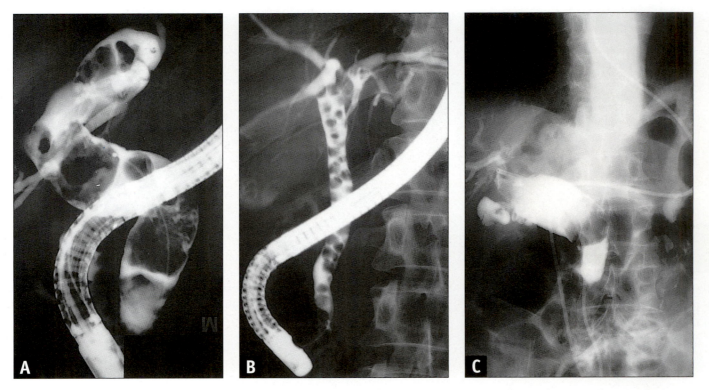

Figure 5-57. After successful sphincterotomy, additional factors may further hinder stone extraction. These include stones larger than 25 mm (**A**), intrahepatic stones, large numbers of stones (**B**), impacted stones, a tortuous or sigmoid bile duct, stones located proximal to a stricture, and a disproportion in the size of the distal bile duct compared with the size of the stone (**C**). (*Courtesy of* Alfred D. Roston, MD, and David L. Carr-Locke, MD.)

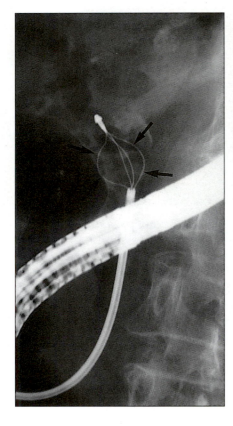

Figure 5-58. Mechanical lithotripsy. With the use of additional endoscopic techniques for extraction of difficult bile duct stones the extraction rate may be as high as 96%. Mechanical lithotripsy employs a modified wire biliary basket device with increased tensile strength and a covering metal sheath attached to a cranking handle. The common bile duct stone is entrapped within a lithotripsy basket (*arrows*). The metal sheath along the lithotripsy basket is passed through the endoscope. After the stone has been engaged, a cranking mechanism closes the basket against the metal sheath, thereby crushing the entrapped stone. There is also air in the biliary tree proximally.

Laser and electrohydraulic lithotripsy depend on local expertise. Successful shockwave focusing may be used with mother-daughter endoscope systems and intraductal/extraductal sonographic or fluoroscopic targeting. Laser lithotripsy clearance range rates range from 80% to 90%. The electrohydraulic lithotripsy clearance rate approaches 86%. Chemical dissolution of bile duct stones is hampered by the catheter delivery systems, which require appropriate contact. Agents such as monooctanoin and methyl-*tert*-butyl ether have been used, and dissolution rates range from 25% to 30%. Other options include placement of a biliary endoprosthesis or nasobiliary catheter. These are temporizing maneuvers, and in the case of cholangitis, may allow for further improvement and subsequent elective therapy. (*Courtesy of* Alfred D. Roston, MD, and David L. Carr-Locke, MD.)

Sphincter of Oddi Dysfunction

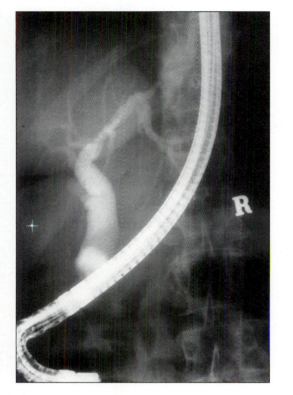

Figure 5-59. Endoscopic retrograde cholangiopancreatography is an important investigation in the study of sphincter of Oddi dysfunction. It excludes the common causes of postcholecystectomy biliary pain such as stone or stricture formation. In some patients, as illustrated in this figure, the bile duct may be dilated without an obvious cause. (*From* Toouli [25]; with permission.)

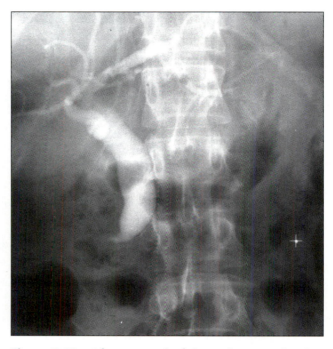

Figure 5-60. After removal of the endoscope, the time to empty contrast from the bile duct into the duodenum is observed. In some patients with suspected sphincter of Oddi dysfunction, contrast may not pass from the bile duct into the duodenum for quite some time. This is a subjective sign, and it is thought that delay in excess of 45 minutes suggests the possibility of sphincter of Oddi dysfunction. This observation has not been shown to objectively correlate with manometry or response to division of the sphincter. (*Courtesy of* James Toouli, PhD.)

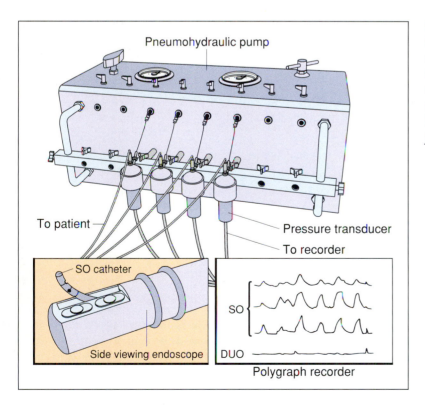

Figure 5-61. The equipment used for manometric measurement from the sphincter of Oddi (SO). Sterile water is perfused through a pneumohydraulic perfusion system via pressure transducers to a triple-lumen catheter. The triple-lumen catheter is inserted into either the bile duct or pancreatic duct via the biopsy channel of a duodenoscope. The rate of perfusion of water through the catheter is 0.125 mL/minute for each lumen. DUO—duodenum. (*Adapted from* Toouli [25].)

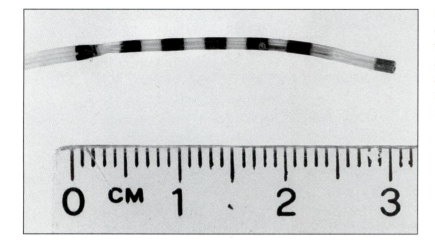

Figure 5-62. Triple-lumen catheter that is used to record sphincter of Oddi manometry. The catheter has three openings that are positioned at 2-mm intervals starting 5 mm from the tip. The lumens are marked; the markings extend proximally at 2-mm intervals and are used by the endoscopist to gauge the depth of insertion of the manometry catheter into either the pancreatic duct or the bile duct. (*Courtesy of* James Toouli, PhD.)

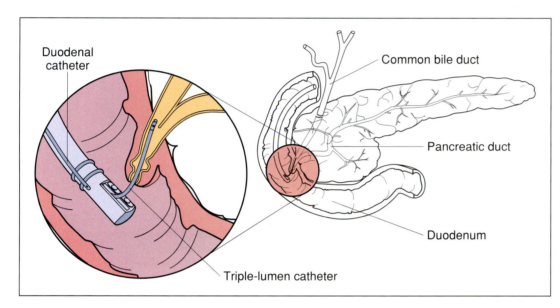

Figure 5-63. Endoscopic manometry is performed with the use of a standard duodenoscope. The manometric catheter is introduced into either the common bile duct or the pancreatic duct to record ductal pressures. It is then withdrawn so that the three recording lumens are situated within the sphincter of Oddi. A separate catheter may simultaneously record duodenal pressure. (*Adapted from* Toouli [25].)

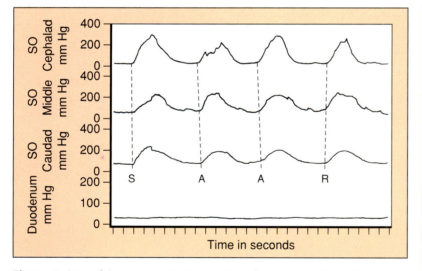

Figure 5-64. This representative tracing shows recordings from the sphincter of Oddi (SO) and duodenum. The sphincter has a low tone on which are superimposed prominent phasic contractions. The contractions are primarily orientated in an antegrade (A) direction. However, in addition, some waves are orientated in a retrograde (R) direction or are simultaneous (S). Simultaneous recording from the duodenum shows that the activity of the sphincter of Oddi is independent of duodenal contractions. (*Adapted from* Toouli [25].)

Normal Sphincter of Oddi Pressures

	Normal		
	Median	**Range**	**Abnormal**
Basal pressure (mm Hg)	15	3–35	>40
Amplitude (mm Hg)	135	95–135	>300
Frequency (number/minute)	4	2–6	>7
Sequences			
Antegrade (%)	80	12–100	
Simultaneous (%)	13	0–50	
Retrograde (%)	9	0–50	>50
CCK 20 ng/kg		Inhibits	Contracts

CCK—cholecystokinin.

Figure 5-65. Normal sphincter of Oddi pressures as recorded by sphincter of Oddi manometry. Abnormal pressures are arbitrarily defined as those in excess of the three standard deviation value. (*Courtesy of* James Toouli, PhD.)

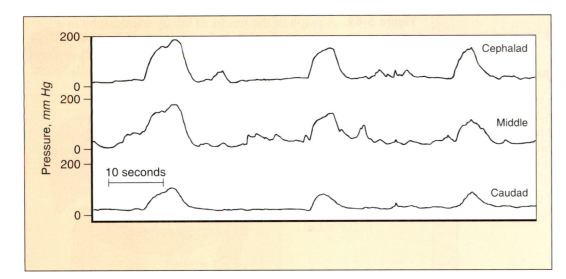

Figure 5-66. Manometrically the sphincter of Oddi is characterized by a low basal pressure on which are superimposed prominent phasic contractions. The contractions occur at a frequency of approximately four per minute and are mainly orientated in an antegrade direction. (*Courtesy of* James Toouli, PhD.)

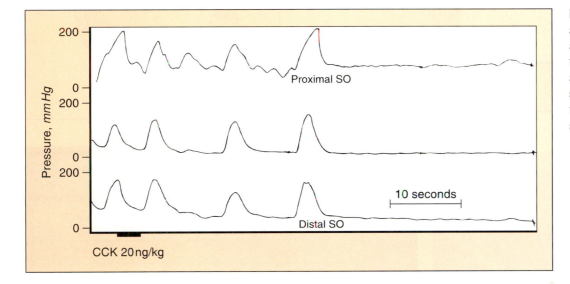

Figure 5-67. The normal response to administration of cholecystokinin (CCK) in a patient during recording from the sphincter of Oddi (SO). The phasic contractions are inhibited and the basal pressure of the sphincter of Oddi falls. These effects are thought to enhance flow of fluid through the sphincter. (*Courtesy of* James Toouli, PhD.)

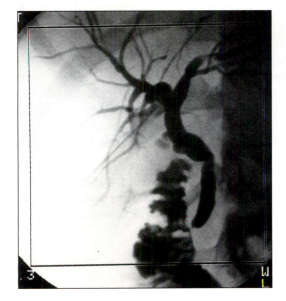

Figure 5-68. Radiograph of a patient who had sphincter of Oddi dysfunction with fixed stenosis of the sphincter. The stenosis is demonstrated by the stricture at the lower end of the bile duct. This patient presented with recurrent pain and abnormal liver enzyme levels. The patient was classified as having type 1 sphincter of Oddi dysfunction and was cured by division of the sphincter. (*Courtesy of* James Toouli, PhD.)

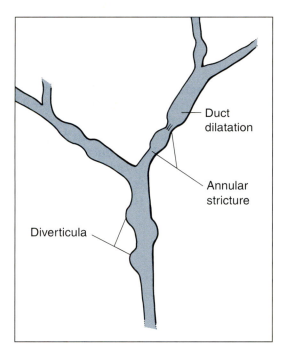

Figure 5-75. Several of the features found on cholangiograms in patients with primary sclerosing cholangitis are schematically depicted. Endoscopic retrograde cholangiopancreatography is the method of choice to examine the biliary tree in these patients. Percutaneous cholangiography is often not able to visualize the biliary tree adequately because of problems identifying sclerotic intrahepatic biliary radicals. Typical findings are multifocal stricturing and irregularity involving both the intrahepatic and the extrahepatic biliary trees. Approximately 20% of the time only intrahepatic ducts will be involved. Strictures are typically diffuse and annular with intervening segments of normal of slightly dilated ducts. Diverticular outpouchings are found in 25% of patients. (*Courtesy of* Keith D. Lindor, MD.)

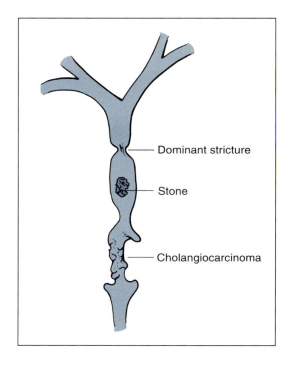

Figure 5-76. This figure illustrates three biliary complications that can lead to recurrent cholangitis and rapidly progressive cholestasis in patients with primary sclerosing cholangitis (PSC). These complications include the formation of a dominant stricture, which is usually due to progression of any one of the many strictures in the biliary tract; the formation of a stone related either to sluggish bile flow and precipitation of cholesterol crystals or, in the setting of recurrent cholangitis, to bacterial deconjugation of bilirubin and precipitation of pigment stones; and lastly, the formation of a cholangiocarcinoma, which is often characterized by longer strictures with overhanging margins and a polypoid appearance. Patients with rapidly progressive jaundice or recurrent cholangitis in the setting of PSC should undergo cholangiography to identify any of these three features. Cholangiography may assist in the resolution of problems related to dominant strictures or biliary stones. The dominant strictures can be dilated and stented, often times with excellent results, and the stones can usually be removed endoscopically. The preferred route for approaching dominant biliary strictures depends upon both the cholangiographic and radiographic appearance. For strictures high in the biliary tree near the liver hilus, when possible, the endoscopic route is preferable, although such strictures may need to be handled percutaneously. Lower strictures should be approached endoscopically. Biliary stone disease occurs in about 25% of patients with PSC, although most stones are confined to the gallbladder [31]. Nevertheless, when cholangitis occurs, one should be certain to exclude choledocholithiasis, which can generally be treated endoscopically. Lastly, cholangiocarcinoma appears in 10 to 15% of patients with PSC, often as the disease becomes advanced [32]. Early detection is desirable, although the management of cholangiocarcinoma complicating sclerosing cholangitis is difficult. Surgery is frequently unsuccessful. Radiation and chemotherapy have not been shown to be useful in most patients. Other than incidentally discovered cholangiocarcinomas at the time of liver transplantation for PSC, many centers now will not perform liver transplantation for these tumors. (*Courtesy of* Keith D. Lindor, MD.)

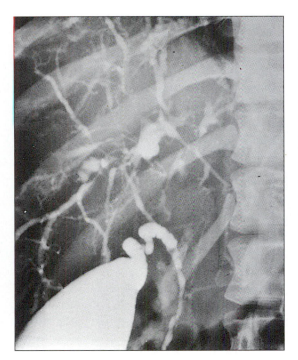

Figure 5-77. Classic cholangiographic appearance of sclerosing cholangitis. Multifocal strictures and intervening cholangiectatic ductal segments are seen. (*Courtesy of* Keith D. Lindor, MD.)

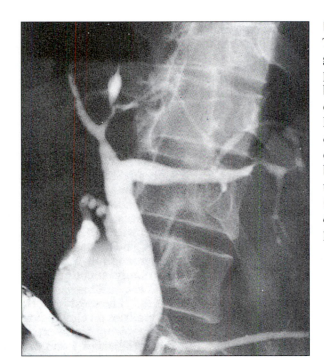

Figure 5-78. This cholangiogram shows pruning and beading of the intrahepatic bile ducts; the extrahepatic bile ducts are unremarkable. (*From* Lindor *et al.* [33]; with permission.)

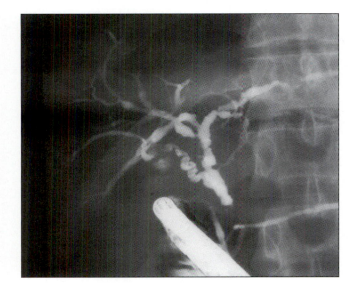

Figure 5-79. ERCP with cholangiogram demonstrating PSC. This 31-year-old policeman was evaluated for intermittent right upper quadrant pain and weight loss. Serial liver tests showed 3-5-fold elevation of alkaline phosphate. A liver biopsy had been performed prior to this cholangiogram and showed a portal tract infiltrate with mild periductal changes suggesting primary sclerosing cholangitis. This cholangiogram demonstrates the typical beading and stricturing of the intrahepatic and extrahepatic biliary tree. A later flexible sigmoidoscopy with biopsy demonstrated ulcerative colitis.

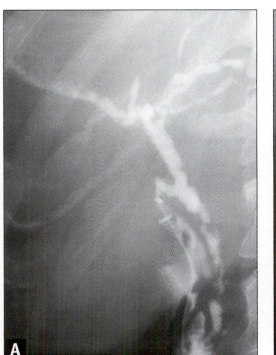

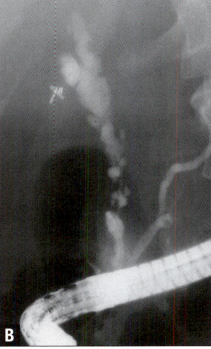

Figure 5-80. Cholangiogram demonstrating PSC. A 30-year-old male medical technologist presented with fatigue and cholestatic abnormalities of liver tests. An episode of right upper quadrant abdominal pain with hyperbilirubinemia associated with an abnormal biliary scintigram not visualizing the gallbladder led to exploratory laparotomy and operative cholangiogram. **A,** An operative cholangiogram demonstrates beading and stricturing of the common bile duct, particularly distally, and also the intrahepatic bile ducts. **B,** ERCP performed 1 year later once again demonstrates beading and stricturing of the distal common bile duct.

A

B

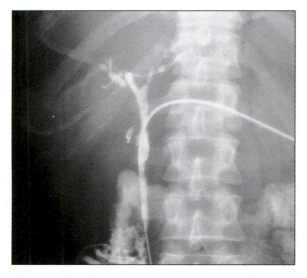

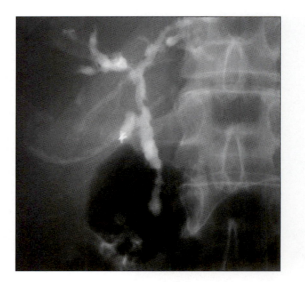

Figure 5-81. Tube cholangiogram with dilation of strictures. The same patient described in Figure 5-80 later underwent percutaneous catheterization of the biliary tree with internal/external tube drainage over the course of 1 year, providing decompression of the biliary tree and resolution of cholestasis.

Figure 5-82. ERCP showing PSC. The same patient described in Figures 5-80 and 5-81 underwent ERCP 2 years after a period of internal/external tube drainage, and changes of primary sclerosing cholangitis are still demonstrated with stricturing of the distal common bile duct and intrahepatic bile ducts. This patient later underwent successful liver transplantation after liver failure ensued.

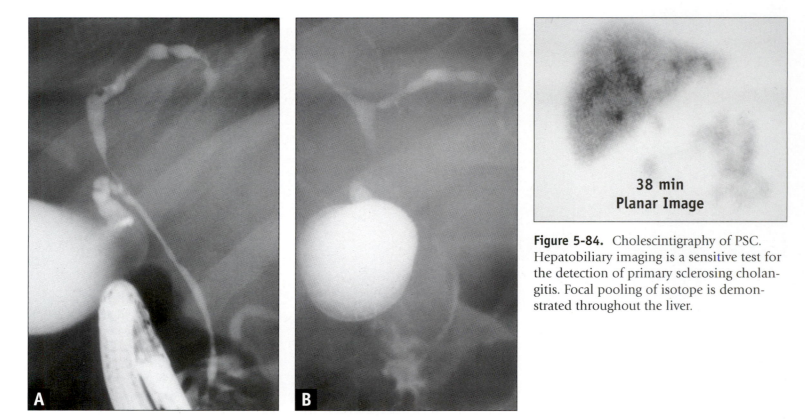

38 min Planar Image

Figure 5-84. Cholescintigraphy of PSC. Hepatobiliary imaging is a sensitive test for the detection of primary sclerosing cholangitis. Focal pooling of isotope is demonstrated throughout the liver.

Figure 5-83. PSC showing diffuse, tight stricturing of the entire common bile duct. A 41-year-old man with known ulcerative colitis and 4 years of stable primary sclerosing cholangitis presented with jaundice and pruritus over a 2-month period. Serum bilirubin was 5.5 mg/dL and alkaline phosphatase 720 U/L. **A,** ERCP demonstrates diffuse, tight stricturing of the entire common bile duct with a particularly tight stricture near the confluence of the right and left hepatic ducts. Injection of contrast preferentially overfills the gallbladder, with only a small amount of contrast passing the tight stricture to fill intrahepatic bile ducts. **B,** The minimal filling of intrahepatic bile ducts is noted on these images with no demonstrated contrast in the area of a tight stricture at the confluence of the right and left hepatic ducts.

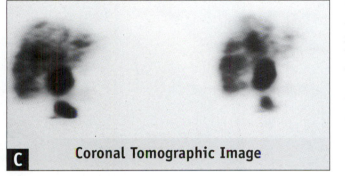

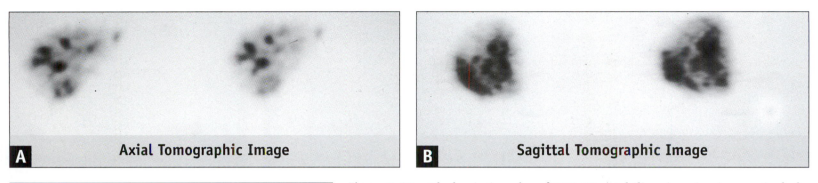

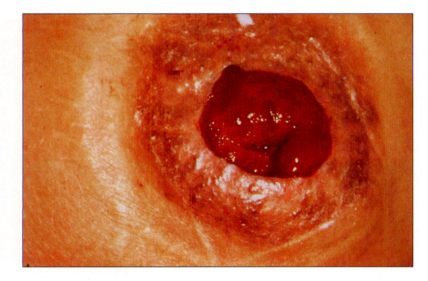

Figure 5-85. Cholescintigraphy of PSC. Hepatobiliary imaging is a particularly sensitive test for the detection of primary sclerosing cholangitis when tomographic techniques are employed. **A**, Axial tomographic image shows irregular focal pooling of isotope compatible with the diagnosis of primary sclerosing cholangitis. **B**, Sagittal tomographic image demonstrates similar findings with more concentrated isotope. **C**, Coronal tomographic image again demonstrates focal pooling of isotope, with all images supporting the diagnosis of primary sclerosing cholangitis rather than diffuse hepatocellular disease.

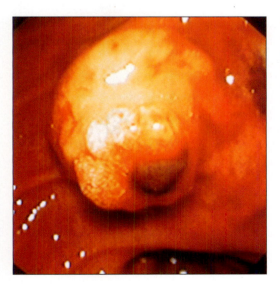

Figure 5-86. Peristomal varices. Peristomal varices may develop in patients with preexisting ulcerative colitis who have undergone a colectomy with an ileostomy [34]. Bleeding can be severe, and no effective local measures are able to control the bleeding. Portocaval shunts have been used, although liver transplantation, if feasible, may be the best way to manage these patients. (*From* Wiesner *et al.* [34]; with permission.)

Biliary Tract Infections and Stone Disease

Figure 5-87. Endoscopy in acute cholangitis. Stone disease remains the most common cause of cholangitis in most large series in the United States. Choledocholithiasis occurs in 8% to 15% of patients undergoing cholecystectomy; the incidence in patients more than 60 years of age is even higher, estimated at 15% to 60% in some series [35]. At endoscopy, the obstructing stone is often seen bulging from the papillary orifice, as in this figure. A recent randomized, controlled trial supports early endoscopic examination and intervention in cases of suspected stone-related acute cholangitis [36]. (*Courtesy of* Wendy Z. Davis, MD, and M. Stanley Branch, MD.)

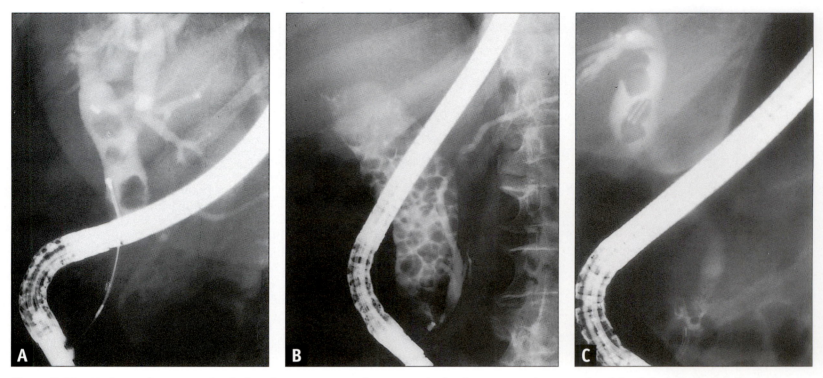

Figure 5-88. Endoscopic retrograde cholangiopancreatography (ERCP) in acute cholangitis. Cholangiography is the gold standard for the diagnosis of choledocholithiasis. **A–C**, Three examples of cholangiograms obtained by ERCP. The choledocholiths are visualized as filling defects as a column of contrast fills the common bile duct. Most stones that originate within the common bile duct are brown pigment stones. Electron microscopy has revealed that such stones are often associated with bacteria [37]. Periampullary diverticula also seem to increase the risk of choledocholith formation, perhaps by serving as a reservoir for intestinal bacteria [38]. The formation of a common bile duct stone around a surgical clip is shown in **panel C**. Foreign bodies, including suture material placed 30 years before the patient presented with common bile duct stones, have often been reported in association with choledocholithiasis [39]. (*Courtesy of* Wendy Z. Davis, MD, and M. Stanley Branch, MD.)

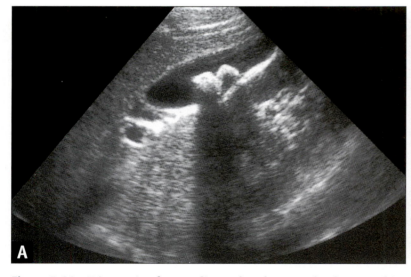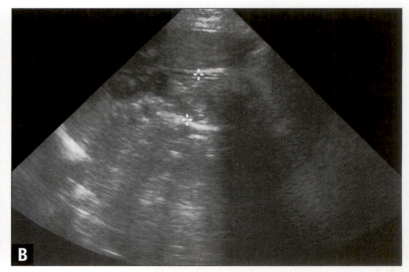

Figure 5-89. Diagnosis of stone disease by ultrasound. Ultrasound is certainly a reasonable early study in the patient presenting with right upper quadrant pain and fever. It is an excellent modality for visualization of gallstones, which appear as echogenic foci, usually mobile, within the gallbladder (**A**). In contrast, the role of ultrasound for diagnosis of common bile duct stones (seen in **panel B** as an echogenic focus within the common bile duct) is less clear. Cited sensitivities of ultrasound for actual visualization of choledocholithiasis range from 18% to 55% [40–42]. When a stone is seen in the duct, however, the finding is highly meaningful, with a positive predictive value of more than 85% [30,31]. A dilated common bile duct on ultrasound is not a reliable indicator of choledocholithiasis; positive predictive values are reported to range only between 34% and 72% [44–47]. (*Courtesy of* Wendy Z. Davis, MD, and M. Stanley Branch, MD.)

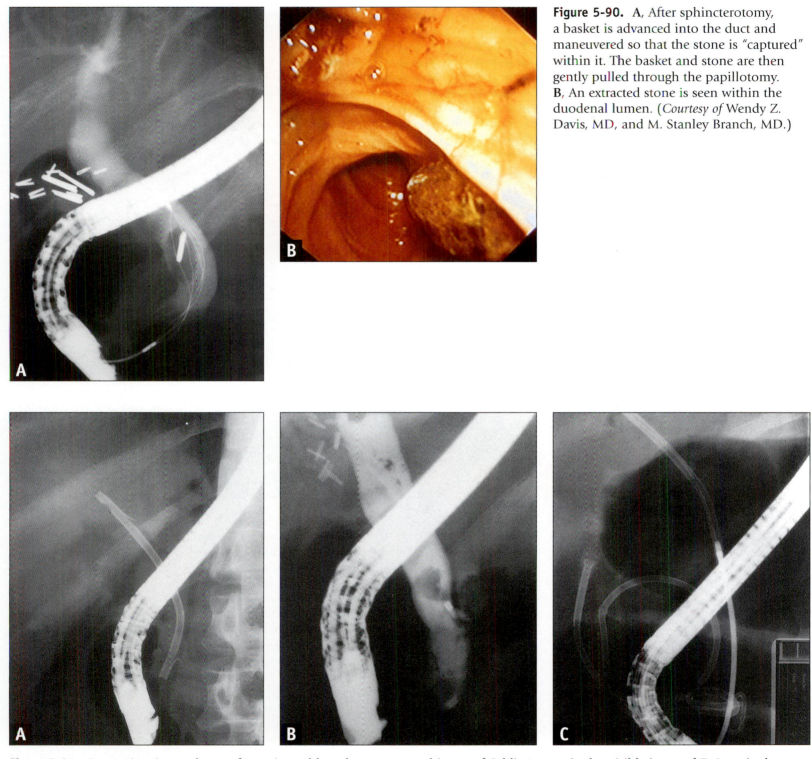

Figure 5-90. **A**, After sphincterotomy, a basket is advanced into the duct and maneuvered so that the stone is "captured" within it. The basket and stone are then gently pulled through the papillotomy. **B**, An extracted stone is seen within the duodenal lumen. (*Courtesy of* Wendy Z. Davis, MD, and M. Stanley Branch, MD.)

Figure 5-91. Stent migration and stone formation. Although stenting can provide excellent drainage in the setting of stones or biliary strictures, occasional migration and loss of adequate drainage occurs. In one large series, migration complicated stent placement in 5% of cases [48]. **A–C**, In the cholangiograms shown here, the stents have moved into the proximal duct from their original position across the sphincter of Oddi. A stone is also visible in **panel B**. Impaired drainage and the indwelling foreign body can result in symptoms of cholangitis. In **panel C**, a Soehendra stent remover (Wilson-Cook Medical, Winston-Salem, NC) has been placed up the duct to engage and extract the migrated stent. (*Courtesy of* Wendy Z. Davis, MD, and M. Stanley Branch, MD.)

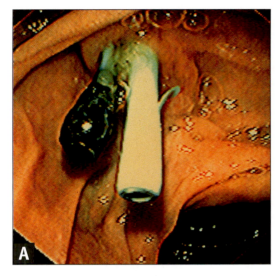

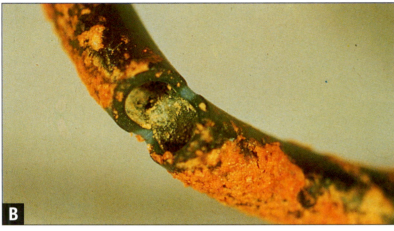

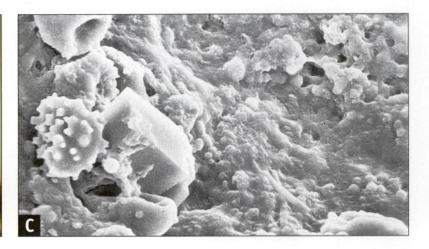

Figure 5-92.   Stent occlusion. Plastic stents are efficacious for short-term management but have a tendency to clog when left in situ for several months. One large study found the median patency of plastic stents to be only 126 days (the range was 7 to 482 days) [49]. **A–B**, The endoscopic appearance and ex vivo appearance of a clogged plastic stent are shown. Investigations have revealed that biofilm, an organic matrix of bacteria and their extracellular products, is primarily responsible for the phenomenon of stent occlusion [50,51]. **C**, An electron micrograph of biofilm is shown. Preliminary studies have suggested that eliminating side holes from stents, impregnating them with silver, or treating stent patients with aspirin or doxycycline may prolong stent survival [52–54]. Results from definitive clinical trials are not yet available. Patients with occluded plastic stents may present with fulminant cholangitis, requiring urgent stent exchange. (*Courtesy of* Wendy Z. Davis, MD, and M. Stanley Branch, MD.)

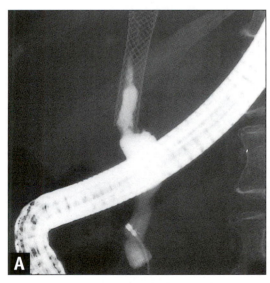

Figure 5-93.   Endoscopic treatment of metal stent occlusion. Expandable metal stents are often placed in malignant strictures or other settings where a permanent stent is required. Obstruction of metal stents due to sludge is uncommon [55]; however, tumor ingrowth causes significant difficulties. **A**, An occluded metal stent is seen on cholangiogram. In one study, 33% of patients with metal stents experienced stent occlusion; the majority presented with cholangitis. Median metal stent patency was 273 days, with a range of 14 to 363 days [49]. A plastic stent placed through the metal stent in this setting can restore biliary drainage, although use of the plastic stent does not provide an ideal solution. **B–C**, The cholangiographic appearance of plastic stents placed through metal stents is shown. A recent retrospective study at Duke University Medical Center examined all patients who underwent placement of plastic stents through indwelling metal stents. A total of 28 plastic stents were placed through metal stents. Five patients received single plastic stents; four of these were functional at the time of the patient's death (27 to 216 days after insertion). Ten other patients received a total of 22 plastic stents: 15 of these became occluded or migrated, 13 were replaced by another endoscopic plastic stent, and 2 required percutaneous management. The median time to occlusion or migration was 60 days [56]. (*Courtesy of* Wendy Z. Davis, MD, and M. Stanley Branch, MD.)

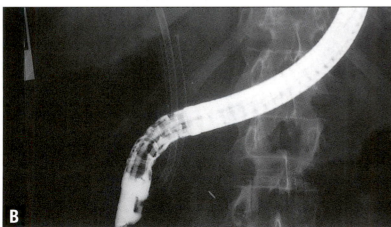

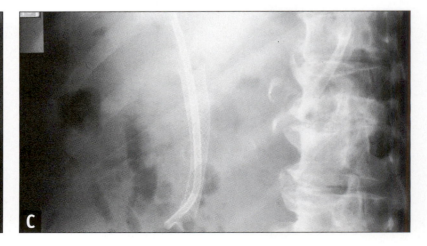

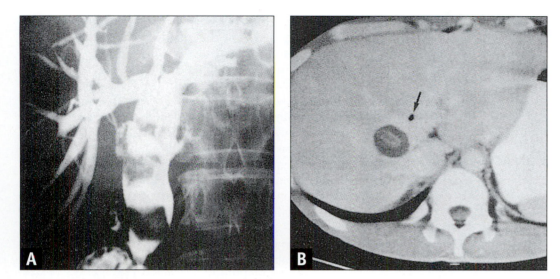

Figure 5-94. Endoscopic retrograde cholangiopancreatography (ERCP), CT, and histopathology in Oriental cholangiohepatitis. Oriental cholangiohepatitis, or recurrent

pyogenic cholangitis, is defined by recurrent episodes of abdominal pain, fever, and jaundice associated with intrahepatic and extrahepatic bile duct stones. The syndrome is common in Southeast Asia; in Hong Kong, it is the most common disease of the biliary tract [57]. With the influx of Asian immigrants, the disease is being seen with increasing frequency in the United States. The presentation is usually a dramatic illustration of Charcot's triad. Cholangiographic findings may include prominent filling defects and marked dilation of intrahepatic and extrahepatic systems; more peripheral intrahepatic ducts taper abruptly (**A**). On CT scan (**B**), a cystically dilated common duct with indwelling stone is seen; pneumobilia is shown at the *arrow*. (*From* Lim [58]; with permission.)

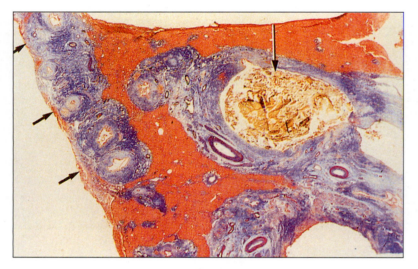

Figure 5-95. A portion of resected liver is shown. A pigmented stone occupies the lumen of a dilated bile duct (*long arrow*); marked fibrosis of adjacent small bile ducts is also seen (*short arrows*). Bile cultures yielded enteric bacteria, chiefly *Escherichia coli*. Attacks may respond to antibiotic therapy alone, but generally stones must be removed and optimal biliary drainage restored to allow recovery. In one report, sphincterotomy provided up to 7 years of remission [57]. Despite aggressive endoscopic and surgical intervention, the disease may recur; papillary stenosis, incomplete clearance of stones, or parasitic reinfestation (discussed later in this chapter) all may contribute to recrudescence of disease. (*From* Lim [58]; with permission.)

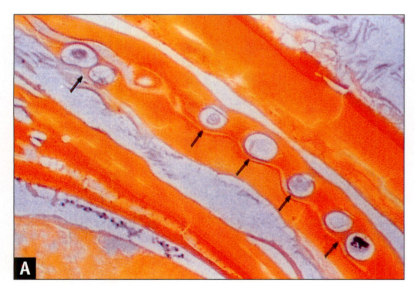

Figure 5-96. Pathophysiology of Oriental cholangiohepatitis and the role of parasitic infection. The cause of Oriental cholangiohepatitis is probably multifactorial; inadequate diet and sanitary conditions, bactibilia, and parasitic infestation are all associated with the syndrome. Clearly, many patients with the disease have parasitic infestation; the presence of *Clonorchis sinensis* or *Ascaris lumbricoides* within the biliary tree causes periductular inflammation, fibrosis, and stricturing, all of which contribute to bile stasis and intrahepatic stone formation. Histologic examination of stones in this setting has revealed evidence of the parasites [58]. **A**, The eggs of *C. sinensis* (*arrows*) are seen embedded in a pigmented stone.

(*Continued on next page*)

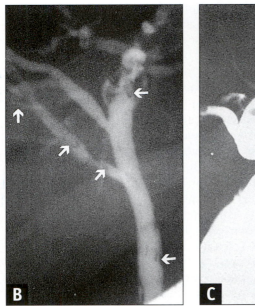
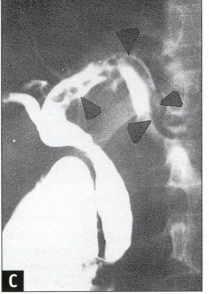

Figure 5-96. *(Continued)* **B,** The cholangiographic appearance of clonorchiasis is depicted; note the intraductal filling defects (*arrows*) and the blunting and irregularity of the terminal intrahepatic branches. **C,** The linear filling defect in the left hepatic duct (*arrows*) represents an ascaride. Treatment of patients known to have clonorchiasis with praziquantel will result in eradication of previously seen filling defects in serial cholangiograms; however, dilation and ductal irregularities persist [59]. Despite the clear association of some cases with parasitic infection, infestation alone likely is not adequate to produce the syndrome of recurrent cholangiohepatitis. Ong and colleagues found that patients with the syndrome had only a marginally higher infestation rate than patients in a general clinic population [60]. Colonization of the biliary tree by enteric bacteria also seems necessary to produce symptoms. It has been suggested that bacterial production of beta-glucuronidase, with subsequent increased hydrolysis of bilirubin, favors formation of calcium bilirubinate stones [57]. (**A,** *From* Lim [58]; with permission. **B,** *From* Leung *et al.* [59]; with permission. **C,** *From* Khuroo *et al.* [57]; with permission.)

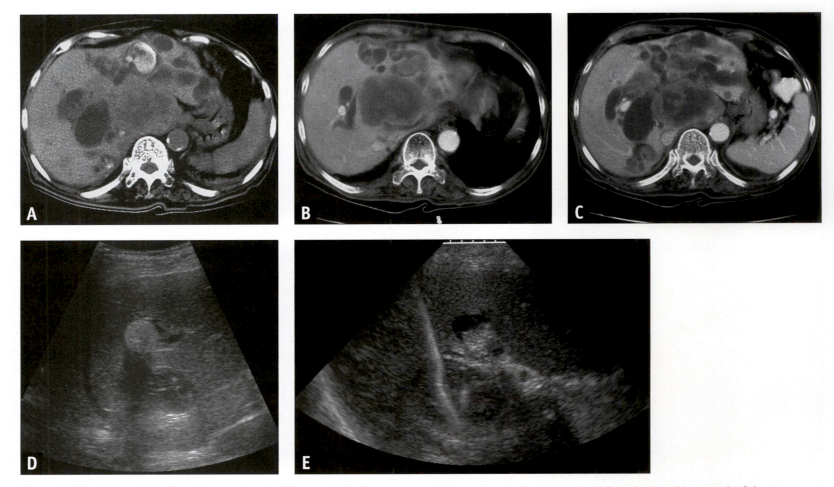

Figure 5-97. Oriental cholangiohepatitis. **A,** CT scan of the liver demonstrates multiple intrahepatic defects and stones, with one prominent stone in the anterior aspect of the liver. **B,** A large, negative shadow within the central portion of the liver is compatible with a large intrahepatic abscess. **C,** Further CT images inferior demonstrate multiple defects and stones within the liver as well as the large hepatic abscess that extends inferiorly. **D,** Ultrasound of the same patient demonstrates a large stone within the liver with the characteristic posterior acoustical shadowing. **E,** Under ultrasound guidance, a catheter is seen inserted transhepatically into the abscess cavity. Copious amounts of purulent material were drained from this abscess cavity. (*Courtesy of* Brooke Jeffrey, MD.)

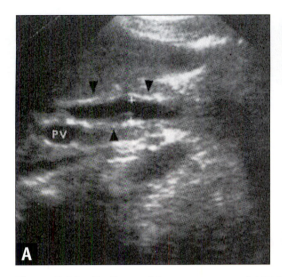

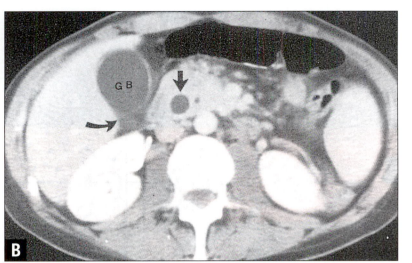

Figure 5-98. Radiographic appearance of AIDS cholangiopathy. Biliary tract disease is being reported with increasing frequency in the AIDS population. Abdominal pain and laboratory evidence of cholestasis are common clinical features that may prompt further investigation. Both ultrasound and CT may demonstrate cholangiographic abnormalities. **A,** This ultrasound depicts dilation (13 mm) and thickening (*arrowheads*) of the common bile duct in a case of cholangitis associated with cryptosporidiosis. **B,** This CT scan shows thickening of the gallbladder (GB) wall, pericholecystic fluid (*curved arrow*), and dilation of the common bile duct (*straight arrow*). PV—portal vein. (*From* Teixidor *et al.* [61]; with permission.)

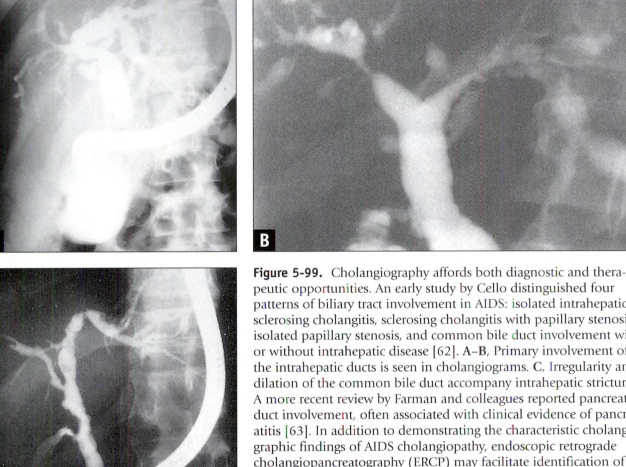

Figure 5-99. Cholangiography affords both diagnostic and therapeutic opportunities. An early study by Cello distinguished four patterns of biliary tract involvement in AIDS: isolated intrahepatic sclerosing cholangitis, sclerosing cholangitis with papillary stenosis, isolated papillary stenosis, and common bile duct involvement with or without intrahepatic disease [62]. **A–B,** Primary involvement of the intrahepatic ducts is seen in cholangiograms. **C,** Irregularity and dilation of the common bile duct accompany intrahepatic strictures. A more recent review by Farman and colleagues reported pancreatic duct involvement, often associated with clinical evidence of pancreatitis [63]. In addition to demonstrating the characteristic cholangiographic findings of AIDS cholangiopathy, endoscopic retrograde cholangiopancreatography (ERCP) may facilitate identification of an associated infectious organism via bile cultures and biliary biopsy specimens. Patients with papillary stenosis also may respond to endoscopic sphincterotomy; in one small series, sphincterotomy relieved abdominal pain in six of seven AIDS patients with papillary stenosis [64]. Another study found that sphincterotomy provided lasting relief of abdominal pain in all 20 patients thus treated [65]. (**A,** *Courtesy of* Wendy Z. Davis, MD, and M. Stanley Branch, MD. **B,** *From* Farman *et al.* [63]; with permission. **C,** *From* Bouche *et al.* [64]; with permission.)

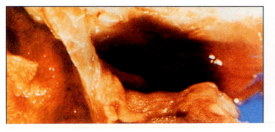
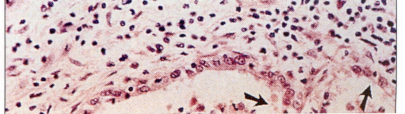

33. Lindor KD, Wiesner RH, MacCarty RL, *et al.*: Advances in primary sclerosing cholangitis. *Am J Med* 1990, 89:73–80.

34. Weisner RH, LaRusso NF, Dozois RR, *et al.*: Peristomal varices after proctolectomy in patients with primary sclerosing cholangitis. *Gastroenterology* 1988, 95:1036–1042.

35. NIH Consensus Conference Statement. *Am J Surg* 1993, 165:387–548.

36. Lai ECS, Mok FPT, Tan ES, *et al.*: Endoscopic biliary drainage for severe acute cholangitis. *N Engl J Med* 1992, 326:1582–1586.

37. Banez VP, Leung JWC: Endoscopic management of gallstone disease. In *Annual of Gastrointestinal Endoscopy*. Edited by Cotton PB. London: Current Science; 1990:79–89.

38. Skar V, Lotveit T, Osnes M: Juxtapapillary duodenal diverticula predispose to common bile duct stones. *Scand J Gastroenterol* 1989, 24:202–204.

39. Ormann W: A thread as a nidus of common bile duct calculus-findings during endoscopic lithotripsy. *Endoscopy* 1989, 21:191–192.

40. Mitchell SE, Clark RA: A comparison of computed tomography and sonography in choledocholithiasis. *AJR Am J Roentgenol* 1984, 142:729–733.

41. Shea JA: Preoperative evaluation of the biliary tract. *Surg Clin North Am* 1985, 65:47–58.

42. Cronan JJ: Ultrasound diagnosis of choledocholithiasis: A reappraisal. *Radiology* 1986, 161:133–134.

43. Blackbourne LH, Earnhardt RC, Sistrom CL, *et al.*: The sensitivity and role of ultrasound in the evaluation of biliary obstruction. *Am Surg* 1994, 60:683–690.

44. Van der Hul RL, Plaisier PW, Hamming JF, *et al.*: Detection and management of common bile duct stones in the era of laparoscopic cholecystectomy. *Scand J Gastroenterol* 1993, 28:929–933.

45. Hollis RA: Predictors of common bile duct abnormalities in patients undergoing ERCP prior to laparoscopic cholecystectomy [Abstract]. *Am J Gastroenterol* 1993, 88:1531.

46. Steele RJC, Park K, Gilbert F: Prediction of common bile duct stones: The importance of ultrasonic duct visualization [Abstract]. *Gut* 1991, F285:51–52.

47. Graham SM, Flowers JL, Scott TR, *et al.*: Laparoscopic cholecystectomy and common bile duct stones—the utility of planned perioperative ERCP and sphincterotomy: Experience with 62 patients. *Ann Surg* 1993, 218:61–67.

48. Johanson JF, Schmalz MJ, Geenen JE: Incidence and risk factors for biliary and pancreatic stent migration. *Gastrointest Endosc* 1992, 38:341–346.

49. Davids PH, Groen AK, Rauws EA, *et al.*: Randomized trial of self-expanding metal stents versus polyethylene stents for distal malignant biliary obstruction. *Lancet* 1992, 340:1488–1492.

50. Speer AG, Cotton PB, Rode J, *et al.*: Biliary stent blockage with bacterial biofilm; a light and electron microscopy study. *Ann Intern Med* 1988, 108:546–553.

51. Leung JW, Ling TKW, Kung JLS, *et al.*: The role of bacteria in the blockage of biliary stents. *Gastrointest Endosc* 1988, 34:19–22.

52. Leung JWC, Lau GTC, Sung JJY, *et al.*: Decreased bacterial adherence to silver-coated stent material: An in vitro study. *Gastrointest Endosc* 1992, 38:338–340.

53. Smit JM, Out MMJ, Groen AK, *et al.*: A placebo controlled study on the efficacy of aspirin and doxycycline in preventing clogging of biliary endoprostheses. *Gastrointest Endosc* 1989, 35:485–489.

54. Coene PPW, Groen AK, Cheng J, *et al.*: Clogging of biliary endoprostheses: A new perspective. *Gut* 1990, 31:913–917.

55. Cotton PB: Endoscopic management of biliary strictures. In *Annual of Gastrointestinal Endoscopy*. Edited by Cotton PB. London: Current Science; 1993:107–121.

56. Mundorf JB, Newcomer MK, Jowell PS, *et al.*: Plastic-through metal: Do plastic stents provide satisfactory decompression of occluded metal mesh stents? [Abstract]. *Gastrointest Endosc* 1995; 41:407.

57. Khuroo MS, Dar MY, Yattoo GN, *et al.*: Serial cholangiographic appearances in recurrent pyogenic cholangitis. *Gastrointest Endosc* 1993, 39:674–679.

58. Lim JH: Oriental cholangiohepatitis: Pathologic, clinical, and radiologic features. *AJR Am J Roentgenol* 1991, 157:1–8.

59. Leung JWC, Sung JY, Banez VP, *et al.*: Endoscopic cholangiopancreatography in hepatic clonorchiasis—a follow-up study. *Gastrointest Endosc* 1990, 36:360–363.

60. Ong GB: A study of recurrent pyogenic cholangitis. *Arch Surg* 1962, 84:199–225.

61. Teixidor HS, Godwin TA, Ramirez EA: Cryptosporidiosis of the biliary tract in AIDS. *Radiology* 1991, 180:51–56.

62. Cello J: Acquired immunodeficiency syndrome cholangiopathy: Spectrum of disease. *Am J Med* 1989, 86:539–546.

63. Farman J, Brunetti J, Baer JW, *et al.*: AIDS-related cholangiopancreatographic changes. *Abdom Imaging* 1994, 19:417–422.

64. Bouche H, Housset C, Dumont J-L, *et al.*: AIDS-related cholangitis: Diagnostic features and course in 15 patients. *J Hepatol* 1993, 17:34–39.

65. Benhamou Y, Caumes E, Gerosa Y, *et al.*: AIDS-related cholangiopathy—critical analysis of a prospective series of 26 patients. *Dig Dis Sci* 1993, 38:1113–1118.

66. Hasan FA, Jeffers LJ, Dickinson G, *et al.*: Hepatobiliary cryptosporidiosis and CMV infection mimicking metastatic cancer to the liver. *Gastroenterology* 1991, 100:1743–1748.

67. Cockerill III FR, Hurley DV, Malagelada JR, *et al.*: Polymicrobial cholangitis and Kaposi's sarcoma in blood product transfusion-related AIDS. *Am J Med* 1986, 80:1237–1241.

68. Ho F, Snape WJ, Venegas R, *et al.*: Choledochal fungal ball—an usual cause of biliary obstruction. *Dig Dis Sci* 1988, 33:1030–1034.

69. Noack KB, Osmon DR, Batts KP, *et al.*: Successful orthotopic liver transplantation in a patient with refractory biliary candidiasis. *Gastroenterology* 1991, 101:1728–1730.

70. Patel SA, Borges MC, Batt MD, *et al.*: Trichosporon cholangitis associated with hyperbilirubinemia, and findings suggesting primary sclerosing cholangitis on ERCP. *Am J Gastroenterol* 1990, 85:84–87.

71. Yamashita Y, Takahashi M, Kanazawa S, *et al.*: Parenchymal changes of the liver in cholangiocarcinoma: CT evaluation. *Gastrointest Radiol* 1992, 17:161–166.

72. Fan ZM, Yamashita Y, Harada M, *et al.*: Intrahepatic cholangiocarcinoma: Spin-echo and contrast-enhanced dynamic MR imaging. *Am J Roentgenol* 1993, 161:313–317.

73. Pitt HA, Dooley WC, Yeo CJ, *et al.*: Malignancies of the biliary tree. *Curr Probl Surg* 1995, 32:1–90.

74. Coons H: Metallic stents for the treatment of biliary obstruction. A report of 100 cases. *Cardiovasc Intervent Radiol* 1992, 15:367–374.

75. Iwai N, Yanagihara J, Tokiwa K, *et al.*: Congenital choledochal dilatation with emphasis on pathophysiology of the biliary tract. *Ann Surg* 1992, 215:27–30.

76. Tanaka K, Nishimura A, Yamada K, *et al.*: Cancer of the gallbladder associated with anomalous junction of the pancreatobiliary duct system without bile dilatation. *Br J Surg* 1993, 80:622–624.

77. Rosen CB, Nagorney DM, Wiesner RH, *et al.*: Cholangiocarcinoma complicating primary sclerosing cholangitis. *Ann Surg* 1991, 213:21–25.

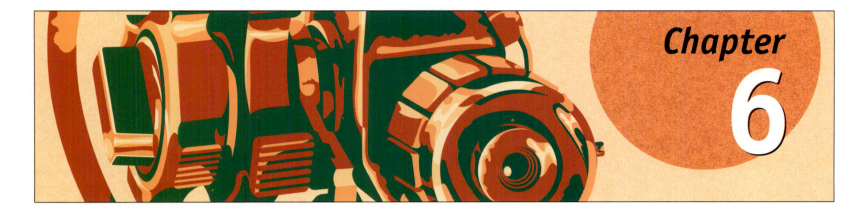

Pancreas

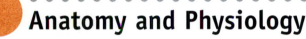

Anatomy and Physiology

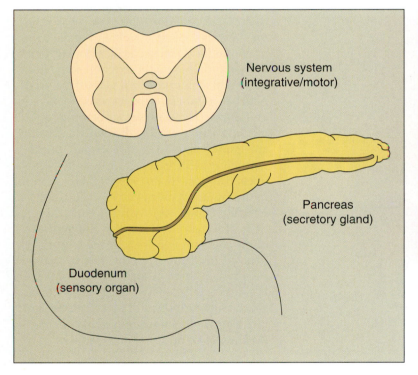

Figure 6-1. Pancreatic control system. Most pancreatic exocrine secretion is controlled through three systems. The duodenum and gastrointestinal tract act as the primary sensory organs for pancreatic function; the sensory information is relayed through nervous and hormonal mechanisms. The nervous system includes portions of the central nervous system, sensory and motor divisions of the autonomic nervous system, and an intrapancreatic nervous system. The nervous system is critical for integration of sensory and hormonal information and stimulation of pancreatic secretion. The pancreas is the glandular structure wherein all stimulatory pathways converge on the ductal and acinar cells. (*Courtesy of David C. Whitcomb, MD.*)

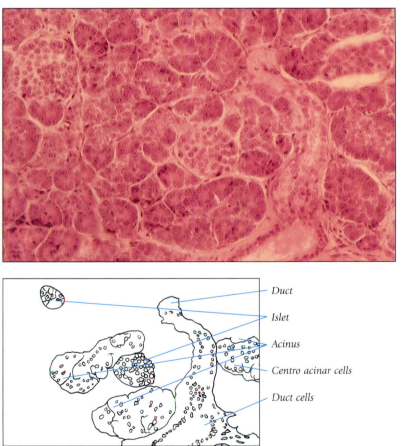

Figure 6-2. Overview of the pancreatic gland. The pancreatic gland contains three major types of cells. The *duct* cells make up about 10% of the pancreas and secrete solutions rich in bicarbonate. The *acinar* cells comprise over 80% of the pancreas and they synthesize and secrete pancreatic enzymes. The *islet* cells make up about 10% of the pancreas and form the endocrine portion of the pancreas. The four major types of islet cells secrete the hormones insulin, glucagon, somatostatin, and pancreatic polypeptide. (*Courtesy of David C. Whitcomb, MD.*)

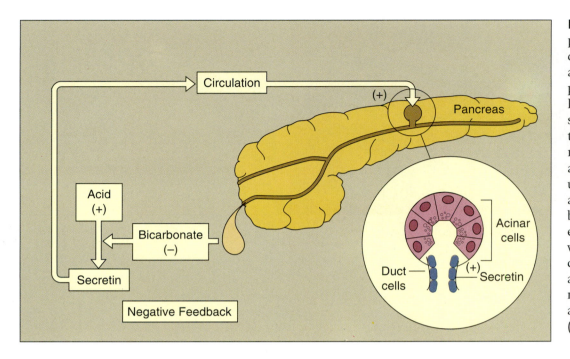

Figure 6-3. Neurohormonal control of pancreatic bicarbonate secretion. The pancreas plays a major role in neutralizing acidic chyme. The event, or stimulus, is the presence of duodenal acid, and the physiologic response is the pancreatic duct cells' secretion of bicarbonate, which enters into the duodenum and neutralizes the duodenal acid. The mechanism of sensation, amplification, and modulation is not fully understood, but the hormone secretin plays a central role. Thus, when the duodenum becomes acidic, secretin is released from endocrine cells in the duodenal mucosa, where it enters the blood stream. Pancreatic duct cells respond by secretion of bicarbonate-rich fluid until the duodenal pH is neutral, thus eliminating the stimulus and completing a negative feedback loop. (*Courtesy of* David C. Whitcomb, MD.)

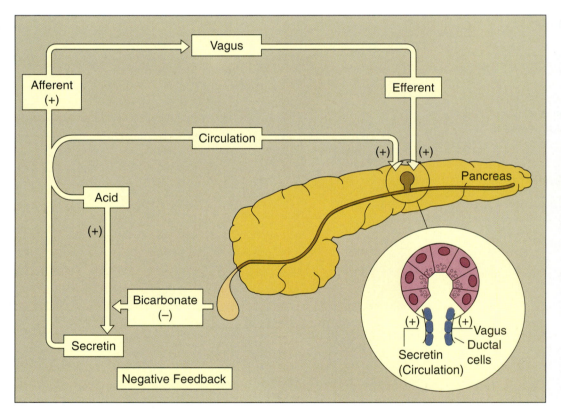

Figure 6-4. The vagus and bicarbonate secretion. The parasympathetic nervous system probably plays a major role in pancreatic bicarbonate secretion. This view is based on the observation that stimulation of the vagal trunk produces pancreatic bicarbonate secretions approaching peak secretion seen after a meal, and that acute transection of the vagus markedly diminishes the response to secretin. The afferent (sensory) vagal fibers may also be important in sensing the duodenal acidity and amplifying the effect of secretin, possibly through secretin receptors on afferent vagal fibers. This view is also supported by studies in the rat that demonstrate blockade of the effects of "physiologic" plasma concentrations of secretin with selective elimination of the afferent vagal fibers by the sensory neurotoxin capsaicin. As the dose of secretin increases, however, a larger fraction of the response is independent of the vagus nerve, suggesting recruitment of other mechanisms, including direct stimulation of ductal cells. (*Courtesy of* David C. Whitcomb, MD.)

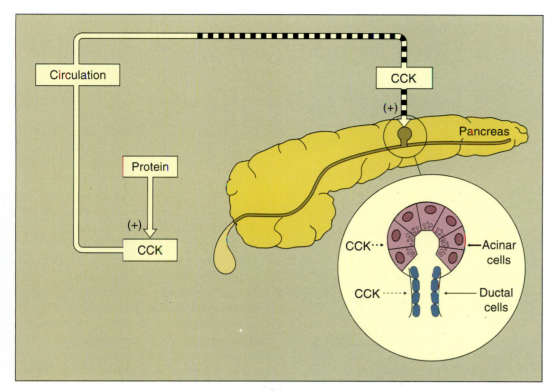

Figure 6-5. Actions of cholecystokinin (CCK). CCK is released by a meal, stimulates pancreatic enzyme secretion, and augments bicarbonate secretion. Blocking the effects of CCK with specific CCK-A receptor blockers inhibits pancreatic enzyme secretion by more than 80%, suggesting that CCK plays a major role in stimulating pancreatic secretion. (*Courtesy of* David C. Whitcomb, MD.)

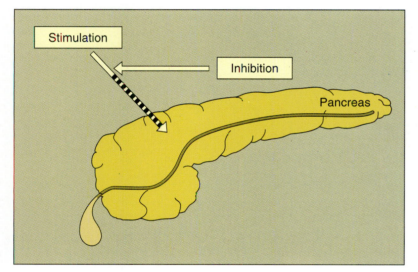

Figure 6-6. The physiologic role of inhibitory peptides and the pathophysiologic consequence of impairing their action have not been fully determined. It appears, however, that the inhibitory neuropeptides actively modulate pancreatic secretion during a meal because immunoneutralization of the inhibitory peptides, somatostatin, pancreatic polypeptide, or peptide YY, results in a 30% to 40% increase in pancreatic output. Two inhibitory peptides that have been widely studied are somatostatin and pancreatic polypeptide. (*Courtesy of* David C. Whitcomb, MD.)

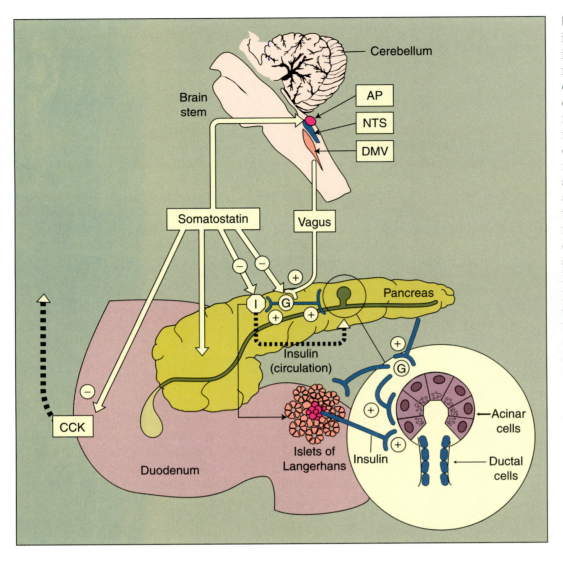

Figure 6-7. Somatostatin inhibits pancreatic secretion at multiple sites. Somatostatin inhibits pancreatic secretion by inhibiting release of stimulatory peptides (*eg*, cholecystokinin) through inhibitory actions at central nervous system sites, by modulating intrapancreatic ganglia, by inhibiting release of acetylcholine at the presynaptic endplate, and possibly by inhibition of insulin release, which is required for active secretion. Although somatostatin receptors are also found on pancreatic acinar cells, these receptors appear to modulate growth rather than to inhibit enzyme secretion directly. The widespread distribution of somatostatin and its multiple receptor types has made it difficult to determine the exact physiologic role of somatostatin. The powerful effect on inhibiting pancreatic secretion at multiple sites, however, and the clinical availability of somatostatin and long-acting somatostatin congeners (*eg*, octreotide) emphasizes the importance of this system. AP—area postrema; DMV—dorsal motor nucleus of the vagus; NTS—nucleus of the tractus solitarius. (*Courtesy of* David C. Whitcomb, MD.)

Acute Pancreatitis

Etiologies of Acute Pancreatitis

Obstructive Causes

Gallstones

Ampullary/pancreatic cancer

Worms in pancreatic duct—ascaris

Choledochocele

Periampullary duodenal diverticula

Foreign body obstructing duct

Pancreas divisum with obstruction of accessory papilla

Hypertensive sphincter of Oddi

Toxins

Ethyl alcohol

Methyl alcohol

Scorpion toxin

Organophosphorus insecticides

Major Drugs that Cause Pancreatitis

With rechallenges

Alpha methyl dopa

5-Aminosalicylate

Azathioprine/6 mercaptopurine

Cimetidine

Furosemide

Metronidazole

Pentamidine

Sulfa drugs

Sulindac

Tetracycline

Valproic acid

Erythromycin

With consistent Latencies

Acetaminophen

(dDI)

Estrogens

Metabolic Causes

Hypercalcemia—rare

Hypertriglyceridemia—type I, type IV, type V

Inherited (Hereditary) Pancreatitis

Autosomal dominant—abnormal gene or chromosome 7g

Associated with chronic pancreatitis and cancer of the pancreas

Infectious Causes of Acute Pancreatitis

Viruses

Mumps

Cytomegalovirus

Herpes

Hepatitis A, B, C

Bacteria

Mycobacteria (tuberculosis, *Mycobacterium-avium* complex)

Leptospirosis

Fungi

Cryptococcus, Candida, coccidioidomycosis

Parasites

Ascaris, Clonorchis, Pneumocystis

Vascular/Hypotension

Atherosclerotic emboli

Ischemia—hypoperfusion

Vasculitis—systemic lupus erythematosus, polyarteritis

Traumatic Causes of Acute Pancreatitis

Blunt trauma

Penetrating trauma

Postoperative

Endoscopic retrograde cholangiopancreatography

Sphincter of Oddi manometry

Idiopathic

Figure 6-8. Causes of acute pancreatitis.

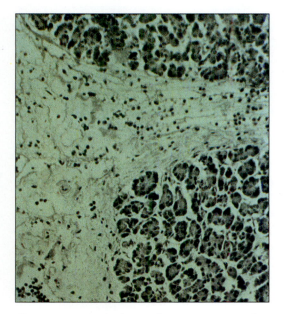

Figure 6-9. Pathology of acute interstitial pancreatitis. There are two main types of acute pancreatitis: interstitial and necrotizing. Interstitial (or edematous) pancreatitis is shown in this photomicrograph. Interstitial pancreatitis is usually associated with clinically mild disease [1]. (*Courtesy of* William M. Steinberg, MD.)

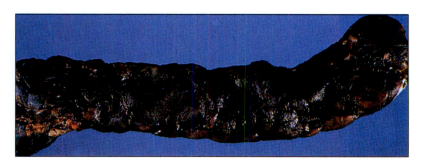

Figure 6-10. Pathology of necrotizing pancreatitis. Extensive ischemic-hemorrhagic necrosis is present in this gross pathology specimen (*From* Klatt [2]; with permission.)

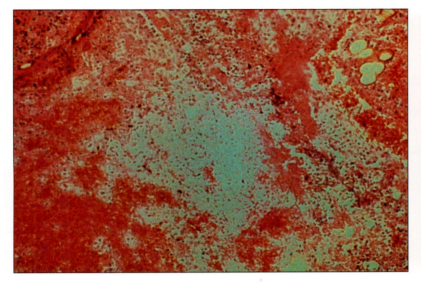

Figure 6-11. Pathology of necrotizing/hemorrhagic pancreatitis. Extensive hemorrhagic necrosis is present. This type of pancreatitis is associated with anemia due to pancreatic hemorrhage and a high mortality rate. Elastase may play a role in hemorrhage. (*From* American Gastroenterological Association [AGA] Collection; with permission.)

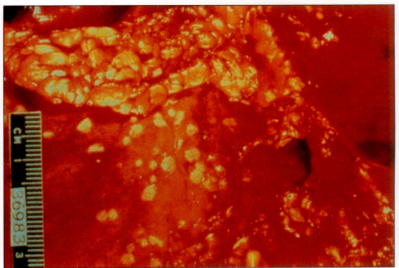

Figure 6-12. Fat necrosis. Fat necrosis seen at surgery is associated with peripancreatic release of lipase, with hydrolysis of triacylglycerols (triglycerides) to toxic fatty acids. (*From* American Gastroenterological Association [AGA] Collection; with permission.)

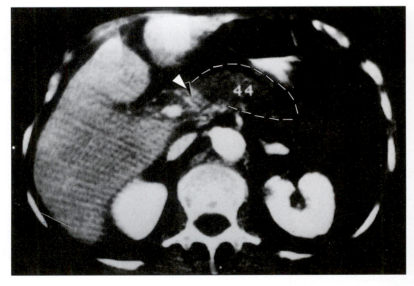

Figure 6-13. Bolus contrast-enhanced computed tomography (CT) in severe acute pancreatitis. A major unsettled issue in the pathophysiology of acute pancreatitis is why most cases are mild and self-limited whereas some progress to the more severe, potentially lethal end of the spectrum of disease. Impairment of the pancreatic microcirculation leading to tissue ischemia may be an important factor in determining the extent of injury and necrosis of the pancreas and the ultimate severity of the disease process. A clinical correlate of this tissue ischemia may be failure of the pancreas to enhance in density on CT after intravenous injection of a bolus of a CT contrast agent in patients with more severe acute pancreatitis. (*Arrowhead*—Normally enhancing tissue in neck of pancreas; *outlined area*—Nonenhancing body and tail of the pancreas.) (*Courtesy of* James H. Grendell, MD.)

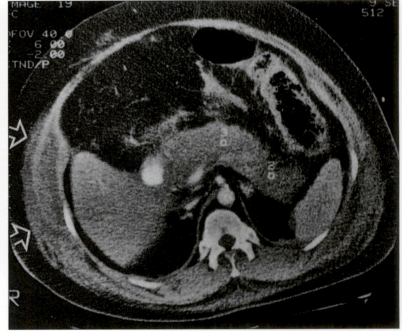

Figure 6-14. Dynamic computed tomography (CT) scan of the pancreas performed by injecting large doses of intravenous contrast rapidly (bolus injection) and scanning the pancreas with thin cuts. This CT scan shows poor perfusion of the pancreas. The presence of poor perfusion on CT scan has about a 90% predictive value of predicting necrosis at surgery; however, only about 60% of patients with necrosis on CT scan have a severe course clinically [3,4]. (*Courtesy of* William M. Steinberg, MD.)

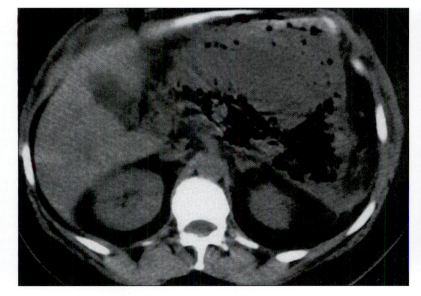

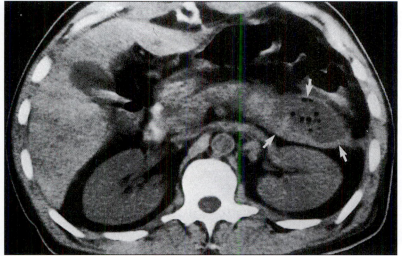

Figure 6-15. Computed tomography (CT) demonstrating the "massive phlegmon" of catastrophic or necrotizing pancreatitis. This particular patient underwent surgical intervention and marsupialization of the retrogastric area. Of those patients who do not require surgical intervention, but have evidence of a massive phlegmon on CT, approximately 70% will undergo evolution to fluid collections and early pseudocyst formation. This particular group of patients with radiologic grade C or D pancreatitis on CT may comprise only 10% to 15% of all patients with pancreatitis, but may be the source of at least 80% of the total morbidity and mortality of necrotizing pancreatitis, pancreatic sepsis, and abscess formation. (*Courtesy of* Stephen B. Vogel, MD.)

Figure 6-16. A computed tomography (CT) scan of the pancreas indicating gas bubbles within the substance of the pancreas. This suggests pancreatic abscess secondary to gas-producing organisms; however, sterile necrosis with microcommunication with the gut can lead to this CT finding. Only with a fine-needle aspirate can one diagnose an abscess with assurance. (*From* Freeny and Lawson [5]; with permission.)

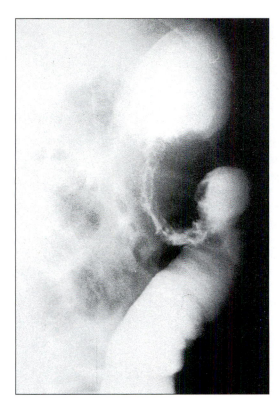

Figure 6-17. An example of colonic obstruction due to pancreatitis. This tends to occur on the left side of the colon. Necrosis and fistulization of the colon can also occur as a late complication. (*From* Huizinga *et al.* [6]; with permission.)

Emergency Endoscopic Retrograde Cholangiopancreatography Plus Sphincterotomy for Biliary Pancreatitis

121 Patients randomized
59 ERCP + ES
62 conventionally

	ERCP + ES	Conventional
Severe (*n*=53)		
Comp	6/25 (24%)	17/28 (61%)
Mort	1/25 (4%)	5/28 (18%)
Mild (*n*=68)		
Comp	4/34 (12%)	4/34 (12%)
Mort	0	0

Figure 6-18. United Kingdom randomized study comparing emergency endoscopic retrograde cholangiopancreatography (ERCP) (within 72 hours of admission) with endoscopic sphincterotomy (ES) with stone removal versus conventional conservative management in biliary pancreatitis. Results show that complications (Comp) and mortality (Mort) are reduced in the ERCP + ES group in severe gallstone pancreatitis (as defined by the modified Glasgow criteria). In those predicted to have mild disease (by the Glasgow criteria), the ERCP + ES group fared the same as those treated conservatively. (*Adapted from* Neoptolemos *et al.* [7].)

Endoscopic Retrograde Cholangiopancreatography in Acute Gallstone Pancreatitis			
	Emergency	**Conservative**	**P value**
All patients			
	n=97	*n*=98	
Complications	18%	29%	0.07
Mortality	5%	9%	0.400
Biliary stone patients			
	n=64	*n*=63	
Complications	16%	33%	0.030
Cholangitis	0%	12%	0.001
Mortality	2%	8%	0.090

Figure 6-19. This Hong Kong study randomized 195 patients to emergency endoscopic retrograde cholangiopancreatography (ERCP) within 24 hours of admission versus no emergency ERCP, although most patients in this group received a subsequent ERCP [8]. If a stone was found, it was removed. About two thirds of the total group had gallstones as the etiology. In this subgroup of biliary stone patients, removing gallstones by emergency ERCP reduced complications, especially cholangitis. Mortality was also reduced, but this was not statistically significant. This study and the one summarized in Figure 6-18 indicated that it is relatively safe to perform emergency ERCP in acute pancreatitis. Proven utility of ERCP is in the removal of suspected gallstones in patients with severe pancreatitis or in those in whom cholangitis is suspected; however, a more recent study suggests that ERCP may not necessarily improve outcome in biliary pancreatitis [8]. Thus, additional studies are needed to settle this issue. (*Courtesy of* William M. Steinberg, MD.)

Chronic Pancreatitits

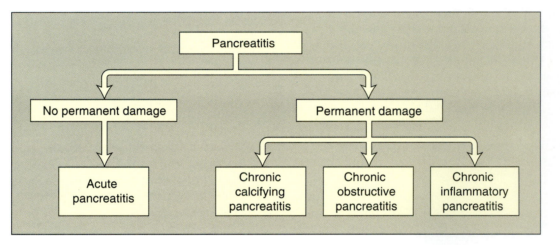

Figure 6-20. Marseilles-Rome classification. The tremendous variability of symptoms and diversity of etiologies have made classification of chronic pancreatitis difficult, and a variety of systems have been developed to classify chronic pancreatitis. The most recent international symposium [9], in 1988, defined three forms of chronic pancreatitis based on morphologic criteria: chronic calcifying pancreatitis, chronic obstructive pancreatitis, and chronic inflammatory pancreatitis. Chronic calcifying pancreatitis is defined by the presence of calcified stones within the pancreatic ductal system, and usually results from long-standing alcohol abuse. Chronic obstructive pancreatitis is defined as downstream obstruction of the main pancreatic duct with upstream dilation; stones are infrequently seen with this condition. Chronic inflammatory pancreatitis is defined by a relative lack of either calcification or dilation of the main pancreatic duct. This classification system is not useful in most clinical situations. (*Courtesy of* Christopher E. Forsmark, MD, and Phillip P. Toskes, MD.)

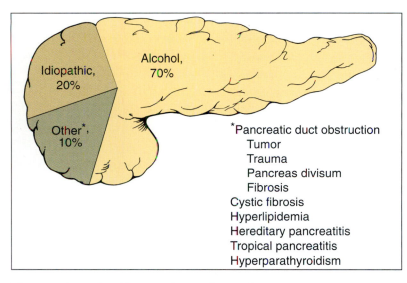

Figure 6-21. Classification by etiology. Chronic pancreatitis may also be classified by its presumed cause. Chronic alcoholism accounts for approximately 70% of all cases of chronic pancreatitis. Prolonged and substantial abuse is generally required to produce chronic pancreatitis, and most (but not all) patients who present with an episode of acute pancreatitis caused by alcohol consumption already have chronic pancreatic damage. Chronic obstruction of the pancreatic duct may also produce chronic pancreatitis, such as that caused by tumors, trauma, pseudocysts, inflammation and fibrosis (such as after a severe episode of acute pancreatitis), pancreas divisum (with associated minor papilla stenosis), and even after prolonged endoscopic stenting of the pancreatic duct. After traumatic injury to the pancreatic duct (such as after a motor vehicle accident or a stab wound), chronic pancreatitis may develop within a few months. Pancreas divisum commonly occurs as a normal variant (in 10% of the population), and most patients remain asymptomatic. This variant occurs after nonfusion of the two pancreatic buds during development, so that most pancreatic secretion in the dorsal segment drains through the minor papilla rather than the major papilla. A small subset of patients have both pancreas divisum and obstruction at the minor papilla, which may produce both acute relapsing pancreatitis or, more rarely, chronic obstructive pancreatitis. Hyperlipidemia, particularly when the serum triglycerides are above 1000 mg/dL, may produce both acute and chronic pancreatitis. Tropical chronic pancreatitis, probably caused by malnutrition and toxic products in the diet, is rare in the United States. Cystic fibrosis is an important cause of chronic pancreatitis in children, although with improved pulmonary care these patients may live to adulthood. Despite careful evaluation, about 20% of patients (in some studies as high as 30%) have no specific identifiable etiology, and are thus classified as having idiopathic chronic pancreatitis. (*Courtesy of* Christopher E. Forsmark, MD, and Phillip P. Toskes, MD.)

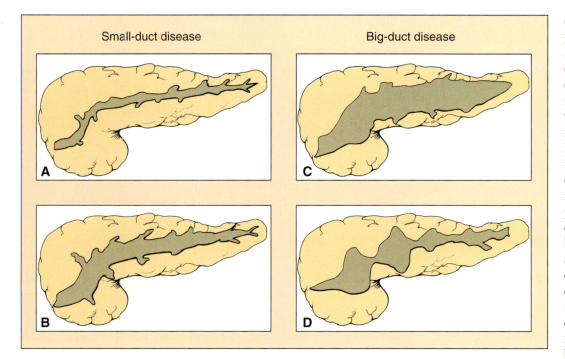

Figure 6-22. Classification by pancreatic duct morphology. The abnormalities demonstrated in the pancreatic duct by endoscopic retrograde pancreatography (ERP) or inferred by findings using computed tomography are the most clinically useful means to classify chronic pancreatitis. This system divides patients into two major groups: big-duct disease, characterized by substantial abnormalities of the main pancreatic duct (particularly dilation, intraductal stones, and strictures), and small-duct disease (or chronic pancreatitis with minimal change), where abnormalities of the main pancreatic duct are absent and changes are limited to the smaller side branches of the duct or the pancreatic parenchyma. In general, patients with big-duct disease have more advanced chronic pancreatitis, often with associated exocrine and endocrine insufficiency (steatorrhea and diabetes mellitus), and commonly have alcoholic chronic pancreatitis. Patients with small-duct disease tend to have less advanced disease and more commonly have idiopathic chronic pancreatitis or early stages of alcoholic chronic pancreatitis. The distinction between these two groups of patients is usually straightforward after the diagnosis of chronic pancreatitis is made; the distinction carries significant therapeutic implications (*see* section on Treatment). **A–B**, examples of small-duct disease are presented. **A**, A nondilated main pancreatic duct with clubbing and dilation of the side branches; **B**, a mildly dilated main duct with abnormal side branches. **C–D**, changes of big-duct disease. **C**, Markedly dilated main pancreatic duct; **D**, end-stage "chain-of-lakes" appearance. (*Courtesy of* Christopher E. Forsmark, MD, and Phillip P. Toskes, MD.)

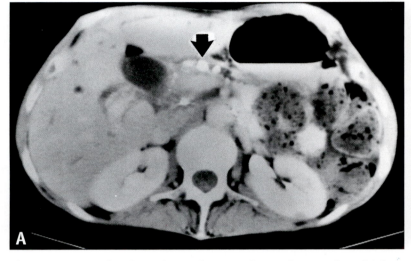

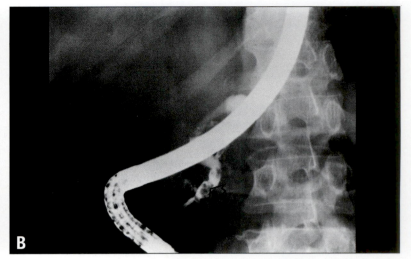

Figure 6-23. Pathophysiology. The specific mechanism by which alcohol produces chronic pancreatitis is unknown, but it does appear to require substantial alcohol ingestion over at least 6 to 12 years. Various physiologic abnormalities have been documented in both animal models and in humans, including a direct toxic effect of pancreatic acinar cells, stimulation of pancreatic secretion, interference with normal intracellular protein trafficking, and the promotion of the formation of protein plugs within the ductal system. These plugs often become calcified, producing pancreatic ductal stones. Whether these stones contribute to the pathogenesis of alcoholic chronic pancreatitis by obstructing the pancreatic ducts is unknown. They may merely be a marker of alcoholic chronic pancreatitis rather than its cause. **A,** Multiple calcified stones within the pancreatic duct on a computed tomography scan (arrow). **B,** A stone within the main pancreatic duct at endoscopic retrograde pancreatography (filling defect within the dye column in the main pancreatic duct [*arrow*]).

The specific mechanism by which other causes of chronic pancreatitis produce pancreatic injury is also unknown. For example, it is unclear if conditions that obstruct the pancreatic duct produce damage by mere obstruction or if additional insults (such as low-grade infection, activation of pancreatic digestive enzymes, inflammation, or high pressure within the obstructed duct) are required. (*Courtesy of* Christopher E. Forsmark, MD, and Phillip P. Toskes, MD.)

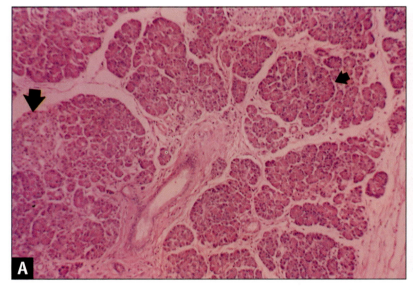

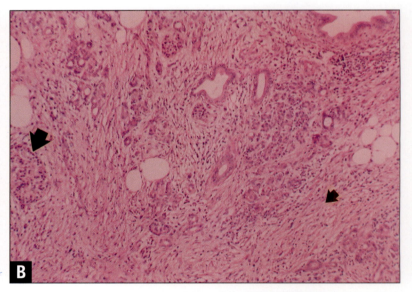

Figure 6-24. Histology. Regardless of the specific cause of chronic pancreatitis, the histologic result is similar. Pancreatic inflammation, together with progressive fibrosis, leads to destruction of the acinar cells either focally or diffusely, producing exocrine insufficiency and steatorrhea. Intraductal concretions and stones may form, which may block the flow of pancreatic secretions and augment the damage. Inflammation involving pancreatic nerves is also commonly found. The endocrine tissue (the islets of Langerhans) is typically spared until late in the disease process, making diabetes mellitus a late complication. **A,** Normal pancreatic tissue is demonstrated with a normal acinar architecture (*small arrow*) and islets of Langerhans (*large arrow*). **B,** Changes of chronic pancreatitis include destruction of acinar tissue with replacement by fibrosis (*small arrow*), but the islets remain intact (*large arrow*). (*Courtesy of* Christopher E. Forsmark, MD, and Phillip P. Toskes, MD.)

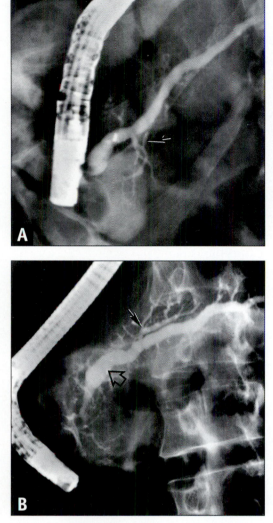

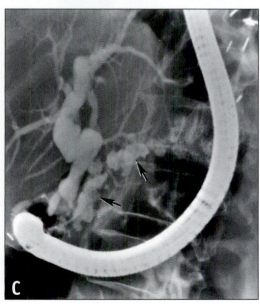

Figure 6-25. Tests of structure: endoscopic retrograde pancreatography (ERP). The most sensitive diagnostic test for chronic pancreatitis that relies on structural changes is ERP. The diagnosis of chronic pancreatitis is based on changes in both the main pancreatic duct and the side branches. The Cambridge criteria [10] define those changes in the main duct suggestive of chronic pancreatitis as dilation, narrowing or stricture formation, irregular contour, associated filling of cavities or pseudocysts, or filling defects (pancreatic duct stones). Side-branch changes include shortening, dilation, and clubbing. At its most advanced stages, the "chain-of-lakes" appearance of alternate dilation and strictures is characteristic of chronic pancreatitis. In advanced chronic pancreatitis these marked changes in the main pancreatic duct (big-duct disease) are common; therefore, ERP is an extremely accurate test. In less advanced disease (small-duct disease), however, the changes are often inadequate to be diagnostic of chronic pancreatitis [11]. **A,** Mild changes with minimal dilation of the pancreatic duct and clubbing of the side branches (*arrow*). **B,** More advanced changes with moderate dilation of the main duct (*large arrow*) and coexistent changes in the side branches (*small arrow*). **C,** Advanced disease, with a characteristic "chain-of-lakes" appearance of the pancreatic duct (*arrows*). Substantial evidence now exists that a significant proportion of patients with histologically proven chronic pancreatitis will have normal or only minimally abnormal results of pancreatograms [12,13]. In addition, various other conditions may mimic the pancreatographic changes of chronic pancreatitis, including normal aging, a recent attack of acute pancreatitis, pancreatic carcinoma, and findings after pancreatic duct stenting [11]. The reported sensitivity of ERP for chronic pancreatitis is 67% to 93%, with specificities ranging from 89% to 100% [14]. These results are generated from studies evaluating patients with more advanced disease, so they are clearly overestimates of true sensitivity and specificity. ERP may also be used to develop therapeutic rather than diagnostic information. In particular, ERP can document main-duct dilation, which is a prerequisite for consideration of surgical duct decompression (Puestow's procedure). ERP can also be useful in differentiating pancreatic malignancy from chronic pancreatitis, both by morphologic criteria and by obtaining cytology from pancreatic duct strictures.

In addition to the abnormalities already described, ERP may document pancreas divisum. This variant anatomy, wherein the bulk of pancreatic secretion drains through the minor papilla, occurs in 10% of the population; in the vast majority of patients, it does not lead to pancreatic disease. In a small minority of patients, obstruction to flow at the minor papilla may produce either acute pancreatitis or chronic pancreatitis. This can be definitively established if the dorsal ductal system is dilated or has changes of chronic pancreatitis, or if a hormonal stimulation test (discussed later) is abnormal. In the absence of these diagnostic criteria, it should not be assumed that this variant is producing the chronic abdominal pain. (*Courtesy of* Christopher E. Forsmark, MD, and Phillip P. Toskes, MD.)

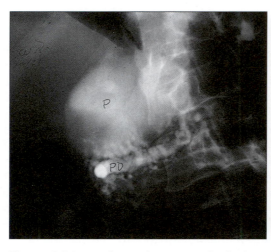

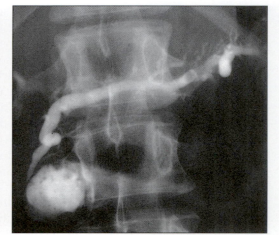

Figure 6-26. Endoscopic retrograde cholangiopancreatography (ERCP) demonstrating a dilated pancreatic duct and a huge pseudocyst in the area of the body of the pancreas. At surgery only the pseudocyst could easily be identified and drained. The preoperative ERCP, however, suggested that drainage of the pseudocyst into a Roux-en-Y would continue to drain the body and tail of the pancreas. (*Courtesy of* Stephen B. Vogel, MD.)

Figure 6-27. Endoscopic retrograde cholangiopancreatography (ERCP) demonstrating a dilated pancreatic duct in a patient with chronic pancreatitis and a small pseudocyst in the head and uncinate process of the pancreas, communicating with the main pancreatic duct. Longitudinal pancreatojejunostomy adequately decompressed the small pseudocyst. (*Courtesy of* Stephen B. Vogel, MD.)

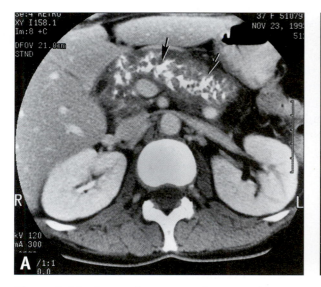

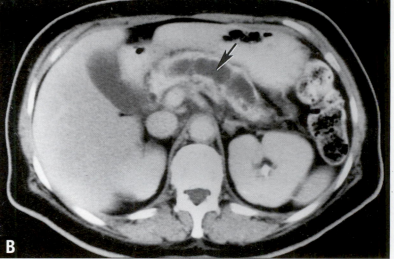

Figure 6-28. Tests of structure: Computed tomography (CT). Findings on CT that suggest chronic pancreatitis include diffuse calcification, ductal dilation, gland atrophy, irregular contour, and associated pseudocysts [14]. CT is less accurate than endoscopic retrograde pancreatography for the diagnosis of chronic pancreatitis, although the new spiral CT technology allows improved resolution of small structures, such as the pancreatic duct, and appears more accurate than earlier scanning methods. **A,** Diffuse pancreatic calcification (*arrows*). **B,** Markedly dilated pancreatic duct (*arrow*) with atrophy of the pancreas. MR imaging has not been evaluated systematically, although the newer "turboflash" technology and use of oral contrast agents has markedly improved the image quality of scans of the pancreas. (*Courtesy of* Christopher E. Forsmark, MD, and Phillip P. Toskes, MD.)

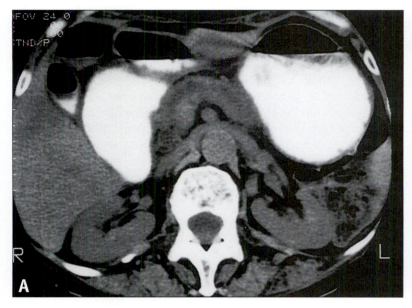
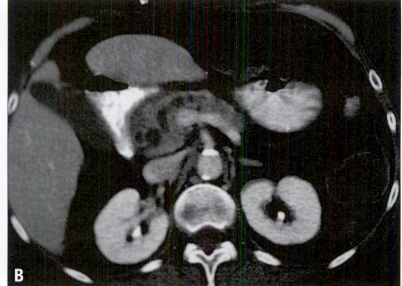

Figure 6-29. A–B, High-resolution spiral computed tomography with fine cuts through the pancreas adequately demonstrates pancreatic duct dilatation, even down to the ampulla, as well as demonstrating chain-of-lakes abnormalities. (*Courtesy of* Stephen B. Vogel, MD.)

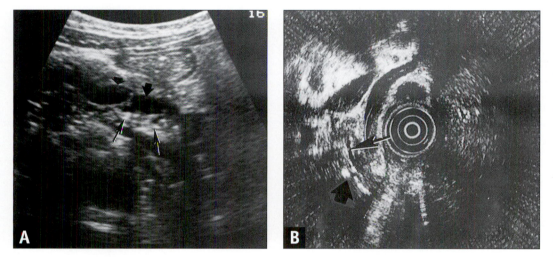

Figure 6-30. Tests of structure: ultrasonography. Ultrasound is an inexpensive, noninvasive diagnostic test that does not submit the patient to ionizing radiation. It is limited by its poor sensitivity (60%–70%) and inability to image the pancreas in the presence of overlying intestinal gas. Characteristic ultrasound findings include gland atrophy, diffuse calcifications, dilation of the pancreatic duct, and an increase in echogenicity with a heterogeneous pattern [14]. Conversely, ultrasound is quite useful in the detection of pancreatic pseudocysts. **A,** Pancreatic calcifications on conventional ultrasonography (*thin arrows*) and a dilated, segmented pancreatic duct (*thick arrows*). Endoscopic ultrasonography has only begun to be evaluated for use in chronic pancreatitis, but early results are promising. **B,** Endosonographic image of the body of the pancreas with a visible pancreatic duct (*thin arrow*) and calcifications within the gland (*thick arrow*). The circular target structure in the center is the instrument. (*Courtesy of* Christopher E. Forsmark, MD, and Phillip P. Toskes, MD.)

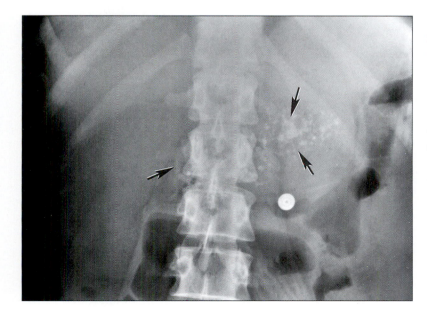

Figure 6-31. Tests of structure: plain abdominal radiograph. The finding of diffuse pancreatic calcification is a specific marker of chronic pancreatitis, but it is only seen in far-advanced disease. Focal calcification is not diagnostic of chronic pancreatitis, and may be seen in a number of other diseases. Although patients with alcoholic chronic pancreatitis will commonly develop diffuse calcifications (70% of patients after 15 years of observation), patients with idiopathic pancreatitis do so only rarely (20%–40% after 15 years of follow-up) [15]. The low sensitivity of plain radiographic limits their use as a diagnostic tool. This figure demonstrates diffuse pancreatic calcification (*arrows*). (*Courtesy of* Christopher E. Forsmark, MD, and Phillip P. Toskes, MD.)

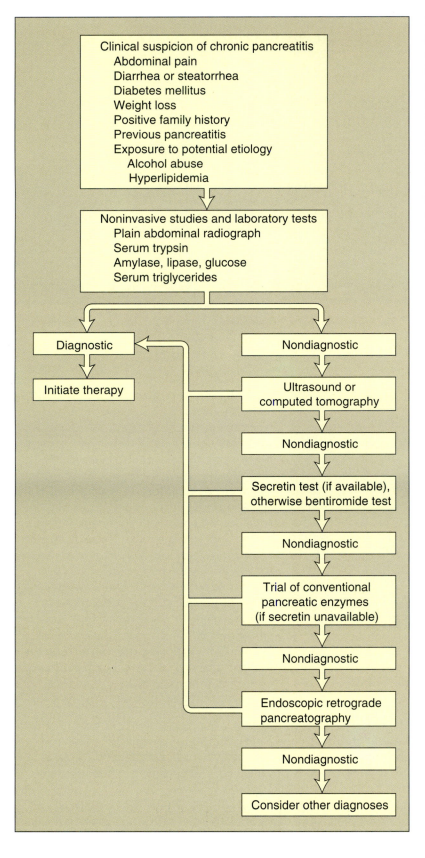

Figure 6-32. Strategy for diagnosis. The overall diagnostic strategy should take into account the relative accuracy, cost, and risks of each diagnostic test. In its advanced form, chronic pancreatitis can be confirmed by a variety of diagnostic tests, so that overall cost and risk of diagnostic tests should be the major concern. In patients with less advanced disease, the accuracy, and in particular, the sensitivity of the diagnostic test become more important. All of this must be tempered by the availability of the variety of diagnostic tests, in particular, the fact that direct hormonal stimulation tests are not universally available. In centers where direct hormonal stimulation tests are not available, a trial of conventional (*ie*, nonenteric-coated) pancreatic enzymes should be considered as a therapeutic trail in patients without major abnormalities of the pancreatic duct because all other diagnostic tests are less sensitive. (*Courtesy of* Christopher E. Forsmark, MD, and Phillip P. Toskes, MD.)

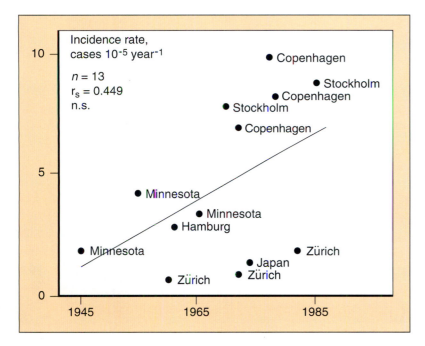

Figure 6-33. Incidence and prevalence. The only prospective study to evaluate the incidence and prevalence of chronic pancreatitis was performed in Copenhagen. It noted an incidence of 8.2 new cases per 100,000 population per year and a prevalence of 27.4 cases per 100,000 population [16]. A number of other studies [17] have estimated incidence of less than 2 per 100,000 population to 10 per 100,000 population. Although it might seem these discrepancies could be explained by the rate of alcohol consumption in the population studied, this does not appear to be the case. All these studies are flawed in that they only identify the patients with more advanced disease or those who have sought medical attention. A substantial number of patients with less advanced disease (small-duct disease) and less severe symptoms were obviously not counted; the true incidence and prevalence of chronic pancreatitis is probably substantially higher than these studies would suggest. (*Adapted from* Worning [17].)

Treatment of Pain

Remove inciting process

Discontinue consumption of alcohol

Treat hyperlipidemia

Treat complications

Pseudocyst

Duodenal obstruction

Common bile duct obstruction

Analgesics

Non-narcotic

Narcotic

Suppress pancreatic secretion

Pancreatic enzymes

Investigational agents

Modify neural transmission

Celiac plexus block

Relieve pancreatic ductal obstruction

Endoscopic stents (?)

Surgery

Remove pancreas through partial or complete surgery

Figure 6-34. Treatment of pain, an overview. The available treatment strategies are outlined in this table. Cessation of consumption of alcohol is a prudent step in patients with alcoholic chronic pancreatitis, but the effect on pancreatic damage is quite variable. Although stopping alcohol consumption may allow for recovery of some pancreatic function, in many patients the disease progresses despite sobriety, albeit possibly at a slower pace. Analgesics are usually required, and many patients require narcotics. The risk of addiction to such drugs is present, and is a particular problem in patients with a history of addictive behavior (chronic alcoholism or drug abuse) and in patients with little social support. Despite the risk of addiction (< 20% overall), adequate pain control should be the primary concern.

Treatments that reduce pancreatic secretion may relieve pain by reducing pancreatic pressure or by other as yet unknown mechanisms. These form the basis for medical therapy of pain, and are discussed in detail in the following figures. Attempts to block neural transmission by celiac axis block are generally ineffective in chronic pancreatitis or are of only short-lived duration, making this technique of little utility for the long-term management of these patients. The effectiveness of surgical therapy in selected patients is discussed in subsequent figures. (*Courtesy of* Christopher E. Forsmark, MD, and Phillip P. Toskes, MD.)

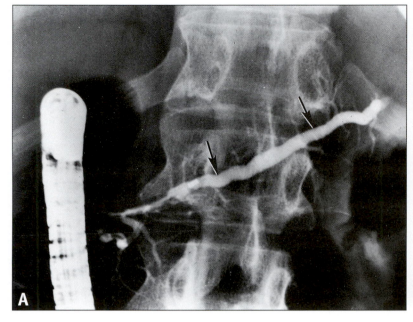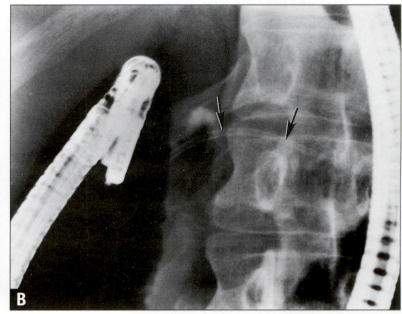

Figure 6-35. Endoscopic treatment. Endoscopic treatment might include dilation of dominant strictures, removal of pancreatic ductal stones, sphincterotomy of the major or minor papilla, or pancreatic duct stenting. None of these techniques have been evaluated in a randomized trial in patients with chronic pancreatitis; in many anecdotal reports, the response rate is equivalent to the placebo response rate (approximately 35%). In addition, pancreatic duct stenting has been documented to produce chronic pancreatitis in both animal models and in humans [11,18]. Endoscopic therapy thus seems to be most amenable in patients with large obstructing pancreatic duct stones or dominant downstream strictures with upstream dilation, but the utility of endoscopic therapy in these conditions is unproven, and its use should be investigated in larger clinical trials. **A**, An injection through the minor papilla in a patient with pancreas divisum, which fills an abnormal dorsal duct (*arrows*). **B**, A stent is being placed into the dilated dorsal duct (*arrows*). (*Courtesy of* Christopher E. Forsmark, MD, and Phillip P. Toskes, MD.)

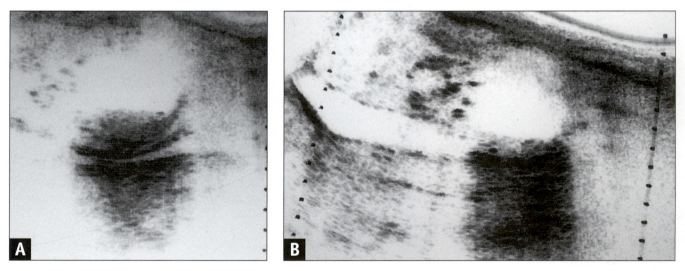

Figure 6-36. A–B, Ultrasound examination of an acutely ill patient demonstrating a pancreatic pseudocyst compressing the vena cava. The patient underwent percutaneous drainage under ultrasound guidance. Follow-up "pseudocystogram" demonstrated no communication with the main pancreatic duct, and the catheter was continued. A recurrent pseudocyst is treated surgically. If persistent percutaneous drainage results in a diminished but continued pancreatic fistula through the catheter (even following therapy with octreotide acetate), then several courses of treatment can be followed. The catheters can be removed following higher dose octreotide acetate treatment. A second surgical option is conversion of an external pancreatic fistula to internal surgical drainage. This is accomplished by changing the percutaneous catheter to a larger catheter preoperatively. This facilitates intra-abdominal identification of the fistulous tract. The tract is then "capped" as it exits the retroperitoneum and is sutured to a Roux-en-Y limb of jejunum. This technique converts the external fistula to internal drainage into the Roux-en-Y limb. (*Courtesy of* Stephen B. Vogel, MD.)

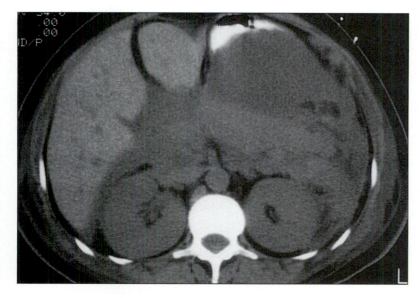

Figure 6-37. Computed tomography demonstrating an acute fluid collection (or early pseudocyst formation) in evolving high-radiologic-grade pancreatitis. In those patients who are symptomatic with either pain, gastric outlet obstruction, or gastroparesis with or without persistent hyperamylasemia, percutaneous drainage often results in rapid resolution of symptoms, and in most cases, normalization of the serum amylase. Continued observation of this fluid collection without intervention may demonstrate evolution of a large retrogastric pancreatic pseudocyst. Additional benefits of percutaneous drainage are the demonstration of bacteria in the fluid and recognition of early abscess formation. These particular patients usually undergo continued percutaneous drainage as long as the clinical course is improving. (*Courtesy of* Stephen B. Vogel, MD.)

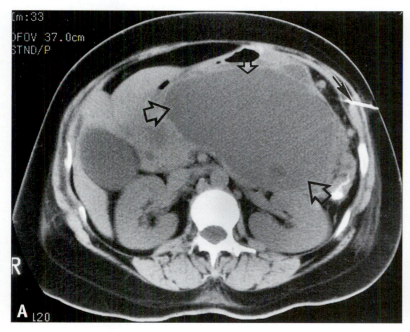

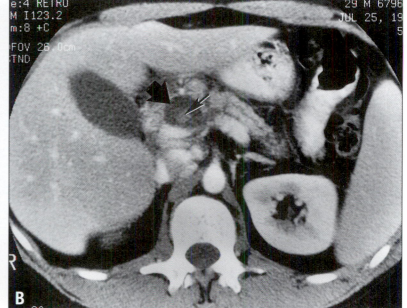

Figure 6-38. Pseudocysts. **A,** A large pseudocyst (*open arrows*), which is being percutaneously drained (*closed arrow*). Pseudocysts that develop in chronic pancreatitis are most commonly caused by duct obstruction, with the formation of a "retention" cyst in the upstream duct or side branch. Unlike the pseudocysts associated with acute pancreatitis, these pseudocysts do not contain activated enzymes, and are usually not a reflection of a necrotizing inflammatory process. These pseudocysts are less likely to produce complications than those associated with acute necrotizing pancreatitis, but they are paradoxically also less likely to resolve. Many of these pseudocysts remain asymptomatic, but they may be complicated by infection, rupture or leak, bleeding, or obstruction of a neighboring hollow viscus (*eg*, duodenum, bile duct, colon, or ureter, among others). Pseudocysts may also worsen chronic pain or even initiate a wasting syndrome.

Recent clinical experience suggests that in patients with pseudocysts smaller than 6 cm, if there is a mature pseudocyst wall on radiographic imaging that does not resemble a cystic neoplasm, minimal symptoms, and no evidence of active alcohol abuse, the risk of complications is extremely small (< 10%). These patients may be safely observed with little risk of serious complication [19,20]. Even larger asymptomatic pseudocysts can be considered for expectant management in this group of patients. Symptomatic pseudocysts or those producing complications require therapy.

Surgical decompression remains the standard criterion for symptomatic pseudocysts with low mortality and little recurrence. Surgical therapy also allows the differentiation of true pseudocysts from cystic pancreatic neoplasms. Percutaneous drainage of symptomatic pseudocysts is usually successful in the short-term, but pseudocyst recurrence is common (although the recurrent pseudocyst may remain asymptomatic!). Percutaneous drainage seems to be particularly effective for infected pseudocysts; however, it is usually ineffective for other complications, such as bleeding, rupture, or leak. Bleeding is a rare event, but carries substantial mortality, often because the bleeding source is a medium-sized artery that has formed a pseudoaneurysm. **B,** A small pseudocyst in the pancreatic head (*thick arrow*) with an arterial pseudoaneurysm within it (*thin arrow*), a condition associated with the potential for massive hemorrhage. Embolization, usually followed by surgical decompression of the pseudocyst and ligation of the bleeding artery, is the treatment of choice. Rupture of a pseudocyst or the development of a leak (pancreaticopleural or other fistula) usually requires preoperative delineation of the anatomy by computed tomography or endoscopic retrograde pancreatography, followed by surgical closure and cyst enterostomy. (*Courtesy of* Christopher E. Forsmark, MD, and Phillip P. Toskes, MD.)

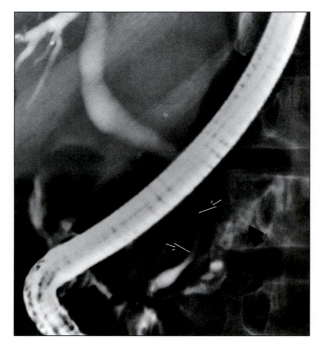

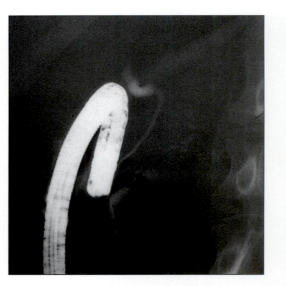

Figure 6-39. Common bile duct stricture. Common bile duct stricture may develop as a consequence of compression by an adjacent pseudocyst or by progressive fibrosis of the head of the pancreas. This figure demonstrates an endoscopic retrograde cholangiopancreatography with changes of chronic pancreatitis (*thick arrows*) and a coexistent smooth stricture of the intrapancreatic common bile duct (*thin arrow*). Symptomatic obstruction of the bile duct usually requires surgical biliary bypass, usually in conjunction with a Peustow procedure. (*Courtesy of* Christopher E. Forsmark, MD, and Phillip P. Toskes, MD.)

Figure 6-40. Endoscopic retrograde cholangiopancreatography (ERCP) in a patient with a known pseudocyst in the head of the pancreas. The tapering of the distal common bile duct may result from either the pseudocyst or from fibrosis in the head of the gland. The pseudocyst does not communicate with the proximal pancreatic duct, but the proximal duct is completely strictured. Computed tomography demonstrated a dilated distal pancreatic duct. Surgical options include either pseudocyst drainage alone or pseudocyst drainage combined with longitudinal pancreatojejunostomy and possibly biliary decompression. At surgery an intraoperative cholangiogram can be performed following pseudocyst decompression to evaluate the distal common bile duct. If the long tapered narrowing is persistent, then simultaneous biliary decompression is indicated. If the common bile duct appears normal following pseudocyst decompression, then either pseudocyst drainage only or pseudocyst drainage combined with a Puestow procedure can be performed. In selected cases an intraoperative "pseudocystogram" can be performed to evaluate whether pseudocyst drainage alone will also decompress the distal dilated pancreatic duct. If no communication is demonstrated between the pseudocyst and the pancreatic duct, then an attempt should be made to drain the distal pancreatic duct independently. (*Courtesy of* Stephen B. Vogel, MD.)

Developmental Anomalies

Anatomic Categorization of Congenital Pancreatic Anomalies and Variants		
Ventral-dorsal ductal malfusion	**Quantitative underdevelopment**	**Atypical ductal configuration**
Pancreas divisum	Agenesis	Ansa
Incomplete pancreas divisum	Hypoplasia	Spiral
Isolated dorsal segment	**Duplication**	Horseshoe
Rotation-migration problems	Ductal	Miscellaneous
Annular pancreas	Total	**Anomalous pancreatobiliary junction**
Ectopic pancreas	Partial—tail, body	**Cystic malformations**
Ectopic papillae	Accessory papilla	Single
		Polycystic

Figure 6-41. Full classification of developmental anomalies of the pancreas. (*Courtesy of* Glen A. Lehman, MD.)

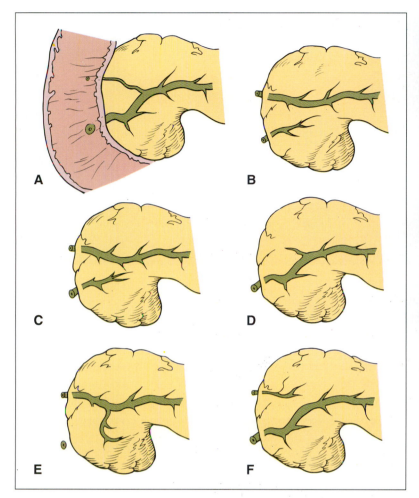

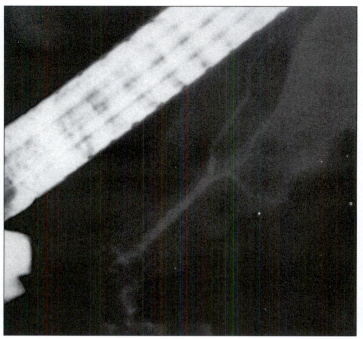

Figure 6-43. Typical ventral ductogram of pancreas divisum showing small ductal system, which terminates in small-caliber branches. (*Courtesy of* Glen A. Lehman, MD.)

Figure 6-42. Variations of pancreatic ductal anatomy, including pancreas divisum. **A,** Most common variant with patent main and accessory ducts and patent major and minor papillae. **B,** Typical pancreas divisum. **C,** Incomplete pancreas divisum. A tiny branch connects the dorsal and ventral portions of the pancreas. **D,** Minor papilla is not patent. **E,** The entire ductal system drains through the minor papilla. **F,** Isolated accessory duct system draining through the minor papilla. (*Courtesy of* Glen A. Lehman, MD.)

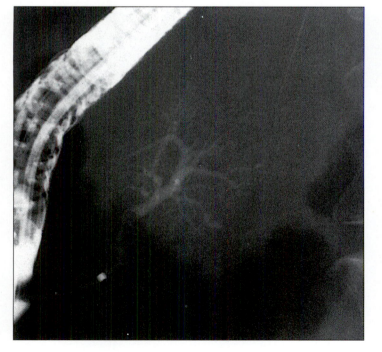

Figure 6-44. Another small, normal ventral ductogram. Slight acinarization has occurred. (*Courtesy of* Glen A. Lehman, MD.)

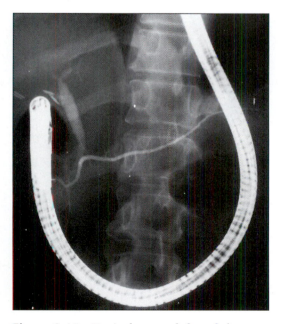

Figure 6-45. Typical normal dorsal ductogram. This is very similar to a standard ductogram obtained through the major papilla. The endoscope is in the long position. The common bile duct is only partially filled. (*Courtesy of* Glen A. Lehman, MD.)

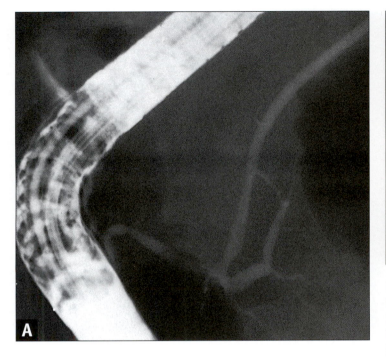

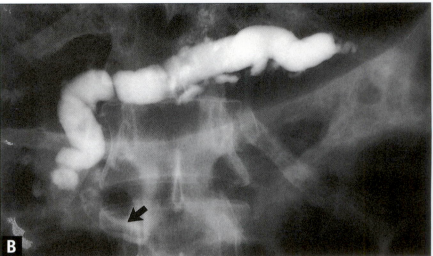

Figure 6-46. **A,** Incomplete pancreas divisum. Note the main duct narrowing over a 5-mm length as it joins the dorsal duct. This narrowing must be differentiated from a pathologic stricture, as is seen with cancer. **B,** Dorsal ductogram obtained through the minor papilla that shows diffuse changes of chronic pancreatitis. The arrow in the lower left corner indicates a tiny ansa ventral branch that connects to the major papilla (*ie,* incomplete pancreas divisum). (*Courtesy of* Glen A. Lehman, MD.)

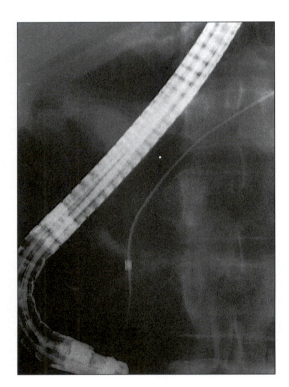

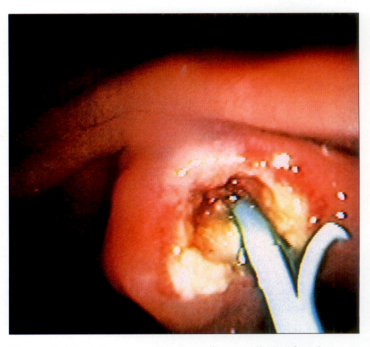

Figure 6-47. Stent placement in the minor papilla. A guidewire has been passed to the tail of the pancreas. A 5-Fr, 2.5-cm length stent has been passed into the minor papilla. (*Courtesy of* Glen A. Lehman, MD.)

Figure 6-48. Minor papilla view after needle knife sphincterotomy. A 5-Fr stent has been placed into the minor papilla; the tissue of the minor papilla has been incised with cautery with a needle knife. (*Courtesy of* Stuart Sherman, MD.)

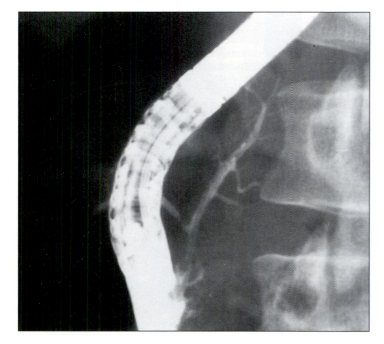

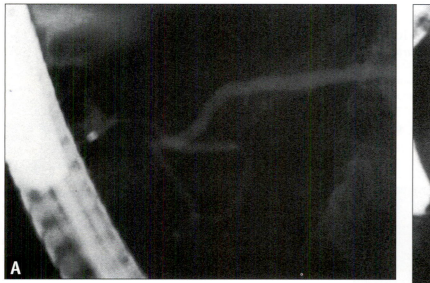

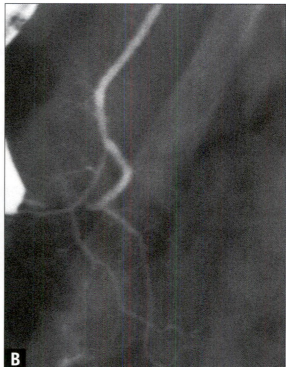

Figure 6-49. Major papilla pancreatogram shows ventral pancreas (of pancreas divisum) combined with annular pancreas. Note branch encircling the endoscope and the descending duodenum. The result of the dorsal pancreatogram was normal. (*Courtesy of* Glen A. Lehman, MD.)

Figure 6-50. Ansa pancreatica. **A,** The main duct has a ventral looping contour. This finding is generally of no clinical significance. **B,** Long branches extend into uncinate process from the main and accessory ducts. This finding is a normal variant. (*Courtesy of* Glen A. Lehman, MD.)

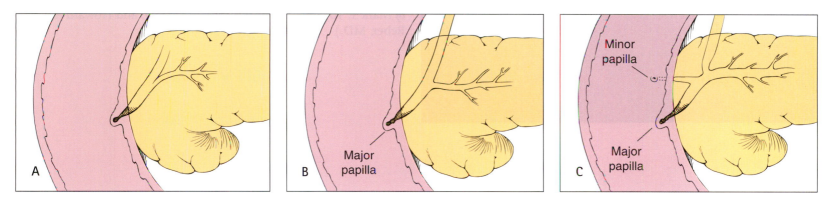

Figure 6-51. Anomalous pancreatobiliary junction. By definition, anomalous pancreatobiliary junction occurs when the common channel is longer than 15 mm, thereby leaving the pancreatobiliary junction upstream from the sphincter of Oddi. Juice from the two ductal systems may intermix or variably be secreted into the alternative duct. This is thought to give rise to pancreatitis or choledochocele. **A,** Long common channel. **B,** The pancreatic duct appears to join the bile duct; the minor papilla is absent. **C,** The bile duct appears to connect into the pancreatic ductal system [21–23]. (*Courtesy of* Glen A. Lehman, MD.)

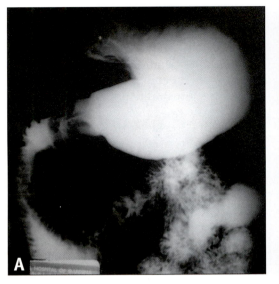

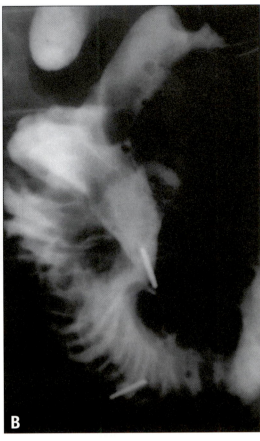

Figure 6-56. Barium studies of the gastrointestinal (GI) tract are not often used to evaluate patients with suspected pancreatic cancer. Because many of these patients present with nonspecific gastrointestinal symptoms, however, an upper GI may be obtained. Findings on upper GI that suggest pancreatic cancer include extrinsic compression, displacement or encasement of the C-loop, mucosal invasion (nodularity or spiculation), or Frostberg's reversed '3' sign. **A,** Widened duodenal sweep and the suggestion of compression of part of the duodenal loop. **B,** Note the reversed '3' sign caused by the nodular compression of the medial duodenal wall by the pancreatic cancer. (*Courtesy of* Barbara Kadell, MD.)

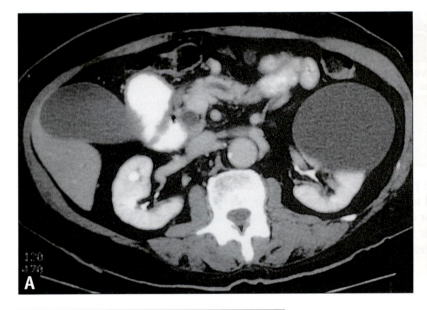

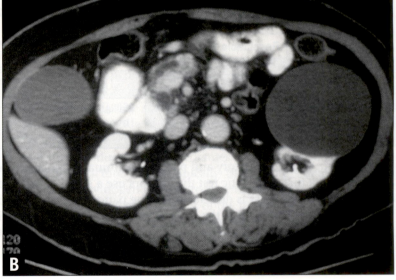

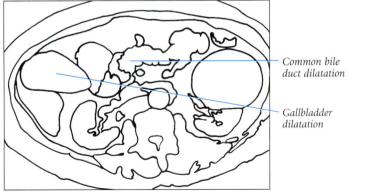

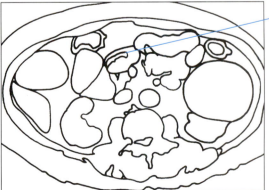

Figure 6-57. Computed tomography scans demonstrating common bile duct and gallbladder dilatation (**panel A**); pancreatic duct dilatation is also evident (**panel B**).

(Continued on next page)

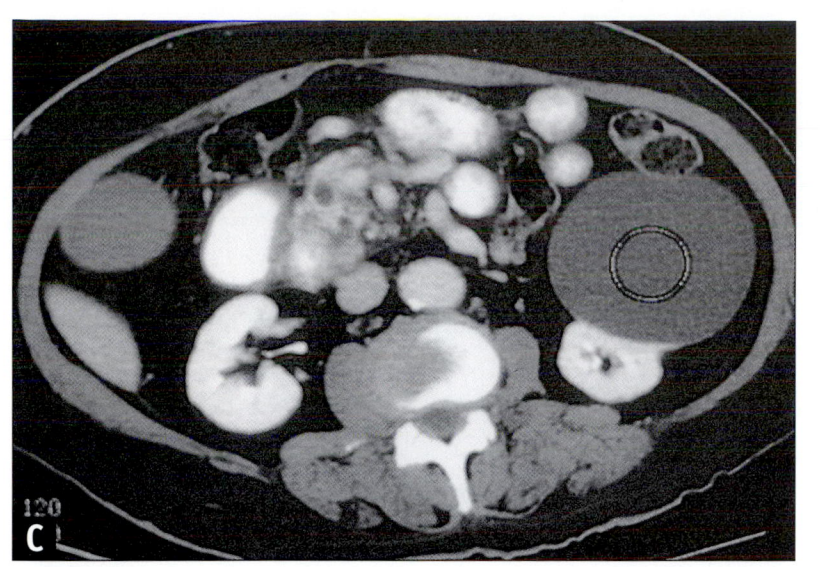

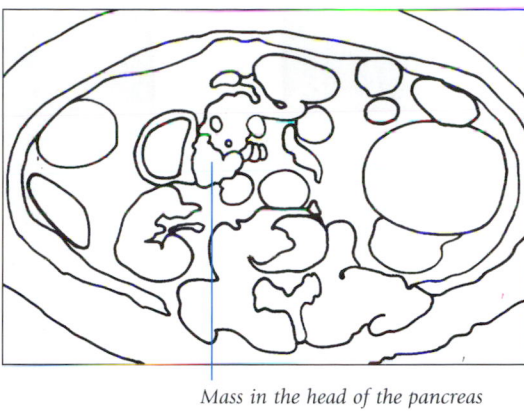

Mass in the head of the pancreas

Figure 6-57. *(Continued)* **C,** Mass in the head of the pancreas. Note the presence of a left renal cyst in all three panels. (*Courtesy of* Barbara Kadell, MD.)

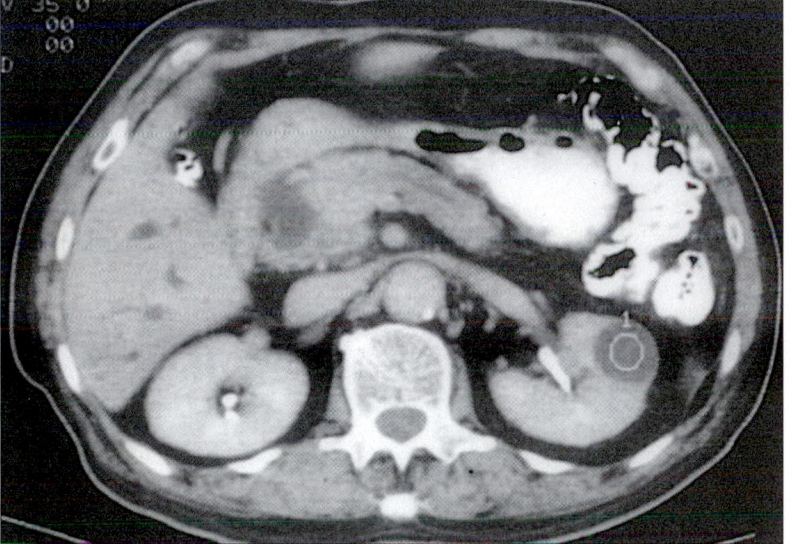

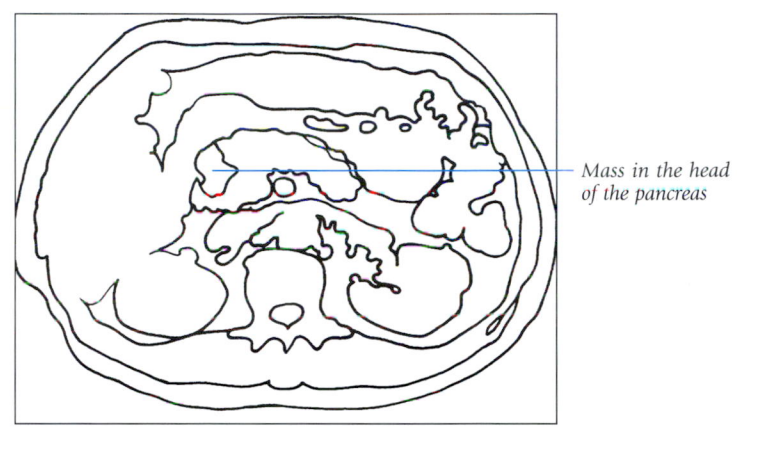

Mass in the head of the pancreas

Figure 6-58. Computed tomography scan demonstrating a mass in the head of the pancreas. (*Courtesy of* Barbara Kadell, MD.)

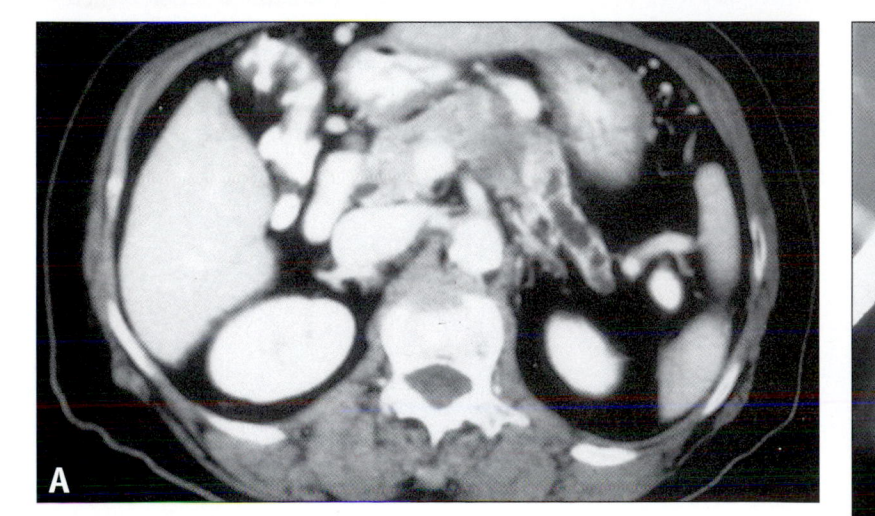

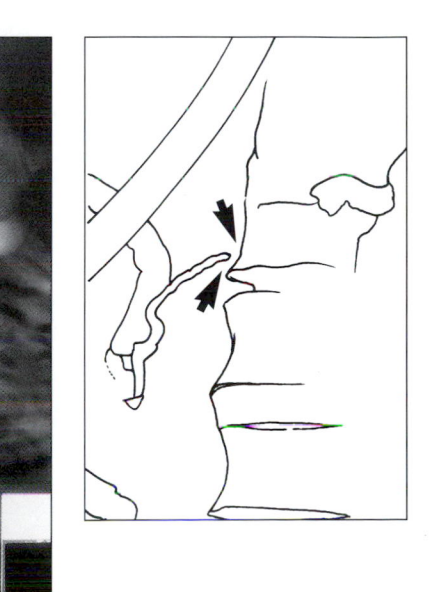

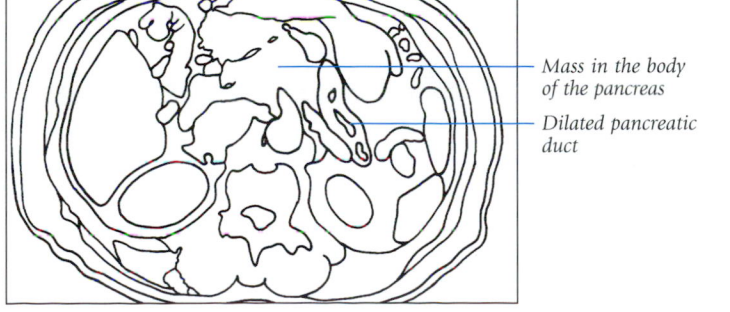

Mass in the body of the pancreas

Dilated pancreatic duct

Figure 6-59. A, Computed tomography scan demonstrates a mass in the body of the pancreas with a dilated pancreatic duct distal to the mass. **B,** Endoscopic retrograde cholangiopancreatography in the same patient showing a stricture (between arrows) in the pancreatic duct with significant distal pancreatic duct dilatation. (*Courtesy of* Barbara Kadell, MD.)

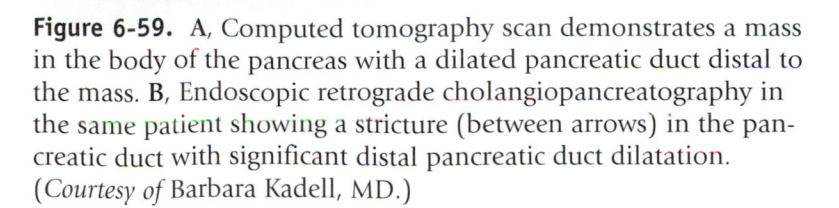

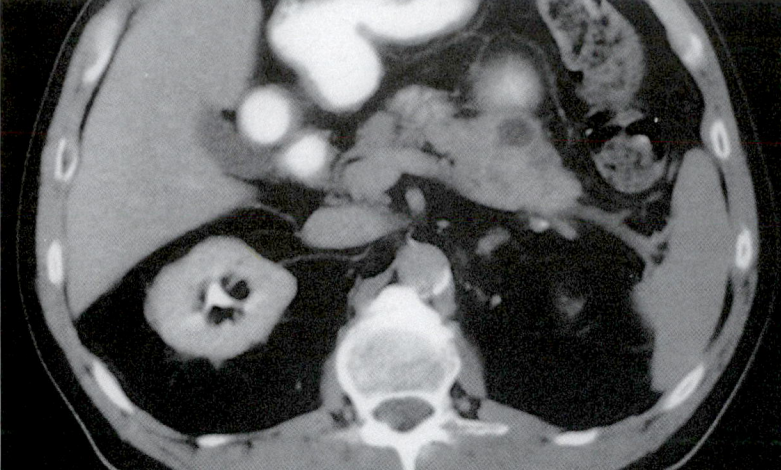

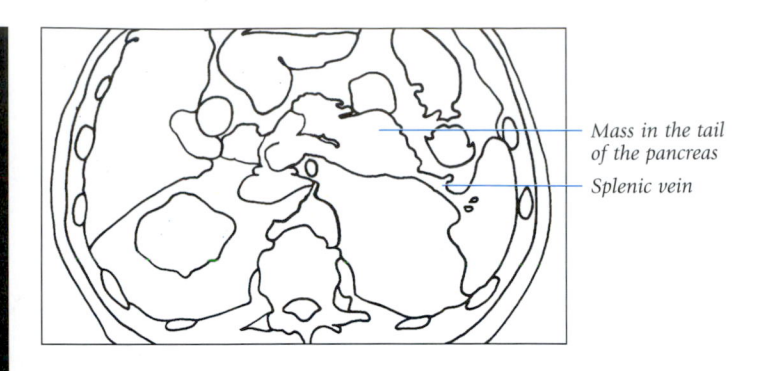

Figure 6-60. Spiral computed tomography scan demonstrating a mass in the tail of the pancreas. (*Courtesy of* Barbara Kadell, MD.)

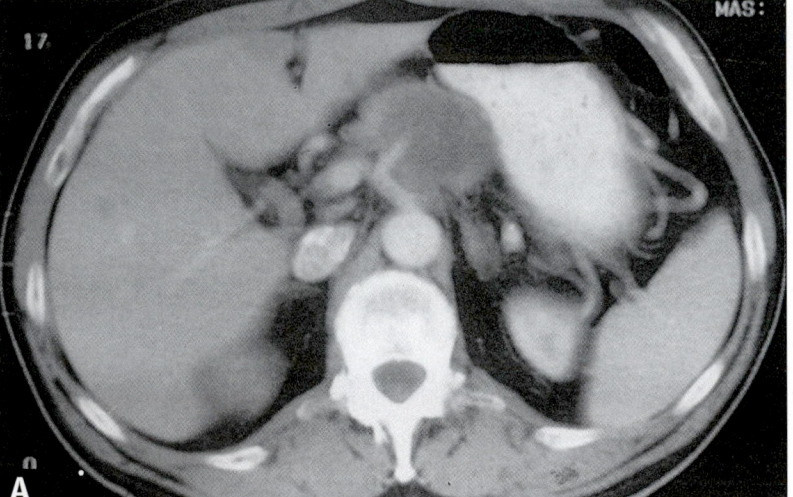

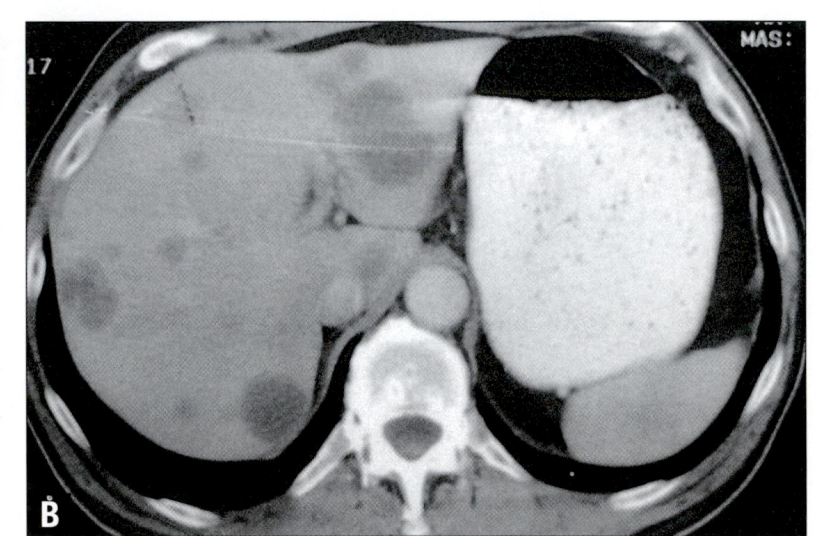

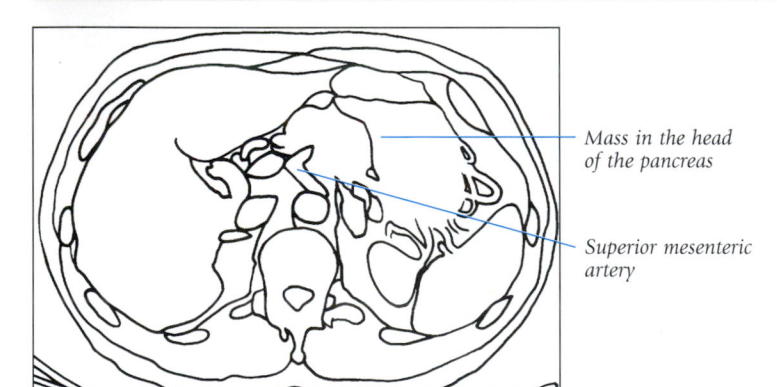

Figure 6-61. **A,** Computed tomography (CT) scan demonstrates encasement of the superior mesenteric artery by a mass in the head of the pancreas. **B,** CT scan of the liver in the same patient showing the presence of multiple liver metastases. This patient's tumors would not be resectable because of involvement of a major vascular structure and the presence of metastatic disease. (*Courtesy of* Barbara Kadell, MD.)

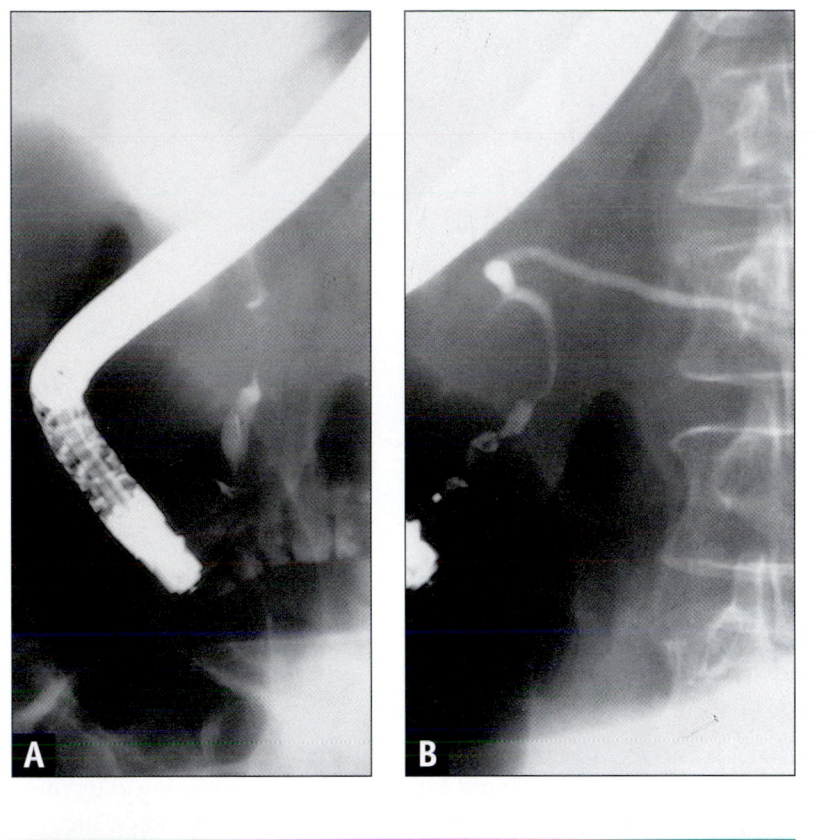

Figure 6-62. **A**, Endoscopic retrograde cholangiopancreatography demonstrating a narrowed intrapancreatic segment of common bile duct. **B**, Pancreatogram in the same patient demonstrating displacement and narrowing of the pancreatic duct within the head of the pancreas. (*Courtesy of* Mark T. Toyama, MD, Amy M. Kusske, MD, and Howard A. Reber, MD.)

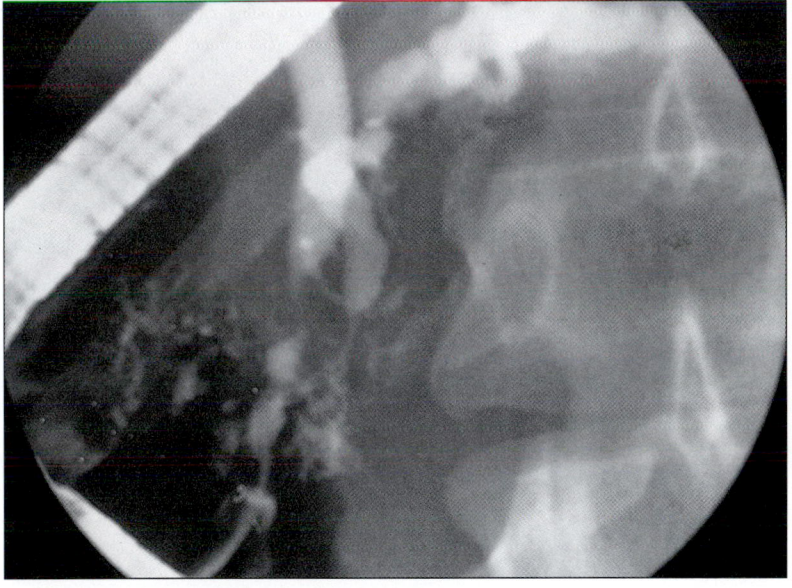

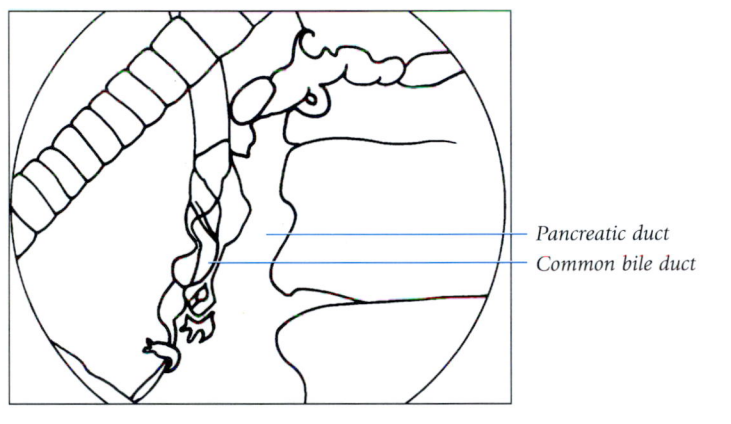

Figure 6-63. Endoscopic retrograde cholangiopancreatography demonstrating the "double duct" sign. Note the narrowing of both the common bile duct and pancreatic duct at the same level within the head of the pancreas, and the distal dilatation in the pancreatic duct. (*Courtesy of* Mark T. Toyama, MD, Amy M. Kusske, MD, and Howard A. Reber, MD.)

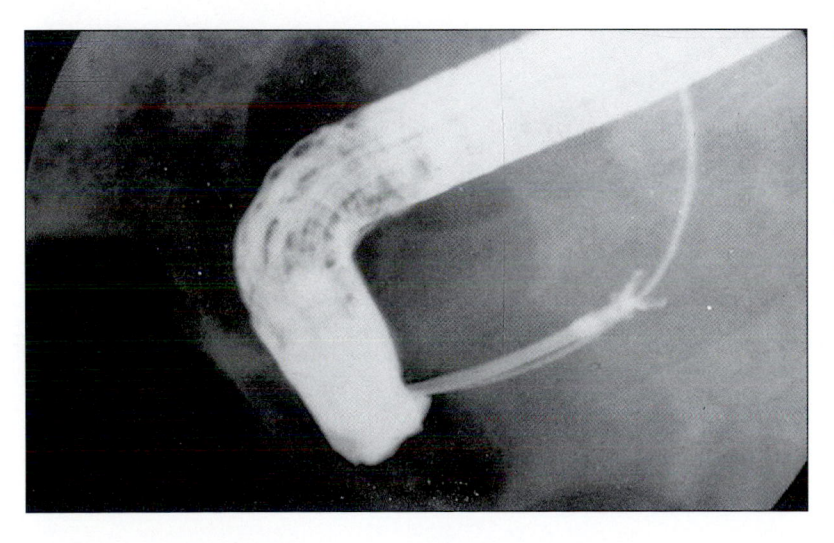

Figure 6-64. Endoscopic retrograde cholangiopancreatography demonstrating biopsy of an intrapancreatic biliary duct stricture. The film shows endoscopic biopsy forceps being passed into the duct to obtain tissue for histologic evaluation. Endoscopy can provide several ways to obtain pancreatic tissue in cases of suspected cancer, including forceps biopsy, needle biopsy, needle aspiration, or intraductal brushings. (*Courtesy of* Mark T. Toyama, MD, Amy M. Kusske, MD, and Howard A. Reber, MD.)

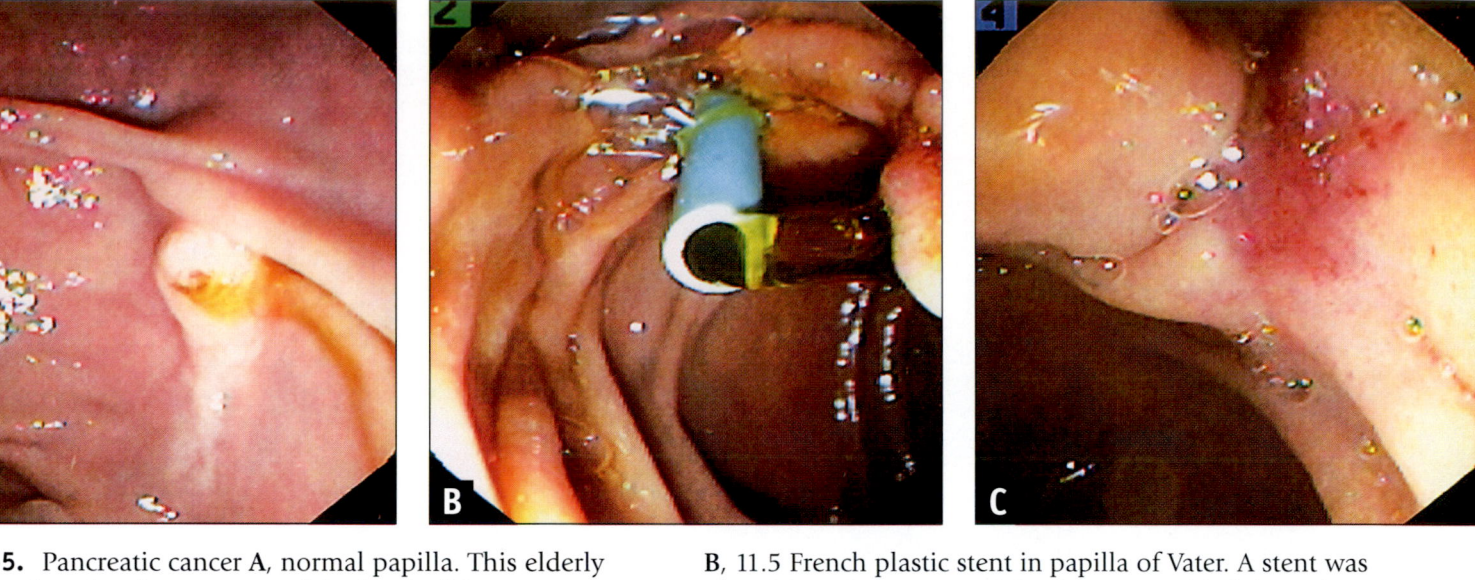

Figure 6-65. Pancreatic cancer **A**, normal papilla. This elderly woman was found to have a mass of the head of the pancreas on CT scan and a dilated biliary tree after undergoing evaluation for abdominal pain and weight loss. She underwent ERCP, which showed an easily identified and normal appearing papilla of Vater. **B**, 11.5 French plastic stent in papilla of Vater. A stent was placed into the common bile duct to provide biliary drainage. **C**, Erythema of duodenal wall secondary to invasive pancreatic adenocarcinoma. Biopsy of this area showed pancreatic cancer. (*Courtesy of* Harvey Young, MD.)

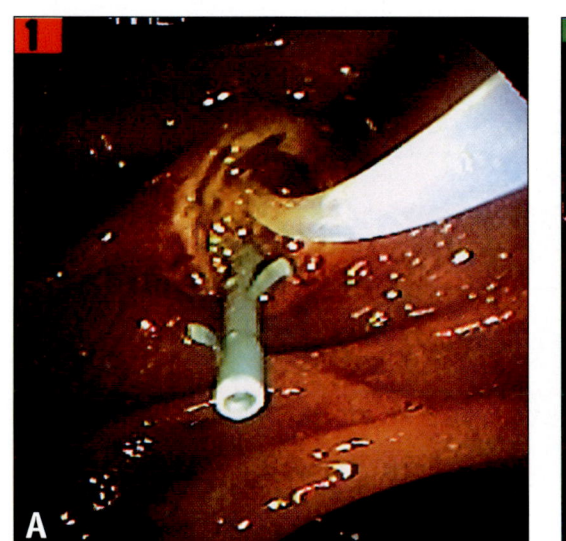

Figure 6-66. Pancreatic cancer invading the common bile duct. **A**, Stent in pancreatic duct and needle knife sphincterotomy. This patient had a pancreatic cancer of the head of the pancreas invading the common bile duct and causing biliary obstruction. A small stent was placed in the pancreatic duct to facilitate safe needle knife sphincterotomy of the papilla. **B**, Wallstent placed in the common bile duct. After successful sphincterotomy, a Wallstent was placed in the common bile duct and provided good bile drainage. (*Courtesy of* Harvey Young, MD.)

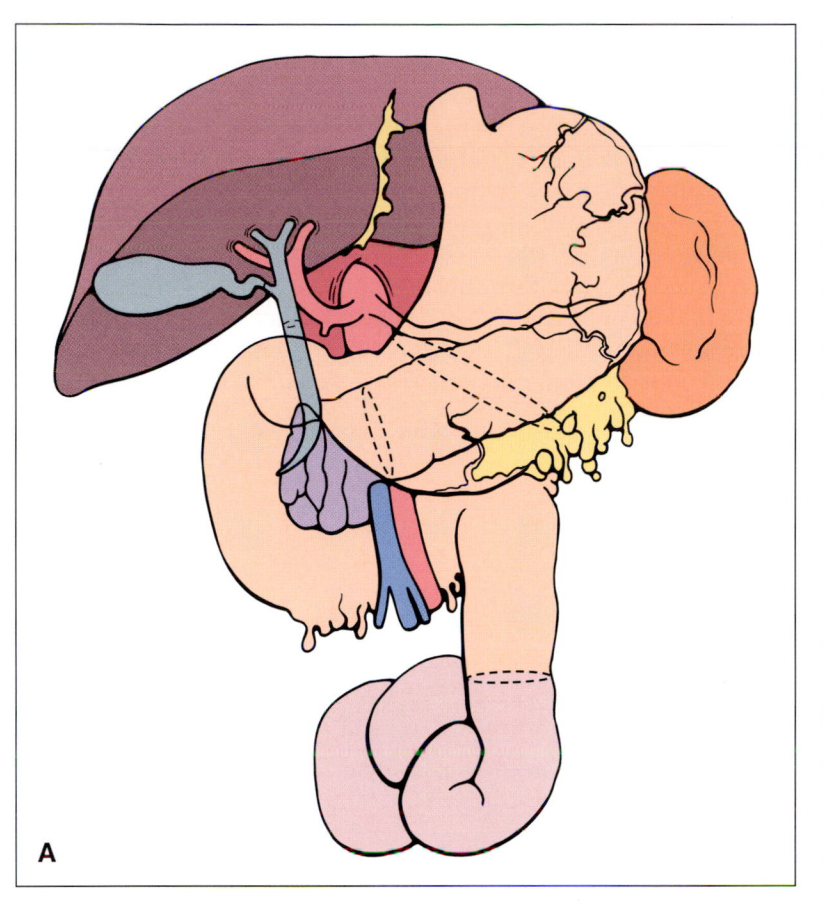

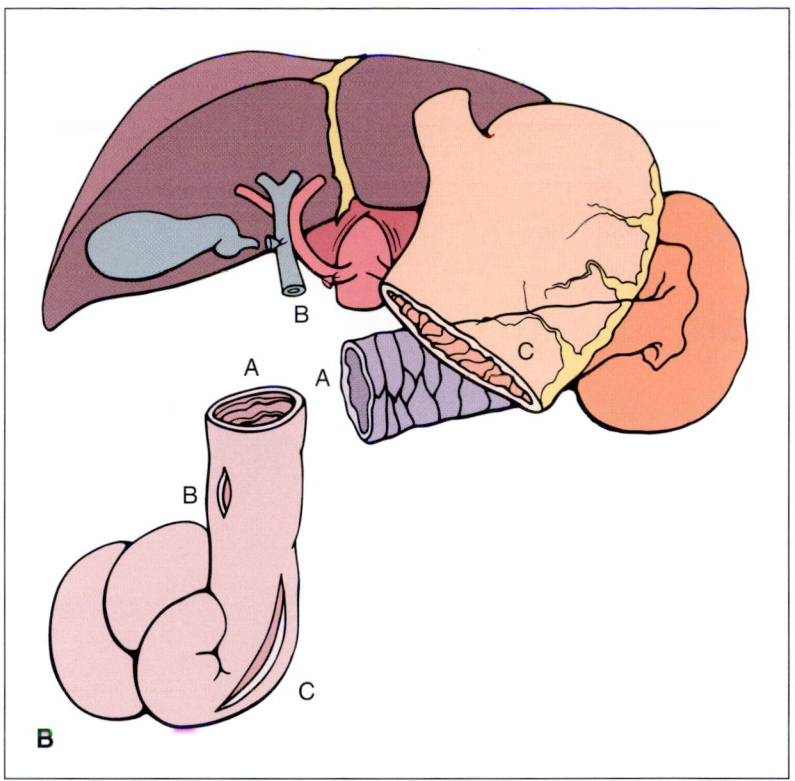

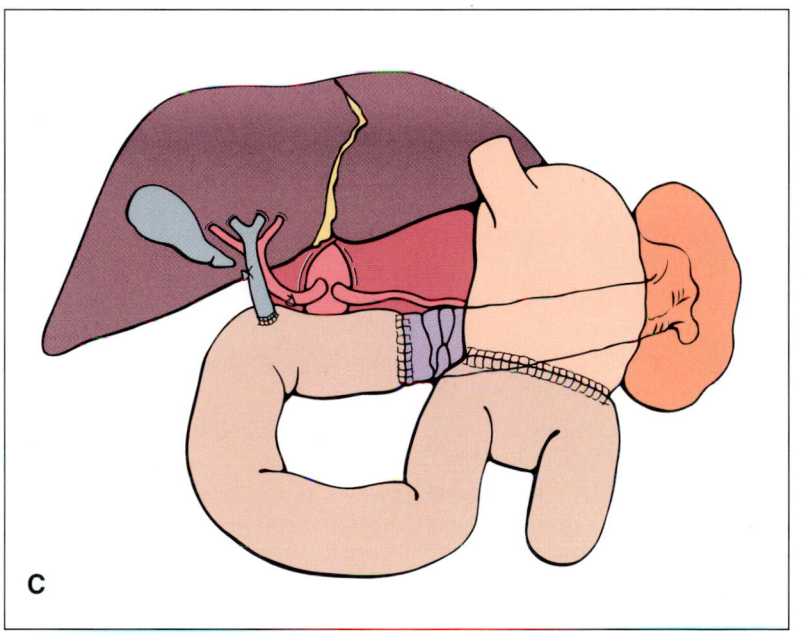

Figure 6-67. The standard Whipple operation, which involves resection of the common bile duct, the gallbladder, the duodenum, and the pancreas to the level of the midbody. **A,** Lines of resection. **B,** Anatomy after resection and before reconstruction (A-A—pancreaticojejunostomy; B-B—choledochojejunostomy; C-C—gastrojejunostomy). **C,** Anatomy after reconstruction.

Pancreatic resection for pancreatic cancer is appropriate only if all gross tumor can be removed with standard resection. The lesion is considered resectable if the following areas are free of tumor: the hepatic artery near the origin of the gastroduodenal artery; the portal and superior mesenteric veins as they pass in front of the uncinate process and behind the body of the pancreas; the superior mesenteric artery, where it courses under the body of the pancreas; and the liver and regional lymph nodes. About 20% of cancers of the head of the pancreas can be resected, but because of local and distant spread, this is rarely possible for lesions of the body and tail. (*Adapted from* Reber [24].)

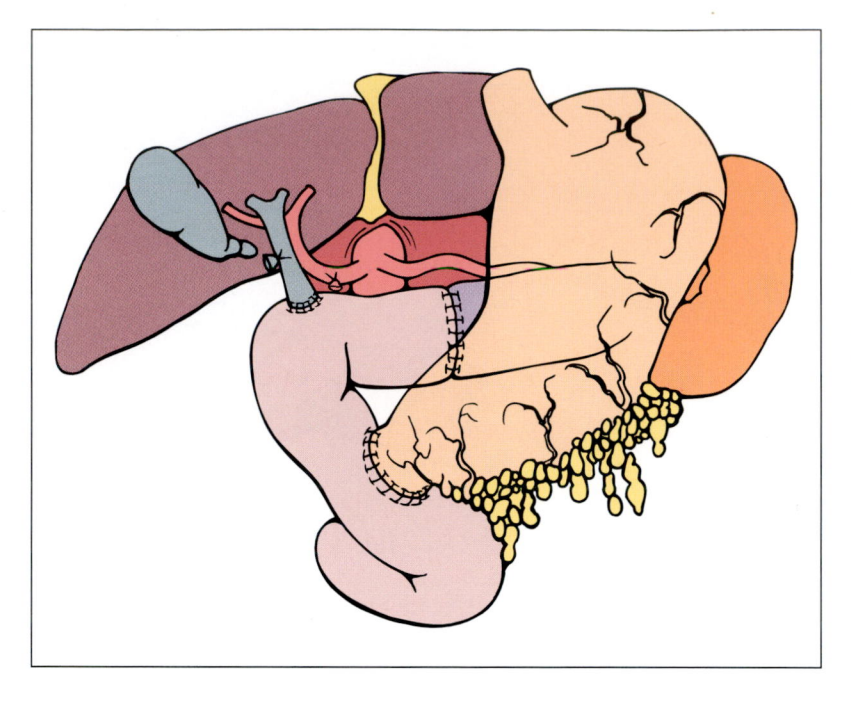

Figure 6-68. Reconstruction after a pancreatoduodenectomy that preserved the pylorus. Instead of the antrectomy that is done with the standard Whipple, the stomach, including the pylorus, is preserved and reanastomosed with the jejunum. This operation was designed as an alternative to the standard Whipple. Many of its proponents argue that it is "more physiologic," therefore patients would have fewer gastrointestinal complaints and nutritional deficits postoperatively compared with the Whipple. No randomized prospective trials have shown this to be true, however. Some believe that this operation may not be adequate when used for malignant tumors, and that the standard Whipple should be performed for all pancreatic cancers. (*Adapted from* Reber [24].)

References

1. Czernobilsky B, Mikat K: The diagnostic significance of interstitial pancreatitis found at autopsy. *Am J Clin Pathol* 1964, 41:35.

2. Klatt EC: Pathology of pentamidine-induced pancreatitis. *Arch Pathol Lab Med* 1992, 116:162–164.

3. Bradley EL, Murphy F, Ferguson C: Prediction of pancreatic necrosis by dynamic pancreatography. *Ann Surg* 1990, 210:495–504.

4. London NJM, Lesse T, Lavelle JM: Rapid bolus contrast enhanced dynamic computed tomography in acute pancreatitis: A prospective study. *Br J Surg* 1991, 78:1452–1456.

5. Freeny PC, Lawson TL: *Radiology of the Pancreas.* New York: Springer-Verlag; 1982:306–398.

6. Huizinga WK, Reddy E, Simjee AE: Pancreatitis and large bowel obstruction. *Dig Dis Sci* 1987, 32:108–109.

7. Neoptolemos JP, Carr-Locke D, James D, *et al.*: Controlled trial of urgent endoscopic retrograde cholangiopancreatography and endoscopic sphincterotomy versus conservative treatment for acute pancreatitis due to gallstones. *Lancet* 1988, 2:979–983.

8. Fan ST, Lai ECS, Mok FPT, *et al.*: Early treatment of acute biliary pancreatitis by endoscopic papillotomy. *N Engl J Med* 1993, 328:228–232.

9. Sarles H, Adler G, Dani R, *et al.*: The pancreatitis classification of Marseilles-Rome 1988. *Scand J Gastroenterol* 1989, 24:641.

10. Axon ATR, Classen M, Cotton PB, *et al.*: Pancreatography in chronic pancreatitis: International definitions. *Gut* 1984, 25:1107–1112.

11. Forsmark CE, Toskes PP: What does an abnormal pancreatogram mean? *Gastrointest Clin North Am* 1995, 5:in press.

12. Hayakawa T, Kondo T, Shibata T, *et al.*: Relationship between pancreatic exocrine function and histologic changes in chronic pancreatitis. *Am J Gastroenterol* 1992, 87:1170–1174.

13. Walsh TN, Rode J, Theis BA, Russell RCG: Minimal change chronic pancreatitis. *Gut* 1992, 33:1566–1571.

14. Neiderau C, Grendell JH: Diagnosis of chronic pancreatitis. *Gastroenterology* 1985, 88:1973–1995.

15. Layer P, Yamamoto H, Kalthoff L, *et al.*: The different courses of early- and late-onset idiopathic and alcoholic chronic pancreatitis. *Gastroenterology* 1994, 107:1481–1487.

16. Copenhagen Pancreatitis Study: An interim report from a prospective epidemiological multicenter study. *Scand J Gastroenterol* 1981, 16:305–312.

17. Worning H: Incidence and prevalence of chronic pancreatitis. In *Chronic Pancreatitis*. Edited by Berger HG, Buchler M, Ditschuneit H, malfertheiner P. Berlin-Heidelberg: Springer-Verlag; 1990:8–14.

18. Gulliver DJ, Edmunds S, Baker ME, *et al.*: Stent placement for benign pancreatic diseases: Correlation between ERCP findings and clinical response. *AJR Am J Roentgenol* 1992, 159:751–755.

19. Vitas GJ, Sarr MG: Selected management of pancreatic pseudocysts: Operative versus expectant management. *Surgery* 1992, 111:123–130.

20. Yeo CJ, Bastidas JA, Lynch-Nyhan A, *et al.*: The natural history of pancreatic pseudocysts documented by computed tomography. *Surg Gynecol Obstet* 1990, 170:411–417.

21. Misra SP, Dwivedi M: Pancreatobiliary ductal union. *Gut* 1990, 31:1144–1149.

22. Mori K, Nagakawa T, Ohta T, *et al.*: Acute pancreatitis associated with anomalous union of the pancreaticobiliary ductal system. *J Clin Gastroenterol* 1991, 13:673–677.

23. Ng WT, Wong MK, Chan YT, Liu K: Clinical application of the study on sphincter of Oddi motor activity in patients with anomalous pancreatobiliary junction. *Am J Gastroenterol* 1992, 87:926–927.

24. Reber HA: The pancreas. In *Principles of Surgery*, edn 6. Edited by Schwartz S. New York: McGraw-Hill; 1994.

Index